Essentials of Pharmacology for Health Occupations, 3rd Edition

Essentials of Pharmacology for Health Occupations, 3rd Edition

RUTH WOODROW, R. N., M. A.

Director, Staff Development
Plymouth Harbor, Inc.
Sarasota, Florida
Former Instructor, Pharmacology
Coordinator, Continuing Education
Sarasota County Technical Institute
Sarasota, Florida

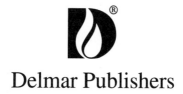

Delmar Publishers

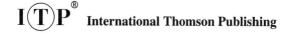 International Thomson Publishing

Albany • Bonn • Boston • Cincinnati • Detroit • London • Madrid
Melbourne • Mexico City • New York • Pacific Grove • Paris • San Francisco
Singapore • Tokyo • Toronto • Washington

NOTICE TO THE READER

The following photos were produced by Chuck Kennedy, photographer, The Chuck Kennedy Group, Inc., Sarasota, Florida: Figures 1.1, 3.2, 4.2, 4.7, 4.8, 4.9, 4.10, 4.11, 4.12, 5.2, 8.1, 8.2, 8.3, 8.4, 8.5, 8.6, 9.1, 9.3, 9.4, 9.5, 14.1, 14.2, and 23.2.

The following figures were drawn by Masako Herman: Figures 2.1, 3.3, 3.4, 4.1, 4.3, 7.1, 8.7, 8.8, 8.10, 8.11, 9.16, 9.17, 9.18, 9.22, and 9.23.

The following figures were drawn by Judy Avery, Commercial Art Department, Sarasota County Vocational-Technical Center, Sarasota, Florida: Figures 3.1, 18.1, and 20.1.

Visual Identification Guide Courtesy: Medical Economics

Cover design courtesy: Brucie Rosch

Delmar Staff

Publisher: Susan Simpfenderfer
Acquisitions Editor: Marion Waldman
Project Editor: William Trudell
Art and Design Coordinator: Rich Killar

Production Coordinator: Cathleen Berry
Marketing Manager: Darryl L. Caron
Editorial Assistant: Sarah Holle
Marketing Assistant: Lynne Rittner

COPYRIGHT © 1997
By Delmar Publishers
a division of International Thomson Publishing Inc.

The ITP logo is a trademark under license

Printed in the United States of America

For more information, contact:

Delmar Publishers
3 Columbia Circle, Box 15015
Albany, New York 12212-5015

International Thomson Publishing Europe
Berkshire House 168-173
High Holborn
London, WC1V7AA
England

Thomas Nelson Australia
102 Dodds Street
South Melbourne, 3205
Victoria, Australia

Nelson Canada
1120 Birchmount Road
Scarborough, Ontario
Canada M1K 5G4

International Thomson Editores
Campos Eliseos 385, Piso 7
Col Polanco
11560 Mexico D F Mexico

International Thomson Publishing Gmbh
Königswinterer Strasse 418
53227 Bonn
Germany

International Thomson Publishing Asia
221 Henderson Road #05-10
Henderson Building
Singapore 0315

International Thomson Publishing - Japan
Hirakawacho Kyowa Building, 3F
2-2-1 Hirakawacho
Chiyoda-ku, 102 Tokyo
Japan

1 2 3 4 5 6 7 8 9 10 XXX 02 01 00 99 98 97 96

Library of Congress Cataloging-in-Publication Data

Woodrow, Ruth.
    Essentials of pharmacology for health occupations / Ruth Woodrow.—3rd ed.
       p. cm.
     Includes index.
     ISBN 0-8273-7022-9 (alk. paper)
     1. Pharmacology.   2. Pharmacology—Examinations, questions, etc.
    3. Allied health personnel.   I. Title.
     [DNLM: 1. Pharmacology.   2. Drug Therapy.   3. Allied Health Personnel.   QV 4 W893e 1996]
RM300.W67 1996
615.5'8—dc20
DNLM/DLC
for Library of Congress   96—18216
                                         CIP

Contents

List of Tables

To my students,
who inspired me by their need,
encouraged me with their questions and comments,
and rewarded me with their success.

Acknowledgments

I wish to express my thanks to all of those who contributed to the original edition as well as the revisions. I especially wish to acknowledge the following individuals whose contributions and advice have been invaluable in the development of this edition.

Contributors

Karen DeHahn, BSN
Former Instructor, Practical Nursing Program
Sarasota County Technical Institute, Florida
Staff Nurse, Venice Hospital, Venice, Florida

Karin Ganns-Lee, MS, RD, LD
Consultant Dietitian, Hillsborough County, Florida

Julie Harman, MSN, ARNP
Former Instructor, Nursing Program, Lansing Community College
Private Practice, Obstetrics and Gynecology, Sarasota, Florida

Ann Holzheimer, RN, MSN
Clinical Nurse Specialist, Hospice of Hillsborough County
Tampa, Florida

Samuel L. Kalush, MD
Cardiovascular Surgeon, Retired
Founder Open Heart Program, Saginaw, Michigan

Barbara Kirkpatrick, M.Ed., RRT
Assistant Professor, Respiratory Care
Manatee Community College, Bradenton, Florida

Consultants

Veronica Foster, R.Ph.
Saginaw, Michigan

Timothy Horvath, R.Ph.
St. Armand's Pharmacy, Sarasota, Florida

Marsha B. Wingate, RN
Pre- and Postoperative Nurse
Cape Surgery Center, Sarasota, Florida

Preface

This book is designed as:

A basic text for nursing students, medical assistant students, and students of other allied health occupations

A continuing education update for practitioners in the health field

Part of a refresher program for practitioners returning to health occupations

A supplemental or reference book for practitioners wishing to extend their knowledge beyond basic training in specific health occupations

The purpose of this book is to provide an extensive framework of knowledge that can be acquired within a limited time frame. It will be especially helpful to students in 1-year training programs with limited time allotted to the study of medications. For those in longer programs, it can be used as the basis for more extensive study. It is appropriate as a required text in training those who will administer medications. It has been especially designed to meet the needs of students in nursing and medical assistant programs. However, students in allied health programs will find the concise format adaptable to their needs also.

This text has been field tested in several classes with students in various health occupations. Students who have already used this book for updating or supplemental education include registered nurses, licensed practical nurses, medical assistants, and paramedics.

Those employed in health occupations now have increased responsibilities for providing the necessary information to patients regarding the safe administration of medications, side effects, and interactions. The quantity of information could be overwhelming and confusing unless presented in a comprehensive and concise manner.

The organization of the text in a concise format eliminates unnecessary detail that may tend to overwhelm or confuse the student. Outdated or infrequently used medications, obsolete information, and complex descriptions are eliminated. The information presented is both factual and functional.

Part I carefully introduces the student to the fascinating subject of drugs, their sources, and uses. Calculations are simplified into two optional, step-by-step processes. *Review questions* at the end of each chapter help the student master the information. Administration checklists allow the student to put the information into practice. Illustrations facilitate the learning process.

Part II organizes the drugs according to classifications, arranged in logical order. Each classification is described, along with characteristics of typical drugs, purpose, side effects, cautions, and interactions. Patient education for each category is highlighted.

Reference tables with each classification list the most commonly prescribed drugs according to generic and trade names, with dosage and available forms.

A worksheet at the end of each chapter helps the student organize the information into outline form. Case studies with each chapter stimulate critical thinking and help the students put into practice the information they have mastered. A comprehensive review quiz for Part I and Part II comes at the end of the book.

An extensive glossary lists and defines terms used in the text. A comprehensive index includes both generic and trade names.

NEW AND REVISED CONTENT

A new chapter has been added, *Drugs and Geriatrics.* Some of the timely topics discussed include drugs which are inappropriate for the elderly. Included are dangerous side effects and mental problems in older adults caused by some drugs.

There have been extensive revisions of the following chapters:

Chapter 16, *Gastrointestinal Drugs* has added many new drugs for the treatment of ulcers, gastroesophageal reflux disease (GERD), and inflammatory bowel disease.

Chapter 17, *Anti-Infective Drugs* includes current tuberculosis protocol, drugs for HIV/AIDS infections and information regarding increased resistance to antibiotics.

Chapter 19, *Analgesics, Sedatives, and Hypnotics* includes improved therapy for control of pain, including *adjuvant analgesics,* as recommended by hospice.

Chapter 20, *Psychotropic Medications, Alcohol, and Drug Abuse* includes new antidepressants, especially the SSRIs; amphetamine and cocaine dangers; and a new drug treatment for alcoholism.

Chapter 24, *Reproductive System Drugs* includes new contraceptive methods, infertility drugs, and new drug therapy for endometriosis and prostate cancer.

Chapter 25, *Cardiovascular Drugs* has added platelet inhibitors and new antihypertensives and antiarrhythmics.

Chapter 26, *Respiratory System Drugs and Antihistamines* has expanded inhalant therapy and added new antihistamines and smoking cessation aids.

In addition, all of the other chapters have been revised and updated. More than 160 new drugs have been added. All of the drug tables have been updated with new drugs and adjusted dosages. Patient education has been expanded. Illustrations have been upgraded and new ones added.

Case studies have been added to all chapters in part II.

Administration checklists have been added in part I.

The Glossary has been expanded to include 25 new terms and definitions.

The *Instructor's Guide* has been improved and expanded to include:

- Review quiz for every chapter, with answers
- Alternate Comprehensive Exam Part II with answers
- Answers to two Comprehensive Review Exams (in textbook)
- Answers to 36 Case Studies (in textbook)

TO THE STUDENT STUDYING PHARMACOLOGY

Other students, such as you, have helped me put this book together. They have learned that the study of medications can be a fascinating one. They tell me that this book has helped them develop confidence and competence in dispensing medications and information about drugs to their patients. You will find this is only the beginning, a framework upon which you will build a vast store of useful knowledge.

Students have told me that the objectives, review questions, worksheets, and case studies were tremendously helpful to them. Organization is the key to acquiring large quantities of information. You will be amazed at all you have learned when you complete this book.

Keep growing and learning and questioning all of your life.

RUTH WOODROW

PART I

Introduction

CHAPTER 1

Consumer Safety and Drug Regulations

OBJECTIVES

Upon completion of this chapter, the student should be able to:

1. Explain what is meant by drug standards.
2. Name the first drug law passed in this country for consumer safety, and give the year it was passed.
3. Summarize the provisions of the Federal Food, Drug, and Cosmetic Act of 1938, and identify the government agency that enforces the act.
4. Interpret what is meant by USP/NF
5. Summarize the provisions of the Controlled Substances Act of 1970.
6. Explain what is meant by a DEA number.
7. Define schedules of controlled substances, and differentiate between C-I to C-V schedules.
8. State several responsibilities you have in the dispensing of medications, as a direct result of the three major drug laws described in this chapter.

Your decision to pursue a career in the health field probably took a great deal of thought. No doubt you have questioned whether you will be able to handle the unique situations that arise in a clinic, health care facility, or physician's office. Have you ever stopped to consider the impact *you* will make on the lives of others as a health care worker? Not only can you make a tremendous difference in the efficiency of the facility, but you can have a positive impact on your friends and family, as well as the patient.

It is inevitable that you will receive phone calls and questions about medications, prescriptions, and drug therapy. A great majority of patients are far too inhibited to tell their physician that there are things they do not understand about their medications. They feel much more at ease discussing their questions with the health care worker. Your potential for informing others with knowledgeable answers about medications can be quite an asset!

The key to reaching that potential is having knowledgeable answers. A serious, responsible attitude about all aspects of drug therapy is imperative. Consider yourself a potential prime resource of medication information for your friends, family, and future patients, as you begin to examine the foundations of facts about drugs. It may be necessary for you to clarify some of the layperson misunderstandings about the legalities of dispensing medications. Consider the following misconceptions and facts.

FALLACY	FACT
Only nurses can give medications to patients.	Trained and certified health care workers who may legally give medications include physicians, physician assistants, paramedics, medical office assistants, and practical, vocational, and registered nurses.
Only physicians may write prescriptions.	Dentists, physicians, physician assistants, veterinarians, nurse practitioners, and registered pharmacists may write prescriptions for their specific field of work, within limitations. For example, veterinarians write prescriptions for animal use only.
Prescriptions are required for narcotics only.	Specific drugs ruled illegal to purchase without the use of a prescription include: • Those that need to be controlled because they are addictive and tend to be abused and dangerous (e.g., depressants, stimulants, psychedelics, and narcotics). • Those that may cause dangerous health threats from side effects if taken incorrectly (e.g., antibiotics, cardiac drugs, tranquilizers, etc.).
All drugs produced in the United States are made in federally approved laboratories.	Numerous undercover, illegal laboratories exist and operate within the United States today.

Drug Laws

The matter of dispensing drugs in the United States is specifically addressed by laws passed in the 1900s. Scientific advances, progress, and changes in society in the last century have made it necessary for drug laws to be set for our safety. Although substances have been taken into the body for their effects for centuries, so many are being produced today that *consumer safety* is now a critical issue.

Drug standards are rules set to assure consumers that they get what they pay for. The law says that all preparations called by the same drug name must be of *uniform strength, quality, and purity.*

Because of drug standardization, when you take a prescription to be filled, you are assured of getting the same basic drug, in the same amount and quality, no matter to which pharmacy or to which part of the country you take the prescription to be filled. According to drug standards, the drug companies must not add other active ingredients or varying amounts of chemicals to a specific drug preparation. They must meet the drug standards (federally approved requirements) for the specified strength, quality, and purity of the drug.

Unlike our predecessors, we no longer have to wonder what ingredients, if any (other than sugar and water, or alcohol), are in the "medicinal waters" being sold.

In the market of illegal (illicit) drugs, the lack of enforcement of drug standards is the consumer's danger. With no controls on the quality of illegal drugs (because they are unapproved for safety), many deaths have occurred from overdose. Consider the heroin user, accustomed to very poor-quality heroin, who accidentally overdoses when given a much higher quality of heroin from a new source.

The laws that have evolved to provide consumer safety can be summed up by three major acts. They are described in the order in which they became necessary for consumer safety.

The importance of the timing of this law should be noted. It came about as the answer to a disastrous occurrence in 1937. A sulfa preparation, not adequately tested for safety, was responsible for 100 deaths that year. Thus, the need was recognized for more proof of the safety and effectiveness of new drugs.

1906   PURE FOOD AND DRUG ACT

First government attempt to establish consumer protection in the manufacture of drugs and foods.

Required all drugs marketed in the United States to meet minimal standards of strength, purity, and quality.

Demanded that drug preparations containing morphine have a labeled container indicating the ingredient morphine.

Established two references of *officially* approved drugs. Before 1906, information about drugs was handed down from generation to generation. No official written resources existed. After the 1906 legislation, two references specified the official U.S. standards for making each drug. Those references, listed below, have since been combined into one book, referred to as the USP/NF:

- United States Pharmacopoeia (USP)
- National Formulary (NF)

1938 FEDERAL FOOD, DRUG, AND COSMETIC ACT AND AMENDMENTS OF 1951 AND 1965

Established the Food and Drug Administration (FDA) under the Department of Health and Welfare to enforce the provisions of the act.

Established *more specific* regulations to prevent adulteration of (tampering with) drugs, foods, and cosmetics:

- All labels must be accurate and must include generic names.

- All new products must be approved by the FDA before public release.

- "Warning" labels must be present on certain preparations, for example, "may cause drowsiness," "may cause nervousness," and "may be habit-forming."

- Certain drugs must be labeled with the legend (inscription): "Caution—federal law prohibits dispensing without a prescription." Thus, the term *legend drugs* refers to such preparations. The act also designated which drugs can be sold without a prescription.

- Prescription and nonprescription drugs must be shown to be *effective* as well as *safe*.

1970 CONTROLLED SUBSTANCES ACT

Established the Drug Enforcement Administration (DEA) as a bureau of the Department of Justice to enforce the provisions of the act.

Set much tighter controls on a specific group of drugs: those that were being abused by society; the name of the act indicates that such *substances needed to be controlled*. They include depressants, stimulants, psychedelics, narcotics, and anabolic steroids. The act:

- Isolated the abused and addicting drugs into five levels, or schedules, according to their degree of danger: C-I, C-II, C-III, C-IV, or C-V.

- Demanded security of controlled substances; anyone (e.g., pharmacists, hospitals, physicians, and drug companies) who dispenses, receives, sells, or destroys controlled substances must keep on hand special DEA forms, indicating the exact current inventory, and a 2-year inventory of every controlled substance transaction.

- Set limitations on the use of prescriptions; guidelines were established for each of the five schedules of controlled substances, regulating the number of times a drug may be prescribed in a 6-month period as well as for which schedules prescriptions may be phoned in to the pharmacy, and so on.

- Demanded that each prescriber of these substances register with the DEA and obtain a DEA registration number, to be present on their prescriptions of controlled substances; drug manufacturers must also be registered and identified with their own DEA numbers, as must pharmacists, physicians, veterinarians, and so on.

The five schedules of controlled substances are arranged with the potentially most dangerous at level I and the least dangerous at level V. The lower the number, the stricter the restrictions for control by the DEA. Thus, level I is the strictest.

Drugs are frequently added, deleted, or moved from one schedule to another. If, for example, the DEA determines that drug A is becoming more of a societal problem, with an increased incidence of overdoses, drug A may be moved from the C-IV schedule to C-III. It is extremely important that the health care worker keep informed of any changes in drug scheduling. For the most part, using the most current drug reference book will keep you up to date.

You will recognize the schedule of a particular controlled substance by noting a *C* with either *I, II, III, IV,* or *V* after it. Some references show the capital C with the Roman numeral inside the curve of the C (Ⓘⱽ). Labels on controlled substances are also designated with a C and a Roman numeral to indicate its level of control. Drug inserts (information leaflets accompanying drugs) are also marked with a C and the appropriate schedule number. (See Fig. 1.1 and Table 1.1.)

TABLE 1.1. FIVE SCHEDULES OF CONTROLLED SUBSTANCES

Schedule Number	Abuse Potential and Legal Limitations	Examples of Substances
1, Ⓒ	High abuse potential Limited medical use	heroin, LSD, marijuana, mescaline
2, Ⓒ	High abuse potential May lead to severe dependence Written prescription only No phoning in of prescription by office health worker No refills May be faxed, but original prescription must be handed in to pick up prescription In emergency, physician may phone in, but handwritten prescription must go to pharmacy within 72 hours	morphine, codeine, methadone, Percocet, Tylox, Dilaudid, Ritalin, cocaine
3, Ⓒ	May lead to limited dependence Written, faxed, or verbal (phoned in) prescription, by physician only May be refilled up to five times in 6 months	paregoric, Empirin with codeine, Tylenol with codeine, Fiorinal, steroids
4, Ⓒ	Lower abuse potential than the above schedules Prescription may be written out by health care worker, but must be signed by the physician Prescription may be phoned in by health care worker or faxed May be refilled up to five times in 6 months	Valium, Ativan, chloral hydrate, phenobarbital, Librium, Darvon, Restoril, Ambien
5, Ⓒ	Low abuse potential compared to the above schedules Consists primarily of preparations for cough suppressants containing codeine and preparations for diarrhea (e.g.) paregoric, and opium tincture)	Cheracol syrup, Robitussin-A-C, Expectorant DC, Donnagel-PG, Lomotil

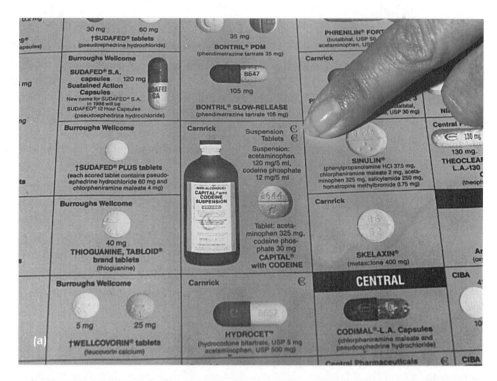

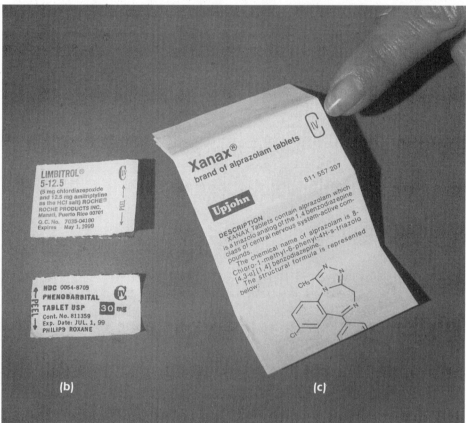

Figure 1.1 Controlled substance schedule numbers appear in a variety of drug information resources, including (a) the Physician's Desk Reference, (b) drug packages, and (c) drug inserts.

FDA and DEA

The increase in the number of drugs produced for marketing brought dangers to the public. The federal Food and Drug Administration was established to assure that some basic standards would be followed. Its responsibilities include:

- Inspecting plants where foods, drugs, or cosmetics are made
- Reviewing new drug applications and petitions for food additives
- Investigating and removing unsafe drugs from the market
- Assuring proper labeling of foods, cosmetics, and drugs

When the need for better control of addictive drugs became urgent, the FDA had its hands full just trying to enforce basic drug standards. It became imperative to set up a new department, the Drug Enforcement Administration, in 1970 to handle all the needs and safety controls for the more dangerous drugs. Thus, the two agencies— FDA and DEA—were established with their own specific areas of drug control.

As a health care worker and an informed citizen, you must be aware of the latest developments concerning these two agencies. Hardly a week goes by without mention of the activities of the FDA or the DEA in the news. You should be able to recognize their separate areas of control.

FDA

Concerned with general safety standards in the production of drugs, foods, and cosmetics

Responsible for approval and removal of products on the market

DEA

Concerned with controlled substances only

Enforces laws against drug activities, including illegal drug use, dealing, and manufacturing

Monitors need for changing the schedules of abused drugs

Health Care Workers and the Law

In some ways, you will be as involved as the physician in observing the restrictions of the drug laws. You will have the responsibility of keeping accurate records of the medications dispensed. You will maintain the supply of drugs at your facility. If you work in a doctor's office, you also will be involved with phoning in prescriptions and securing prescription forms at your facility.

The following guidelines should be followed by the health care worker involved in dispensing medications:

1. Keep a current drug reference book available at all times. You should be able to readily identify substances that must be controlled.

2. Keep controlled substances locked securely. Double-locking is recommended. This means:

   a. Placing the drugs in a locked safety box.

   b. Placing the locked box in a cupboard that is also locked.

3. Conceal prescription pads at your office, clinic, or facility. Do not leave pads out in the open, especially in patient examining rooms. The prescription pads, with the physician's DEA registration number, are a possible source of fraud and drug tampering when forged and used illegally. Keep the pads in a designated location (e.g., a drawer), out of the public areas of the office or nursing station.

4. Keep accurate records of each controlled substance dispensed, received, or destroyed at your facility. These records, as well as the records from the previous 2 years, must be available at all times.

5. Be responsible for keeping up to date with current news of the activities of the FDA and the DEA. Keep informed of any changes in the scheduling of controlled substances.

6. Establish a working rapport with a pharmacist. A local pharmacist is an excellent resource for you when you are unsure of your legal responsibilities with drugs or have any uncertainties about drug therapy.

7. If you work in an office, maintain a professional rapport with the pharmaceutical representatives who leave drug samples there. They are also excellent resources of drug information.

 Check your knowledge of this chapter before going any further.

Chapter Review Quiz

Complete the following statements:

1. The first major U.S. drug law was passed in the year _____ and was called the_____ .

2. USP stands for _____ and is the title of _____ .

3. NF stands for _____ .

4. Which drug law established the USP and NF (which are now one)?

    _____

5. The agency that requires you to keep a record of each controlled substance transaction is the_____ .

6. Prescriptions for schedule C- _____ drugs may be phoned in by the health care worker.

7. How long must you keep an inventory record of each controlled substance transaction at your office? _____

8. Three responsibilities of the FDA include:

    _____

    _____

    _____

9. What types of drugs are listed in the C-V schedule?

    _____

10. What method is recommended for securing the controlled substances at your office?_____

11. If a patient calls to request a refill of a Percodan (C-II) prescription, how would you reply?

    _____

CHAPTER 2

Drug Names and References

OBJECTIVES

Upon completion of this chapter, the student should be able to:

1. Define the following as they relate to drugs: pharmacology, classification, prototype, action, indication, adverse reaction, precautions, interactions, and contraindications.
2. Differentiate among the following drug names: generic name, official name, trade name, and chemical name.
3. Explain what is indicated by a number included in a drug trade name (e.g., Tylenol No. 3).
4. Define and explain the restrictions of drug sales implied by the following: OTC, legend drug, and controlled substance.
5. List at least two drug references available today.
6. Discuss several characteristics that you consider important in choosing the best drug reference.
7. Identify the types of information listed on drug cards.
8. Define the following side effects: ototoxicity, nephrotoxicity, tinnitus, and photosensitivity.

Pharmacology can be defined as the study of drugs and their origin, nature, properties, and effects on living organisms. We need to know why drugs are given, how they work, and what effects to expect. The thousands of drug products on the market would make this subject difficult to tackle if it were not for:

- Numerous drug references, geared to a variety of levels of readers, from layperson to pharmacist
- Grouping of drugs under broad subcategories
- Continuity in the use of basic identifying terms for the names and actions of drugs

Classifications

Each drug can be categorized under a broad subcategory, or subcategories, called *classifications* (see list below). Drugs that affect the body in similar ways are listed in the same classification. Drugs that have several types of therapeutic effects fit under several classifications. For example, aspirin has a variety of effects on the body. It may be given to relieve pain (analgesic), to reduce fever (antipyretic), or to reduce inflammation of tissues (anti-inflammatory). Therefore, aspirin is categorized under three classifications of drugs (as shown in parentheses).

Another drug, cyclobenzaprine (Flexeril), however, is known to be used for only one therapeutic effect: to relieve muscle spasms. Flexeril, therefore, is listed under only one classification (muscle relaxant).

Examples of some of the other drug classifications are listed below. Are you familiar with any of them already?

adrenergics	cholinergics	hormones
anesthetics	decongestants	hypnotics
antibiotics	diuretics	laxatives
antihistamines	electrolytes	sedatives
antihypertensives	emetics	tranquilizers
antitussives	expectorants	vasoconstrictors
cardiotonics	hematinics	vasodilators

The second part of this text compares the characteristics of the various major drug classifications. In each chapter, as a classification is explained, you will learn what general information to associate with drugs of that classification:

- Therapeutic uses
- Most common side effects
- Precautions to be used
- Contraindications
- Interactions that may occur when taken with other drugs or foods
- Some of the most common product names, usual dosages, and comments on administration

You will also be given a prototype of each classification. A *prototype* is a model example, a drug that typifies the characteristics of that classification. Hopefully, each time you learn of a new drug, you will associate the prototype and its characteristics with the new drug, based on its classification.

You can find the classification, as well as the various names of the drug, by referring to a drug reference book.

Identifying Names

Four terms apply to the various titles of a drug:

1. *Generic name.* Common or general name assigned to the drug; differentiated from trade name by initial lowercase letter; never capitalized
2. *Trade name.* The name by which a pharmaceutical company identifies its product; is copyrighted and used exclusively by that company; can be distinguished from generic name by capitalized first letter and is often shown on labels and references with the symbol ® after the name (for "registered" trademark)
3. *Chemical name.* The exact molecular formula of the drug; usually a long, very difficult name to pronounce and of little concern to the health care worker
4. *Official name.* Name of the drug as it appears in the official reference, the *USP/NF*; generally the same as the generic name

The use of generic and trade names for drugs can be compared to the various names of grocery products. Two examples of generic names are orange juice and detergent. Corresponding trade names are Sunkist, Bird's Eye, Tropicana, and Minute Maid, and Cheer, Tide, All, and Fab. While there is only one generic name, there may be many trade names.

When a company produces a new drug for the market, it assigns a generic name to the product. After testing and approval by the FDA, the drug company gives the drug a trade name (often something short and easy to remember when advertised). For 17 years, from the time the company submitted a new drug application (NDA) to FDA for approval, the company has the exclusive right to market the drug. Once approved, the drug is listed in the USP/NF by an official name, which is usually the same as the generic name. When 17 years have passed, and the patent has expired, other companies may begin to combine the same chemicals to form that specific generic product for marketing. Each company will assign its own specific trade name to the product.

Compare the names of the following two drugs:

Generic Name	Chemical Name	Trade Name (Drug Company)
tetracycline hydrochloride	4-dimethylamino-4,12 aocta-hydro-3,6,10,12,12a penta-hydroxyl-6-methyl-1,11-dioxi-2 naphthacenecarbo-xamide hydrochloride	Achromycin V (Lederle Labs) Sumycin (Apothecon) Tetracycline HCL (Richlyn)*
propoxyphene hydrochloride	alpha-4-dimethylamino-3-methyl-1-2,2-diphenyl-2 butanol, proprionate hydrochloride	Darvon (Eli Lilly) Propoxyphene HCL (Rexall)*

*Some companies simply elect to market the product by the generic name.

PATIENT EDUCATION

Patients may ask you about the difference between generic and trade (brand) name products. Generally, trade name products are more expensive, although the basic active ingredients (drug contents) are the same as in the generic. The higher price helps to pay for advertisements promoting the trade name. (Can you think of certain trade names that are heavily advertised in television commercials?)

For this reason it is economically wise to compare prices of over-the-counter (OTC) products that have the same generic components and strengths. For example, several cough syrups may have exactly the same contents, but the prices may vary widely.

Concerning prescription drugs, most states have enacted legislation encouraging physicians to let pharmacists substitute less expensive *generic equivalents* for prescribed brand name drugs. Specific provisions of *drug substitution laws* vary from state to state.

The physician may indicate "no substitutions" on the prescription, usually indicated by a DAW (dispense as written). Often physicians have preferences for certain products. Even though the drug contents are the same, the "fillers," or ingredients that are used to hold the preparation together, may be slightly different. This difference in fillers may affect how quickly the drug dissolves or takes effect. Dyes in some products may alter effects in some sensitive patients by leading to an allergic response.

Many products are combinations of several generic components. You will recognize this when you see several generic names (not capitalized) and corresponding amounts listed under one trade name (capitalized). Examples are:

Trade Name	*Generic Name and Amount*
Darvocet-N-100	acetaminophen, 650 mg
	propoxyphene napsylate, 100 mg
Darvon Compound-65	aspirin, 227 mg
	propoxyphene HCL, 65 mg
	caffeine, 32 mg
Ornade	chlorpheniramine, 8 mg
	isopropanolamine iodide, 2.5 mg
	phenylpropanolamine, 50 mg

It should be noted that a number may be part of the trade name. The number often refers to an amount of one of the generic components and helps to differentiate it from an almost identical product. Identify the significance of the numbers in comparing the following trade names:

Trade Name	*Generic Name and Amount*
Empirin	aspirin, 325, mg
Empirin No. 1	aspirin, 325 mg
	codeine phosphate, 7.5 mg
Empirin No. 2	aspirin, 325 mg
	codeine phosphate, 15 mg

Empirin No. 3   aspirin, 325 mg
                          codeine phosphate, 30 mg
Empirin No.4   aspirin, 325 mg
                          codeine phosphate, 60 mg

While one of the products is plain aspirin, the other four have a controlled substance, codeine, added. *The larger the number, the greater the amount of controlled substance present.* Other trade names including numbers that can also be written in this way include:

Fiorinal #1, #2, #3
Tylenol #1, #2, #3, #4

Many drug errors have occurred because the trade name was misinterpreted for the number of tablets to be given. So . . .

  Check your knowledge of this chapter before going any further.

> *Be certain you can clearly read and understand the order!*

Another type of drug error involves needless allergic reactions to one of the generic components of a medication. The problem stems from:

Not consulting the patient's chart for the history of allergies before a new medication is ordered or given

Not checking a reference to find out if a medication being ordered or given contains any generic components to which the patient has a known allergy

For example, if a patient has an allergy to aspirin, do not administer the first dose of any new medication to the patient without finding out if the product contains aspirin. Although the doctor is in error for ordering the medication, you are also in error for administering a medication with which you are unfamiliar. The physician is often hurried and pressured in meeting the demands of an office schedule. A proficient health care worker should check the history and chart for known allergies, and pick up any discrepancies. Alertness is the key to safety in any setting.

> *Always keep a drug reference handy, and use it when you are unfamiliar with the generic components of a drug ordered for a patient with known drug allergies. With experience, you will learn and remember the names of products most commonly used at your facility.*

Legal Terms Referring to Drugs

A drug may be referred to by terms other than its classification, generic name, trade name, chemical name, or official name. As mentioned in Chapter 1, the following terms imply the legal accessibility of the drug:

1. *OTC*. Over-the-counter; no purchasing restrictions by the FDA
2. *Legend drug*. Prescription drug; determined unsafe for over-the-counter purchase because of possible harmful side effects if taken indiscriminately; includes birth control pills, antibiotics, cardiac drugs, hormones, etc.; indicated in the Physician's Desk Reference (discussed later in this chapter) by the symbol to the far right of the trade name
3. *Controlled substance*. Drug controlled by prescription requirement because of the danger of addiction or abuse; indicated in references by schedule numbers C-I to C-V (see Chapter 1)

Terms Indicating Drug Actions

Most references follow a similar format in describing drugs. When you research drug information, you will find the following terms as headings under each drug. You will find specific information more quickly if you understand what is listed under each heading.

Indications. A list of medical conditions or diseases for which the drug is meant to be used (e.g., diphenhydramine hydrochloride [Benadryl], is a commonly used drug; indications include allergic rhinitis, mild allergic skin reactions, motion sickness, and mild cases of parkinsonism).

Actions. A description of the cellular changes that occur as a result of the drug. This information tends to be very technical, describing cellular and tissue changes. While it is helpful to know what body system is affected by the drug, this information is geared more for the pharmacist (e.g., as an antihistamine, Benadryl appears to compete with histamine for cell receptor sites on effector cells).

Contraindications. A list of conditions for which the drug should not be given (e.g., two common contraindications for Benadryl are pregnancy or lactating mother).

Warnings and Cautions. A list of conditions or types of patients that warrant closer observation for specific side effects when given the drug (e.g., due to atropinelike activity, Benadryl must be used cautiously with patients who have a history of bronchial asthma, hypertension, or increased intraocular pressure).

Side Effects and Adverse Reactions. A list of possible unpleasant or dangerous secondary effects, other than the desired effect (e.g., side effects of Benadryl include sedation, dizziness, disturbed coordination, epigastric distress, anorexia, and thickening of bronchial secretions). This listing may be quite extensive, with as many as 50 or more side effects for one drug. Because it is difficult to know which are most likely to occur, choose a reference book that

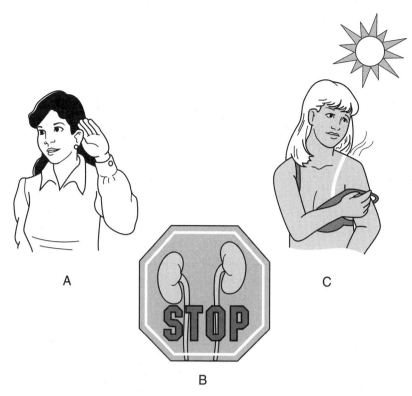

A

B

C

Figure 2.1 *Side effects or adverse reactions can include (a) ototoxicity, (b) nephrotoxicity, and (c) photosensitivity.*

underlines or italicizes the most common side effects. Certain drugs may have side effects with which you are not familiar. Note the definitions of the following three side effects associated with specific antibiotics (see Fig. 2.1):

- Ototoxicity causes damage to the eighth cranial nerve, resulting in impaired hearing or ringing in the ears (tinnitus). Damage may be reversible or permanent.
- Nephrotoxicity causes damage to the kidneys, resulting in impaired kidney function, decreased output, and renal failure.
- Photosensitivity is an increased reaction to sunlight, with the danger of intense sunburn.

Interactions. A list of other drugs or foods that may alter the effect of the drug, and usually should not be given during the same course of therapy (e.g., monoamine oxidase [MAO] inhibitors will intensify the effects of Benadryl; you will find MAO inhibitors listed under interactions for many drugs; the term refers to a group of drugs that have been used for the treatment of depression; it has been found that they can cause serious blood pressure changes, and even death, when taken with many other drugs and some foods).

Other headings often listed under information about a drug include "How Supplied" and "Usual Dosage." "How Supplied" lists the available forms and strengths of the drug. "Usual Dosage" lists the amount of drug considered safe for administration, the route, and the frequency of administration. For example:

How supplied: tablets (tabs): 20 mg and 40 mg; suppository: 20 mg
Usual dosage: 10 mg orally every 4 h (q4h)

For a listing of common abbreviations regarding drug administration and medication orders, see Tables 4.1 and 5.1.

Drug References*

The Physicians' Desk Reference (PDR) is one of the most widely used references for drugs in current use. It is an old standby found in every medical setting: offices, clinics, hospital units, pharmacies, and so on. As the name indicates, however; it is geared to the physician. Many new choices of references are available today. Four are compared here, including the *PDR*. You must find the reference most suitable for you, one that you can interpret quickly and easily. By becoming knowledgeable about the drugs you administer, you may prevent possible drug errors from occurring.

Physician's Desk Reference (PDR)†

Pro	*Con*
Distributed to practicing physicians; single hardback volume	Geared for physicians and pharmacists
Several supplements published throughout the year, with revised information or descriptions of new products introduced after the previous edition went to press	Lengthy descriptions
	Difficult to sort out what is most important to remember
	No easily identified nursing implications
All drugs cross-referenced, by several color-coded indexes, according to one of the following:	Includes many code numbers in the description of "How Supplied " making it difficult to interpret
• Company that makes the drug (white, "Manufacturers' Index")	Contains only those drugs that manufacturers pay to have incorporated; incomplete with regard to OTC drugs, making it necessary to buy PDR OTC book
• Trade and generic names (pink, "Product Name Index")	
• Drug classification (blue, Product Category Index)	
Includes photographs of many drugs for product identification	
Includes a list of all U.S. Poison Control Centers, with addresses and phone numbers	
Includes a description of substances used for medical testing (green, "Diagnostic Product Information"), for example, barium, X-ray dyes, substances used for allergy testing	

*References listed here were used to compile the information in this book.
†Published annually by Biomedical Information Corp., New York, New York.

*United States Pharmacopeia/Dispensing Information (USP/DI)**

Pro	*Con*
Two paperback volumes (and six updates on new drugs per year):	No photographs of drugs
• *Drug Information for the Health Provider,* drug information for the physician; includes up-to-date information on carcinogenicity (studies on the ability of drugs to cause cancer)	Must be purchased, is not distrubuted freely
• *Advice for the Patient*	
Easy-to-read, practical guidelines for the patient	
Stresses most important aspects of the patient's history for the physician to be aware of before prescribing the drug	
Stresses many tips for proper use of medication and what precautions to take	
Includes a pronunciation key for each drug name	

*AHFS Drug Information (American Health-System Formulary Service)****

Pro	*Con*
Distributed to practicing physicians; single paperback volume	Some parts (e.g., "Chemical Information" and "Drug Stability") not necessary for the health care worker
Good, concise information; easy to read	
Arranged by classifications, with a general statement about each classification at the beginning of each section	

Compendium of Drug Therapy†

Pro	*Con*
Distributed to practicing physicians; two hardback volumes:	None
• *Compendium of Patient Information,* helpful patient guidelines for a particular specialty area (e.g., obstetrics, orthopedics, pediatrics, family practice, etc.)	
• *Compendium of Drug Therapy*	
Very easy to read, well arranged	
Index tabs easily separate sections by drug classification	
Includes photographs of drugs	
Includes phone numbers of major pharmaceutical companies and Poison Control Centers	
Includes copies of some drug package inserts	

*Published annually by U.S. Pharmacopeial Convention, Inc., Rockville, Maryland.

**Published annually by the American Society of Health-System Pharmacists, Bethesda, Maryland.

†Published annually by U.S. Biomedical Information Corp., New York, New York.

Other references (e.g., *The Pill Book, Handbook of Nonprescription Drugs*) may be found in bookstores, but they may not contain adequate information for the health care worker. Your school may recommend a specific drug reference other than the four listed in this text. Many new references geared to the nurse or health care worker are currently being published.

Drug Cards

As a student of pharmacology, you may find it helpful to prepare drug cards because there are so many drugs to learn. Many educational programs require drug cards with the curriculum. You may use 3×5- or 5×7-inch index cards stored in a recipe card box or other similar file. Included on the cards should be the information most useful to medical personnel. Although the cards should be updated periodically, using them saves valuable time compared to using the larger drug references. Certain information should be included on the drug card:

1. Generic and trade name of the drug
2. Classification or classifications of the drug
3. Forms in which the drug is available
4. Drug action
5. Indications
6. Side effects
7. Routes of administration
8. Dosage range and customary dosage
9. Any special instructions for giving the medication

In addition to making it easier and faster to locate information on drugs, drug cards constitute an ideal method of becoming more knowledgeable about drugs, classifications, and other pharmaceutical terminology.

Pharmaceutical salespeople and drug company representatives frequently have drug inserts or package brochures that are also useful. Such material can be attached to index cards or filed separately. It is especially important that drug cards be prepared on those drugs used predominantly at your medical facility.

The following is a sample drug card. Note that a number of abbreviations are used to save space. Common abbreviations regarding drug administration and medication orders appear in Tables 4.1 and 5.1.

Drug. Nitroglycerin (Nitro-Bid, Nitrostat).

Classification. Vasodilator.

Form. Sublingual tablet, timed-release tablets or capsules, ointment, dermal patches, and IV.

Action. Relaxes smooth muscles, dilates arterioles and capillaries.

Uses. Management of acute angina pectoris episodes.

Side Effects and Toxicities. Headache with throbbing, dizziness, weakness, blurred vision, dry mouth, tachycardia, and postural hypotension.

Route. Sublingual, topical, by mouth (PO), or IV.

Dosage. Sublingual, one tablet under tongue or in buccal pouch, may be repeated three times (×3) if necessary; timed-release capsule, two or three times a day at 8–12-h intervals; ointment, apply to any convenient skin area and spread in thin, uniform layer 1–2 inches, may be applied every 3–4 h (q3–4h) whenever necessary (PRN).

Special Instruction. Severe headache may occur; flushing, dizziness, or weakness is usually transient; if blurred vision or dry mouth occurs, discontinue use.

Check your knowledge of this chapter before going any further.

Chapter Review Quiz

Match the definition with the term:

1. _____ List of conditions for which a drug is meant to be used

2. _____ Subcategories of drugs, based on their side effects on the body

3. _____ Description of the cellular changes that occur as a result of a drug

4. _____ Conditions for which a drug should not be given

a. Contraindications

b. Precautions

c. Indications

d. Prototype

e. Actions

f. Classifications

Refer to the following drug description to answer questions 5–8:

Pyridium®
(phenazopyridine HC1 tablets, USP)
Product of Warner-Lambert, Inc.
Description: Pyridium (phenazopyridine HCl) is a urinary tract analgesic agent, chemically designated 2.6-pyridinediamine, 3-(phenylazo), monohydrochloride.

5. The generic name of the drug is _____ .

6. The chemical name of the drug is _____ .

7. The trade name of the drug is _____ .

8. What is indicated by the ℞ symbol in the upper right corner?

_____

9. List four drug references:

_____

_____

10. Explain the difference between these two medication orders:

a. Give two Empirin, PO.

b. Give one Empirin #2, PO.

_____

_____

CHAPTER 3

Sources and Bodily Effects of Drugs

OBJECTIVES

Upon completion of this chapter, the student should be able to:

1. *Identify the four sources of drugs.*
2. *Differentiate between the following: drug actions and drug effects, systemic effects and local effects, loading dose and maintenance dose, and toxic dose and lethal dose.*
3. *Define the following processes as they are related to the passage of drugs through the body and give conditions that may decrease the effectiveness of each: absorption, distribution, metabolism, and excretion.*
4. *Define the following terms: selective distribution, toxicity, placebo, synergism, potentiation, and antagonism.*
5. *List several variables that may affect the action of drugs.*
6. *Identify the fastest route of drug administration.*
7. *Define the following undesirable drug effects: teratogenic effect, idiosyncrasy, tolerance, dependence, hypersensitivity, and anaphylactic reaction.*

Sources of Drugs

Any chemical substance taken into the body for the purpose of affecting body function is referred to as a *drug*. In earlier times, these substances were found in nature, sometimes accidentally. *Plants* were the primary source of substances used on the human body. Berries, bark, leaves, resin from trees, and roots were found to aid the body and are still very important drug sources today (see Fig. 3.1).

Minerals from the earth and soil also found their way into human use as drugs. Iron, sulfur, potassium, silver, and even gold are some of the minerals used to prepare drugs.

More sophisticated sources of drugs emerged as human beings progressed. Research led to the use of substances from *animals* as effective drugs. Substances

Sources of Drugs:

	Example:	Trade Name:	Classification:
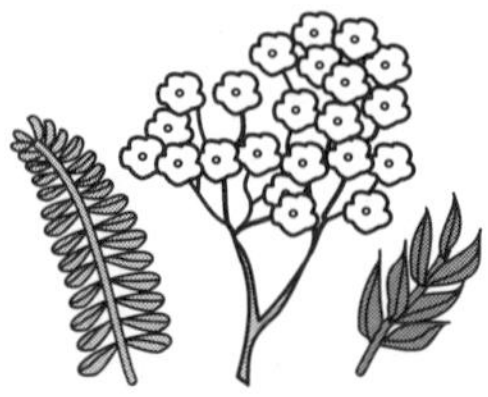 **Plants**	Cinchona Bark	Quinidine	Antiarrhthymic
	Purple Foxglove Plant	Digitalis	Cardiotonic
	Poppy Plant (Opium)	Paregoric, Morphine, Codeine	Antidiarrheal Analgesic Analgesic, Antitussive
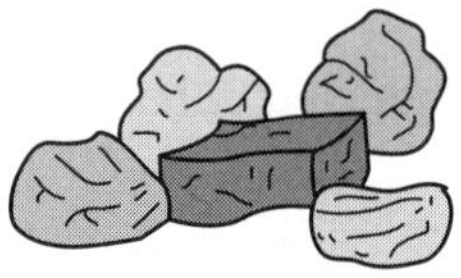 **Minerals**	Magnesium	Milk of Magnesia	Antacid, Laxative
	Zinc	Zinc Oxide Ointment	Sunscreen, Skin Protectant
	Gold	Solganal, Auranofin	Anti-Inflammatory; Used in the Treatment of Rheumatoid Arthritis
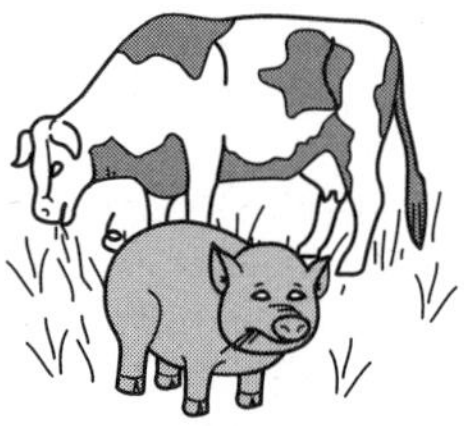 **Animals**	Pancreas of Cow, Hog	Insulin: regular, NPH, PZI	Antidiabetic Hormone
	Stomach of Cow, Hog	Pepsin	Digestive Hormone
	Thyroid Gland of Animals	Thyroid, USP	Hormone
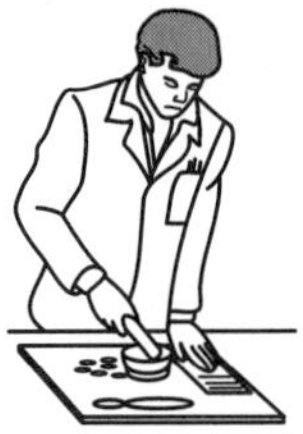 **Synthetic**	Meperidine	Demerol	Analgesic
	Diphenoxylate	Lomotil	Antidiarrheal
	Co-Trimoxazole	Bactrim, Septra	Anti-Infective Sulfonamide; Used in the Treatment of Urinary Tract Infections UTI

Figure 3.1 Sources of drugs. (a) Plant sources; (b) mineral sources; (c) animal sources; (d) synthetic sources.

lacking in the human body can be replaced with similar substances from the glands, organs, and tissues of animals. The origin of drugs from an animal source even now includes human extractions. The pituitary gland from cadavers can be used to make a drug for the treatment of growth disorders.

Finally, chemists use synthetic sources to make drugs to market for human consumption. The *synthetic* (manufactured) sources evolved with human skills in laboratories and advanced understanding of chemistry. Drug compounds are produced from artificial rather than natural substances. This method is probably the most actively pursued source of drugs by major companies today. Competitive research is a big industry in experimenting with chemicals to discover cures for current medical problems. Numerous antibiotics are synthetic or semisynthetic, the results of researchers' meeting the need for better treatment of infections. Someday the cure for cancer or human immunodeficiency virus (HIV) may be found from a synthetic source developed in a laboratory.

Two exciting developments in drug research occurred during the 1980s:

- The Eli Lilly company developed a new insulin that does not require an animal source. Humulin, which is more similar to human insulin than its predecessors, is made from Escherichia coli bacteria and altered DNA (deoxyribonucleic acid) molecules.
- The *Discovery III* space shuttle, launched in August 1984, carried the first nonastronaut space traveler. On board, a researcher conducted experiments with a drug processing machine. The ongoing goal of the space research is to produce a degree of drug purity that cannot be attained under conditions influenced by gravity.

During the 1990s, the emphasis on investigational new drugs (INDs) has been on the development of drugs for the treatment of life-threatening or other very serious conditions, for example, HIV infection/AIDS, various malignancies, and Alzheimer's disease. Three of the many INDs developed in the last decade include:

- Zidovudine (AZT) (Retrovir), which slows the progression of HIV infection in some patients. It is not a cure.
- Interferon (Roferon A), which has been used to treat many different malignancies and also has been used in the management of AIDS-related Kaposi's sarcoma.
- Tacrine (Cognex), which has been used to slow the progression of dementia in some patients with Alzheimer's disease. It is not a cure.

Research continues with these and many other INDs in the treatment of many very serious diseases.

Effects of Drugs

No matter how different the sources, the common characteristic of all drugs is the ability to affect body function in some manner. When introduced into the body, all drugs cause cellular changes (drug actions), followed by some physiological change (drug effect). Generally, drug effects may be categorized as systemic or local:

1. *Systemic effect.* Reaches widespread areas of the body (e.g., acetaminophen (Tylenol) suppository, although given rectally, has the ability to be absorbed and distributed throughout the body to cause a general reduction in fever and pain).

2. *Local effect.* Is limited to the area of the body where it is administered (e.g., dibucaine ointment (Nupercainal), applied rectally, affects only the rectal mucosa to reduce hemorrhoidal pain).

Drug Processing by the Body (Pharmacokinetics)

Within the body, drugs undergo several changes. From start to finish, the biological changes consist of four processes:

1. *Absorption.* Getting into the bloodstream.
2. *Distribution.* Moving from the bloodstream into the tissues and fluids of the body.
3. *Metabolism.* Physical and chemical alterations that a substance undergoes in the body.
4. *Excretion.* Eliminating waste products of drug metabolism from the body.

Many variables affect how quickly or successfully substances go through the body via these four processes. If any of the four processes is hampered, the drug action and effects will be hampered. Note in Table 3.1 conditions that may hamper each process.

Directions for the administration of one drug versus another may vary widely because the physical properties of the drugs may vary widely. The specific directions ("Usual Dosage and Administration," "Contraindications," and "Warnings") that accompany each drug are given to enhance the absorption, distribution, metabolism, and excretion of the drug. For example, directions to "Give on an empty stomach" ensure the most effective means of absorption. "Use cautiously in patients with renal dysfunction" implies possible effects on the excretion of a drug.

TABLE 3.1. PROCESSING OF DRUGS WITHIN THE BODY

Process	Primary Site of Process	Conditions That May Hamper Process
Absorption	Mucosa of the stomach, mouth, small intestine, or rectum; blood vessels in the muscles or subcutaneous tissues; or dermal layers	Incorrect administration may destroy the drug before it reaches the bloodstream or its site of action (e.g., giving certain antibiotics after meals instead of on an empty stomach).
Distribution	Circulatory system, through capillaries and across cell membranes	Poor circulation (impaired flow of blood) may prevent drug from reaching tissues.
Metabolism	Liver	Hepatitis, cirrhosis of liver, or a damaged liver may prevent adequate breakdown of drug, thus causing a buildup of unmetabolized drug.
Excretion	Kidneys, sweat glands, lungs, or intestines	Renal damage or kidney failure may prevent passage of drug waste products, thereby causing an accumulation of the drug in the body.

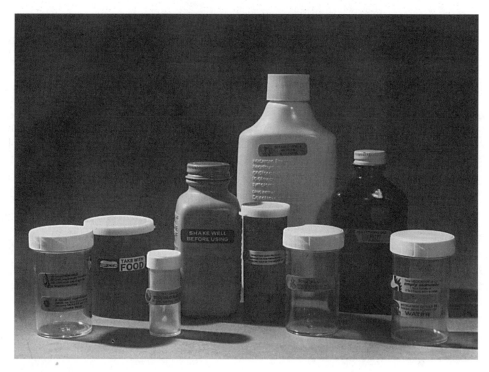

Figure 3.2 Read labels carefully before administration.

"Decrease dose in patients with hepatic dysfunction" implies possible effects on the metabolism of a drug. *Read all labels carefully, and caution the patient to do so also* (see Fig. 3.2).

Absorption

The site of absorption of drugs varies according to the following physical properties of each drug:

1. *pH*. Drugs of a slightly acidic nature (e.g., aspirin and tetracycline) are absorbed well through the stomach mucosa. Drugs of an alkaline pH are not absorbed well through the stomach, but are readily absorbed in the alkaline environment of the small intestine. The antibiotic tetracycline is recommended to be given on an empty stomach so that its pH is not altered. If given in the presence of milk, dairy products, or antacids, it will not be properly absorbed. Oral medications for infants (syrups and solutions) may not be absorbed well after infant feedings. The milk or formula neutralizes the acidity of the stomach. Thus, absorption may be enhanced when the infant is given medications on an empty stomach.

2. *Lipid (fat) solubility*. Substances high in lipid solubility are quickly and easily absorbed through the mucosa of the stomach. Alcohol and substances containing alcohol are soluble in lipids. They are rapidly absorbed through

the gastrointestinal (GI) tract. Substances low in lipid solubility are not absorbed well through the stomach or intestinal mucosa, and are absorbed best when given by a means other than the GI tract. An exception is the drug neomycin, which is not lipid soluble and yet is given orally. It is indicated for suppression of intestinal bacteria before intestinal or bowel surgery, or in the treatment of bacterial diarrhea. By giving neomycin orally, it passes through the GI tract, unable to be absorbed. As a result, it tends to build up and accumulate in the bowel. There, the trapped antibiotic kills the bacteria in the bowel, for the desired effect.

3. *Presence or absence of food in the stomach.* Food in the stomach tends to slow absorption due to a slower emptying of the stomach. If a fast drug effect is desired, an empty stomach will facilitate quicker absorption. On the other hand, giving some medications on an empty stomach is contraindicated. Medications that are irritating to the stomach can be buffered by the presence of food. Directions may indicate "Give before meals" or "Take with food" to decrease side effects (e.g., nausea and gastric ulcers) on the GI tract.

Distribution

The movement of a drug from the bloodstream into the tissues and fluids of the body is also affected by specific properties of the drug. Reaching sites beyond the major organs may depend on the drug's ability to cross a lipid membrane. Some drugs pass the "blood-brain barrier" or the "placental barrier," whereas others do not. You may read about drugs contraindicated for lactating mothers because the drug has the ability to pass through the cell membranes into the milk.

Some drugs have a *selective distribution* (see Fig. 3.3). This refers to an affinity, or attraction, of a drug to a specific organ or cells. For example, amphetamines have a selective distribution to cerebrospinal fluid (CSF). The human chorionic gonadotropin (HCG) hormone, which is used as a fertility drug, has a selective distribution to the ovaries.

By virtue of their properties, some drugs are distributed more slowly than others. Thus, while two drugs may be categorized in the same drug classification, one may be known to act on the cells and achieve the effect more quickly than the other.

Metabolism

When transformed in the liver (biotransformation), a drug is broken down and altered to more water-soluble by-products. Thus, the drug may be more easily excreted by the kidneys.

If hepatic disease is present, a patient may exhibit toxic (poisonous) effects of a drug. This occurs because the drug is not being broken down properly by the inefficient liver. It may accumulate, unchanged by the liver, and may be unable to pass out of the body's excretory system.

It is possible for some drugs to bypass the process of metabolism. They reach the kidneys virtually unchanged and may later be detected in the urine.

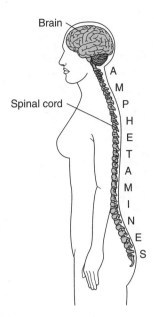

Figure 3.3 Distribution. One example of selective distribution is the attraction of amphetamines to the cerebrospinal fluid.

Excretion

While it is possible for some drugs to be eliminated through the lungs (e.g., exhaled gases and anesthetics) or through perspiration, feces, bile, or breast milk, most are excreted by the kidneys.

If a drug is not excreted properly before repeated doses are given, eventually a cumulative effect may occur. A *cumulative effect* is an increased effect of a drug demonstrated when repeated doses accumulate in the body. If unnoticed, the cumulative effect may build to a dangerous, or toxic, level. This can be of particular concern with the elderly.

Toxicity refers to a condition that results from exposure to either a poison or a dangerous amount of a drug that is normally safe when given in a smaller amount. In drug therapy, the goal is to give just enough of the drug to cause the desired (therapeutic) effect while keeping the amount below the level at which toxic effects are observed.

Digoxin is a cardiac drug that must be given cautiously because of its potential for causing a cumulative effect. Normally, digoxin slows the heart rate, but if the drug accumulates, the heart rate may slow to a dangerously low level. Circulation and renal function must be adequate, or the digoxin will accumulate, leading to digoxin toxicity.

Other Variables

Many variables affect the speed and efficiency of drugs being processed by the body. The physical properties of the drugs themselves and the condition of the body systems have been discussed. Other variables affecting drug action and effect follow.

AGE

Metabolism and excretion are slower in the elderly, and therefore attention must be paid to possible cumulative effects. Children have a lower threshold of response and react more rapidly and sometimes in unexpected ways; therefore, frequent assessment is imperative.

WEIGHT

Generally, the bigger the person, the greater the dose should be. However, there is great individual variation in sensitivity to drugs. Many drug dosages are always calculated on the basis of the patient's weight.

SEX

Women respond differently than men to some drugs. The ratio of fat per body mass differs, and so do hormone levels. If the female is pregnant or nursing, most drugs are contraindicated, or the dosage must be adjusted.

PSYCHOLOGICAL STATE

It has been proven that the more positive the patient feels about the medication he or she is taking, the more positive the physical response. This is referred to as the *placebo effect.*

A *placebo* is an inactive substance that resembles a medication, although no drug is present. For example, a sugar tablet or a saline solution for injection may be used as a placebo.

Placebos are most often used in blind study experiments, in which groups of people are given either a drug or a placebo. The individuals, unaware of which they have been given, are studied for the effects. Often, by virtue of strong belief, the placebo-administered individuals achieve the desired effect associated with the drug they think they have received.

Placebos are occasionally given to patients who are developing a psychological dependence on a drug. Substituting a placebo for the drug may prevent a physical dependence.

It is also possible to have a decreased drug effect when the attitude of a patient toward a medication is negative.

Attitudes toward medicines can also be influenced positively or negatively by cultural or religious beliefs. The caregiver needs to understand the importance of these beliefs to the patient.

> *The significance for you, the health care worker, is to recognize that your attitude regarding a medication may be picked up by the patient and indirectly may affect the patient's response to the drug.*

DRUG INTERACTIONS

Whenever more than one drug is taken, it is possible that the combination may alter the normal expected response of each individual drug. One drug may interact with another to increase, decrease, or cancel out the effects of the other.

The following terms are used to describe drug interactions:

Synergism. The action of two drugs working together in which one helps the other simultaneously for an effect that neither could produce alone. Drugs that work together are said to be synergistic.

Potentiation. The action of two drugs in which one prolongs or multiplies the effect of the other. Drug A may be said to potentiate the effect of drug B.

Antagonism. The opposing action of two drugs in which one decreases or cancels out the effect of the other. Drug A may be referred to as an antagonist of drug B.

It is extremely important for the prescribing physician to know of all medications that a patient is taking in order to prevent undesirable drug interactions. On the other hand, it may be intentionally ordered that two drugs be taken together, because some drug interactions are desirable and beneficial. Compare the following situations, describing both desirable and undesirable drug interactions:

Desirable synergism. Promethazine (Phenergan) (a nonnarcotic sedative) and meperidine (Demerol) (a narcotic analgesic) are very effective in relieving pain. By giving small amounts of each together, pain can be relieved more safely that by giving a large amount of Demerol (which is addictive) by itself.

Undesirable synergism. Sedatives and barbiturates given in combination can depress the central nervous system (CNS) to dangerous levels, depending on the strengths of each.

Desirable potentiation. To build up a high level of some forms of penicillin (an antibiotic) in the blood, the drug probenecid (Benemid) (antigout medication) can be given simultaneously. Benemid potentiates the effect of penicillin by slowing the excretion rate of the antibiotic.

Undesirable potentiation. Toxic effect may result when cimetidine (Tagamet) (a gastric antisecretory) is given simultaneously with Tofranil (an antidepressant). Tagamet potentiates the level of antidepressant concentrations in the blood.

Desirable antagonism. A narcotic antagonist (e.g., naloxone, Narcan) saves lives from drug overdoses by canceling out the effect of narcotics.

Undesirable antagonism. Antacids taken at the same time as tetracycline alter the pH and prevent absorption of tetracycline.

DOSAGE

Different dosages of a drug may bring about variations in the speed of drug action or effectiveness. *Dosage* is defined as the amount of drug given for a particular therapeutic or desired effect. Terms of various dosage levels are:

1. *Minimum dose.* Smallest amount of a drug that will produce a therapeutic effect
2. *Maximum dose.* Largest amount of a drug that will produce a desired effect without producing symptoms of toxicity
3. *Loading dose.* Initial high dose (often maximum dose) used to quickly elevate the level of the drug in the blood (often followed by a series of lower maintenance doses)
4. *Maintenance dose.* Dose required to keep the drug blood level at a steady state in order to maintain the desired effect
5. *Toxic dose.* Amount of a drug that will produce harmful side effects or symptoms of poisoning
6. *Lethal dose.* Dose that causes death
7. *Therapeutic dose.* Dose that is customarily given (average adult dose based on body weight of 150 lb); adjusted according to variations from the norm

You may be familiar with the use of a high loading dose followed by a lesser maintenance dose. If you have taken antibiotics, you may have been instructed to take two tablets or capsules initially and then to take one tablet every 6 hours. It is frequently desirable to give a loading dose of antibiotics to build up a high level and get the process of killing the bacteria started.

ROUTE

The route of administration is probably the most significant factor in the speed of drug action.

The route of drug administration can be compared to the route of travel. In planning a trip from point A to point B, you may have a map that shows several courses of travel to reach the destination. The course you select is optional, depending on your choice for the quickest, cheapest, safest, or most scenic route.

Options for routes of drug administration are much the same. There are a number of methods by which drugs may be given to reach their destination. Sometimes the route selected is based on the degree of speed, cost, or safety of administration. Sometimes there is no choice of routes because some medications can be given only by one route. Often this is because absorption occurs by that route only, or the substance is dangerous or toxic when given by another route. Insulin, for example, may be given only by injection. Much research has been done to produce an oral form of insulin, but attempts have failed because the drug is destroyed by gastric juices.

The most common routes of administration may be grouped into two main categories:

1. *GI tract routes*
   a. Oral (PO)
   b. Nasogastric tube (NG)
   c. Rectal (R)
2. *Parenteral routes*, which include any other than the gastrointestinal tract

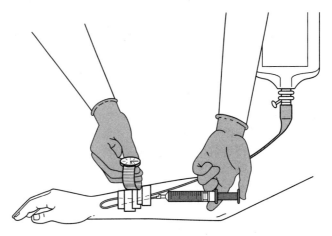

Figure 3.4 Intravenous push or bolus. IV drugs are administered slowly over a specified period of time (usually 1–7 minutes).

    a. Sublingual (SL) or buccal
    b. Injection routes
       i.   Intravenous (IV)
       ii. Intramuscular (IM)
       iii. Subcutaneous (SC)
       iv. Intradermal (ID)
       v. Intracardiac, Intraspinal, Intracapsular*
    c. Topical (T)
       i.   Dermal (D)
       ii. Mucosal
    d. Inhalation

There are advantages and disadvantages in the use of each route. The doctor's choice of a particular route of administration of a drug may depend on (1) desired effects (e.g., fast or slow, local or systemic); (2) absorption qualities of the drug; and (3) how the drug is supplied. Other general points regarding the effect of the route on the drug absorption are as follows:

1. The oral route is the easiest, but the effects are slower because of the time required for disintegration of drugs in the alimentary canal before absorption.
2. The intravenous route is the fastest: Drugs enter the bloodstream immediately. Doses to be given IV are in small amounts; effects are immediate and can be quite dangerous if given in amounts recommended for other routes. Intravenous drugs can be administered by IV push or bolus (a concentrated drug solution) (Fig. 3.4), or they can be diluted and solutions are then infused more slowly by IV drip.

---

*The latter three injection routes are less common and are administered by the physician.

a. IVs are administered by a physician, registered nurse, or paramedic.

b. IV is the best route for treatment of emergencies because of the speed of action.

3. Parenteral routes are the choice when:

a. Patient can take nothing by mouth (NPO).

b. The drug is not suitable for GI absorption.

4. The intramuscular route is fairly rapid because the muscles are highly vascular. If it is desirable to retard the speed of absorption, a drug to be given IM may be added to an oily base.

Unexpected Responses to Drugs

Several other terms must be defined in order to complete your awareness of the bodily effects of drugs. These terms refer to adverse drug effects.

Teratogenic effect. Effect from maternal drug administration that causes the development of physical defects in a fetus.

Idiosyncrasy. Unique, unusual response to a drug. For example, a patient may have an idiosyncrasy to a particular tranquilizer if it causes agitation and excitement rather than tranquillity.

Tolerance. Decreased response to a drug that develops after repeated doses are given. To achieve the desired effect, the drug dosage must be increased or the drug replaced.

Dependence. Acquired need for a drug that may produce psychological and/or physical symptoms of withdrawal when the drug is discontinued.

• Psychological dependence involves only a psychological craving; no physical symptoms of withdrawal other than anxiety.

• Physical dependence exists when cells actually have a need for the drug; symptoms of withdrawal include retching, nausea, pain, tremors, and sweating.

Hypersensitivity. Immune response (allergy) to a drug may be of varying degrees.

• May be mild with no immediate effects; rash may appear after 3–4 days of drug therapy.

• May develop after uneventful previous uses of a drug.

• More likely to exist in patients with other known allergies.

Note: Nausea, vomiting and diarrhea are *not* considered signs of allergies.

Extreme caution should be taken when giving a medication to a patient for the first time, particularly if the patient has a history of other allergies.

Anaphylactic reaction. Severe, possibly fatal, allergic (hypersensitivity) response.

- Signs include itching, urticaria (hives), hyperemia (reddened, warm skin), vascular collapse, shock, cyanosis, laryngeal edema, and dyspnea.
- Treatment includes cardiopulmonary resuscitation (CPR) if indicated and drugs as required: epinephrine (Adrenalin) to raise blood pressure; corticosteroid (Solu-Medrol) to reduce inflammation and the body's immunological response; antihistamine (Benadryl) to suppress histamine, thereby reducing redness, itching, and edema.
- Anaphylaxis has been noted often with the following: antibiotics, especially penicillin; X-ray dyes containing iodides (IVP [intravenous pyelogram] dye, angiogram dye, gallbladder dyes, etc.); foods (shellfish, onions, peanuts, etc.); and insect stings (bees and ants).

Knowledge of any adverse reactions to drugs should be included in the patient's history. This information can be helpful in preventing repeated episodes. Getting an accurate drug history and clearly listing known allergies is a critical function of the health care worker.

Persons who have had an anaphylactic reaction to a substance should always wear a Medic-Alert tag or bracelet to identify the substance to which they are extremely allergic. Persons who have had hypersensitivity reactions to a substance are more at risk for reactions to other substances as well. Allergies should be listed on a card and carried in the wallet of the sensitive individual.

Check your knowledge of this chapter before going any further.

Chapter Review Quiz

Fill in the blanks.

1.

Drug Sources	Example	Trade Name	Classification

2. Drugs that are distributed throughout the body have _____ effects.

3. Drugs whose action is limited to a specific location have _____ effects.

4. As drugs pass through the body, they undergo four processes:

Process	Definition of Process

5. Factors that may affect the passage of drugs through the body:

Process	Primary Site of Process	Conditions Hampering Process

6. If circulation is poor, metabolism faulty, or excretion inadequate, drugs may build up in the system, leading to _____ effects, causing poisonous, or _____ levels of the drug.

7. Variables affecting the efficiency of drug action include _____ , _____ , _____ , and _____ .

Match the term with the definition:

8. Synergism _____ a. Amount of drug required to keep drug level steady

9. Antagonism _____ b. Amount of drug that can cause death

10. Potentiation _____ c. Amount of drug that can cause dangerous side effects

11. Lethal dose _____ d. One drug making the effect of another drug more powerful

12. Toxic dose _____ e. Drugs working together for a better effect

13. Maintenance dose _____ f. Drugs working against each other or counteracting each other's effect

14. Idiosyncrasy _____ a. Acquired need for a drug, with symptoms of withdrawal when discontinued

15. Tolerance _____ b. Unusual response to a drug, other than expected effect

16. Dependence _____ c. Effects on a fetus from maternal use of a drug

17. Teratogenic _____ d. Decreased response after repeated use of a drug, increased dosage required for effect

Fill in the blanks:

18. An allergy or immune response to a drug is called

_____ .

19. Allergic reactions to drugs may be *mild*, with symptoms such as

_____

_____ .

20. Allergic reactions to drugs are more common in patients with

_____ .

21. *Severe* allergic reaction with shock, laryngeal edema, and dyspnea is called

_____ .

22. Treatment of severe allergic reactions include the following three medications in order of administration: _____,

_____ , and_____ .

CHAPTER 4

Medication Preparations and Supplies

OBJECTIVES

Upon completion of this chapter, the student should be able to:

1. Differentiate between various oral drug forms: sublingual tablet versus buccal tablet, solution versus suspension, syrup versus elixir, enteric-coated tablet versus scored tablet, and timed-release capsule versus lozenge.
2. Explain what is meant by parenteral.
3. List four classifications of drugs that are commonly given by the rectal route.
4. Define the following types of injections and explain how they differ in administration and absorption rate: IV, IM, SC, and ID.
5. Compare the IV injections referred to as IV push, IV infusion, and IV piggyback.
6. List and define at least eight drug forms used for topical (both dermal and mucosal) administration.
7. Explain the advantages of administering drugs via a dermal patch.
8. Identify various supplies used in the preparation of medications.

The forms in which drugs are prepared are as numerous as the routes of administration. *Drug form* refers to the type of preparation in which the drug is supplied. Pharmaceutical companies prepare each drug in the form or forms most suitable for its intended route and means of absorption. *Drug form* and *drug preparation* are synonymous. The *PDR* lists the forms available for each drug under the heading "How Supplied." See Table 4.1 for abbreviations of some of the drug forms and routes of administration.

TABLE 4.1. ABBREVIATIONS FOR DRUG ADMINISTRATION

Drug Forms		Routes	
cap	capsule	D	dermal
elix	elixir	ID	intradermal
		IM	intramuscular
gtt	drop	IV	intravenous
supp	suppository	IVPB	intravenous piggyback
susp	suspension	PO, p.o., per os	oral
tab	tablet	R	rectal
ung	ointment	SC, subcu, subq	subcutaneous
		T	topical

A Space-Age Drug Form

Great advances have occurred recently in developing a new drug form that may revolutionize the way a number of drugs are administered. The new drug form is the dermal patch, or *transdermal delivery system*. Dermal patches were taken on the space shuttles during the 1990s for the prevention of nausea. The key to the transdermal system is that the drug molecules are present in a variety of sizes and shapes that allow for absorption through the skin at various rates. Thus, a patch can provide a constant, even flow of a drug over a long period of time—hours or days. The drug, being released at a consistent rate, remains at an effective level in the blood, as opposed to rising and falling, as happens with pills. Advantages of this method of administration include:

- Easy application, with no discomfort or undesirable taste
- Effectiveness for long periods of time, hours for some drugs and days for others
- Consistent blood level of drug, since drug is released at varying rates, rather than all at one time

Dermal patches vary in size, shape, and color (Fig. 4.1). They are most commonly seen today on patients for the prevention of angina. Current marketing of dermal patches also includes others for the prevention of motion sickness (may be applied before traveling), for management of chronic pain (e.g., Duragesic; see Chapter 19), as a smoking deterrent (e.g., Habitrol and Nicoderm), and for estrogen replacement (e.g., Estraderm). Research is ongoing in the development of dermal patches for birth control, high blood pressure, ulcers, allergies, and heart conditions. Probably not all drug molecules will be adaptable to this drug form, but it certainly has opened new doors in the area of drug administration.

Standard Drug Forms

You probably have received medications in many of the standard forms at some time during your life. Each form is defined and listed below according to the routes

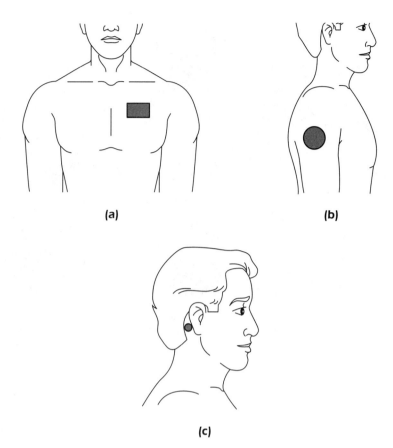

Figure 4.1 *Transdermal drug delivery. Dermal patches vary in size, shape, and color. (a, b) For prevention of angina pectoris, and for management of chronic pain; and (c) for prevention of motion sickness.*

of administration (see Fig. 4.2). As you read in Chapter 3, drugs may be administered through the gastrointestinal (GI) tract or parenterally. GI routes include oral, nasogastric tube, and rectal. Parenteral refers to any route not involving the GI tract, including injection, topical (skin or mucosal), and inhalation routes.

ORAL DRUG FORMS

Oral drug forms include:

Tablet. Disk of compressed drug; may be a variety of shapes and colors; may be coated to enhance easy swallowing; may be *scored* (evenly divided in halves or quarters by score lines) to enhance equal distribution of drug if it has been broken.

Enteric-coated tablet. Tablet with a special coating that resists disintegration by gastric juices. The coating dissolves further down the GI tract, in the enteric, or intestinal, region. Some drugs, such as aspirin, that are irritating to the stomach are available in enteric-coated tablets. To be effective, the coating must never be destroyed by chewing or crushing when it is administered.

Capsule. Drug contained within a gelatin-type container.

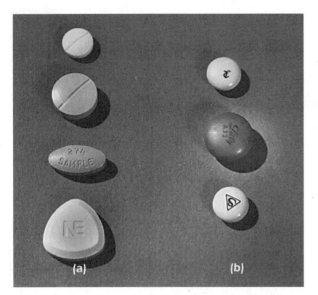 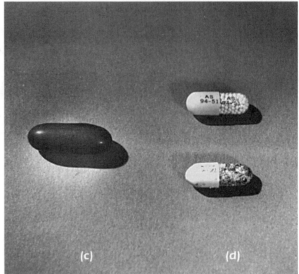

Figure 4.2 Oral drug forms. Tablets and capsules vary in size, shape, and color. (a) Tablets, scored and unscored; (b) enteric-coated tablets; (c) gelatin capsule; (d) timed-release capsules.

- Easier to swallow than noncoated tablets.
- Double chamber may be pulled apart to add drug powder to soft foods or beverages for patients who have difficulty swallowing (unless specifically contraindicated for absorption).

Timed-release (sustained-release) capsule. Capsule containing drug particles that have various coatings (often of different colors) that differ in the amount of time required before the coatings dissolve. This form of drug preparation is designed to deliver a dose of drug over an extended period of time. An advantage of taking a drug in the timed-release form is the decreased frequency of administration. For example, the tranquilizer Valium may be administered in tablet form, 5 mg tid, or in the timed-release form (Valrelease, 15 mg) only once qd. (See Table 5.1 for common abbreviations.) Because of the significance of the various coatings that encapsulate the drug particles, it is important that the small colored pellets *not* be crushed or mixed with foods. Damage to the coatings of drug pellets allows the drug to be released all at one time as it is administered. Such immediate release of drug is a potential overdose. Timed-release capsules should be swallowed whole, with no physical damage to the contents of the capsule.

Lozenge (troche). Tablet containing palatable flavoring, indicated for a local (often soothing) effect on the throat or mouth.

- Patient is advised not to swallow a lozenge; it should be allowed to slowly dissolve in the mouth.
- Patient is also advised *not* to drink liquids for approximately 15 min after administration, to prevent washing of the lozenge contents from the throat or mouth.

Suspension. Liquid form of medication that must be shaken well before administration because the drug particles settle at the bottom of the bottle. The drug is not evenly dissolved in the liquid.

- A cephalosporin (Keflex) suspension is a commonly used antibiotic suspension for children. This form is more easily ingested by children than are capsules of Keflex.

Emulsion. Liquid drug preparation that contains oils and fats in water.

Elixir, fluid extract. Liquid drug forms with alcohol base.

- Should be tightly capped to prevent alcohol evaporation.
- Should not be available to alcoholics.

Syrup. Sweetened, flavored liquid drug form. Cherry syrup drug preparations are common for children.

Solution. Liquid drug form in which the drug is totally evenly dissolved. Appearance is clear, rather than cloudy or settled (as with a suspension).

Many drug forms for the oral route are commonly available over the counter and include thousands of trade name products. The oral route is the easiest and probably the cheapest for administration. It is, however, *not* the route of choice for treatment of emergencies, acute pain, NPO* patients, or patients unable to swallow. Other routes, especially the parenteral routes, produce a more rapid absorption rate and drug effect.

RECTAL DRUG FORMS

Rectal drug forms include:

Suppository. Drug suspended in a substance, such as cocoa butter, that melts at body temperature.

Enema solution. Drug suspended in solution to be administered as an enema.

The rectal route of administration is often the choice if the patient is ordered to have nothing by mouth (NPO) or cannot swallow. The most common classifications of drugs given rectally include sedatives, antiemetics, and antipyretics. A local analgesic effect may also be achieved by this route. In the past, rectal administration of drug solutions was given for general anesthesia, but is not common today.

INJECTABLE DRUG FORMS

Injectable drug forms include:

Solution. Drug suspended in a sterile vehicle.

- Quite often the solutions have a sterile water base and are thus referred to as *aqueous* (aq) (waterlike) solutions.

*See Table 5.1 for common abbreviations.

- Some solutions have an oil base, which tends to cause a more prolonged absorption time. The oily nature of these solutions makes them thick; thus they are referred to as viscous (thick) solutions.

Powder. Dry particles of drugs. The powder itself cannot be injected. It must be mixed with a sterile diluting solution (sterile water or saline solution) to render an injectable solution. This is termed *reconstitution* of a drug. Drugs are supplied undiluted in powder form because of the short period of time they remain stable after dilution.

The various injection routes differ according to the type of tissues into which the drug is deposited and the rate of absorption. Each is briefly defined below:

Intravenous. Injected directly into a vein. Immediate absorption and availability to major organs renders this route a dangerous one. IV drugs are usually administered by physicians, paramedics, or registered nurses. Types of intravenous injections include:

- IV push, a small volume of drug injected through a syringe and needle into the bloodstream.
- IV infusion or IV drip, a large volume of fluids, often with drugs added, which infuses continually into a vein.
- IV piggyback (IVPB), a drug diluted in moderate volume (50–100 ml) of fluid for intermittent infusion at specified intervals, usually q6–8h; the diluted solution is infused (piggyback) into a port on the main IV tubing or into a rubber adapter on the IV catheter (Fig. 4.3).

Intramuscular. Injected into a muscle, by positioning the needle and syringe at a 90-degree angle from the skin (Fig. 4.4). Absorption is fairly rapid due to the vascularity of muscle.

Subcutaneous. Injected into the fatty layer of tissue below the skin by positioning the needle and syringe at a 45-degree angle from the skin (Fig. 4.5). This may be the route of choice for drugs that should not be absorbed as rapidly as through the IV or IM routes.

Intradermal. Injected just beneath the skin, by positioning the needle and syringe at a 15-degree angle from the skin (Fig. 4.6). This route is used primarily for allergy skin testing. Because of the lack of vascularity in the dermis, absorption is slow. The greatest reaction is in the local tissues rather than systemic. When a small amount (0.1-0.2 cc) of drug is injected intradermally, the amount of redness that develops around the injection site can be used to determine whether a person is sensitive to the drug. Tuberculin (TB) skin tests (PPD) are also administered intradermally and the site is inspected 48–72 hours later for hardness (induration) and swelling. Redness (erythema) alone, *without swelling*, does not indicate a positive test result with PPD. The *raised area (induration)* is measured with a special ruler and the number of millimeters (mm) is documented. Check with your local Public Health Department regarding appropriate protocol with a positive PPD test result.

The less common parenteral routes, which are limited to a physician's administration, are:

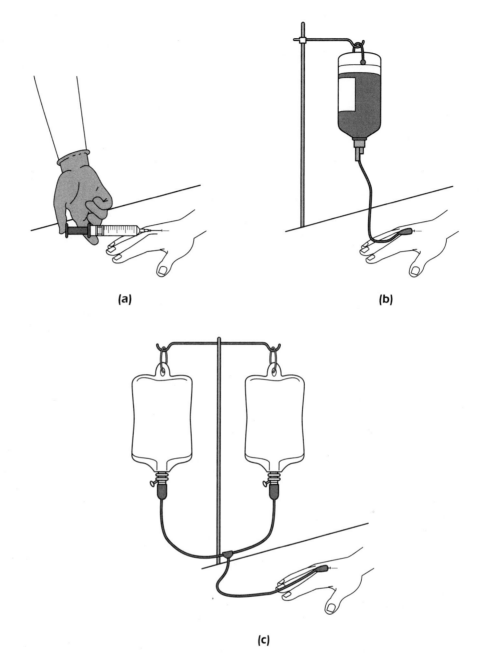

Figure 4.3 Intravenous administration. Different forms of IV injection include (a) IV push; (b) IV infusion (continuous); and (c) IV piggyback (intermittent).

Intracardiac. Injected directly into the heart. This route is used to administer adrenaline as a last resort to resuscitate a patient whose heart has stopped.

Intraspinal. Injected into the subarachnoid space, which contains cerebrospinal fluid (CSF) that surrounds the spinal cord. Drugs injected by this route are frequently anesthetics, which render a lack of sensation to those regions of the body distal to the intraspinal injection.

Intracapsular (intra-articular). Injected into the capsule of a joint, usually to reduce inflammation, as in bursitis. Arthritic or bursitic joints often injected with anti-inflammatory drugs include shoulders, elbows, wrists, ankles, knees, and hips.

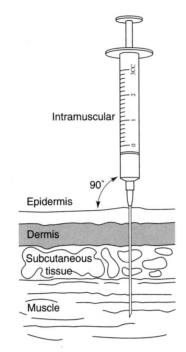

Figure 4.4 Intramuscular injection. Needle is inserted at a 90-degree angle.

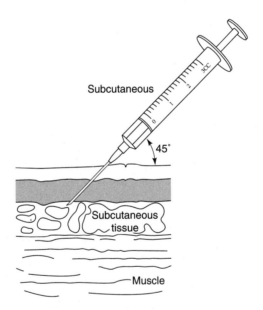

Figure 4.5 Subcutaneous injection. Needle is inserted at a 45-degree angle.

TOPICAL DRUG FORMS

Topical drug forms include drugs for dermal application and drugs for mucosal application. Those for *dermal* application include:

Cream or ointment. A semisolid preparation containing a drug, for external application. **Note:** Creams and ointments are not the same. The dose used differs for each.

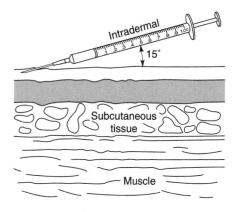

Figure 4.6 *Intradermal injection. Needle is inserted just beneath the skin at a 15-degree angle.*

Rule of thumb: If skin is wet, use cream, if skin is dry, use ointment.

Lotion. A liquid preparation applied externally for treatment of skin disorders. Unlike hand lotions, medicated lotions (e.g., calamine lotion) should be *patted*, not rubbed, on the affected skin.

Liniment. Preparation for external use that is rubbed on the skin as a counterirritant. As such, the liniment creates a different sensation (e.g., tingling or burning) to mask pain in the skin or muscles.

Dermal patch. Skin patch containing drug molecules that can be absorbed through the skin at varying rates to promote a consistent blood level between application times.

Both the dermal patch and ointment are common forms for administration of nitroglycerin. Nitroglycerin is a vasodilator used for the treatment of angina (chest pain related to narrowing of the coronary arteries). The beauty of the external applications of nitroglycerin is their ability to *prevent* angina by the slow, consistent release of the drug over a period of time. Before the external applications became available, nitroglycerin was primarily available in the form of a sublingual tablet to be taken at the time of an angina attack. Now all three forms are used—the tablet, the ointment, and the patch—with the external forms focusing on the prevention of angina. They are applied at regular intervals, as follows:

Ointment: 1–5 inches applied q8h measured and applied on special Appli-Ruler paper (Fig. 4.7)

Dermal patch: one patch (available in varied doses) q24h*

Other drug preparations considered topical are those that are applied to *mucosal membranes.* Some are administered for local effect (at the site of application) and, in other cases, a systemic effect is desired. The *mucosal drug forms* include:

Eye, ear, and nose drops (gtt). Drugs in sterile liquids to be applied by drops (referred to as instillation of drops).

*See Table 5.1 for common abbreviations.

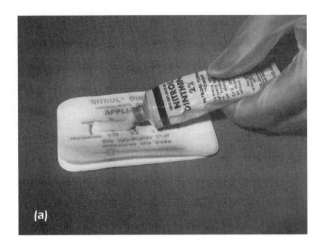
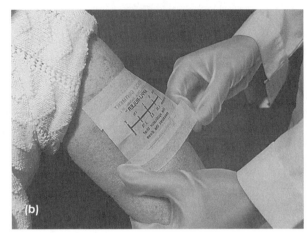

Figure 4.7 Topical administration. Dermal application includes creams and liquids placed on the skin. (a) Nitroglycerin ointment is measured on Appli-Ruler paper. (b) Paper containing ointment is applied to the skin.

Eye ointment. Sterile semisolid preparation, often antibiotic in nature, for oph-thalmic use only.

Vaginal creams. Medicated creams, often of antibiotic or antifungal nature, that are to be inserted vaginally with the use of a special applicator.

Rectal and vaginal suppositories. Drug suspended in a substance, such as cocoa butter, that melts at body temperature, for local effect. Some rectal supposito-ries are also used for systemic effects (Fig. 4.8).

Douche solution. Sterile solution, often an antiseptic such as povidone iodine solution and sterile water, used to irrigate the vaginal canal.

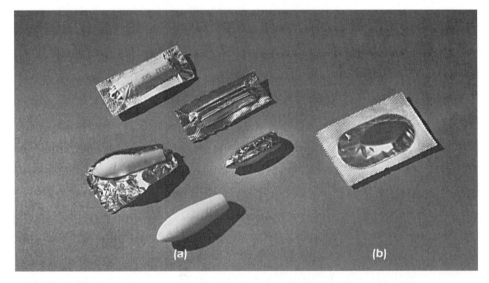

Figure 4.8 Topical administration via mucous membranes. Suppositories come in various shapes and sizes, for example, (a) rectal suppositories, wrapped in foil and unwrapped; and (b) vaginal suppository, wrapped in foil.

Buccal tablet. Tablet that is absorbed *via the buccal mucosa* in the mouth.
- Patient is told *not* to swallow tablet; it is to be placed between the cheek and gums, and allowed to dissolve slowly.
- Not commonly used today.

Sublingual tablet. Tablet that is absorbed via the mucosa under the tongue.
- Patient is told not to swallow tablet; it is to be placed under the tongue and allowed to dissolve slowly.
- The most common sublingual tablet is nitroglycerin. Given for the treatment of angina, this drug reaches the bloodstream immediately via the sublingual capillaries. Angina may be relieved within 1–5 min after sublingual nitroglycerin is administered.

INHALABLE DRUG FORMS

The drug forms used for the inhalation route include:

Spray or mist. Liquid drug forms that may be inhaled as fine droplets via the use of spray bottles, nebulizers, or metered dose inhalers.
- In the hospital setting, respiratory therapists instill a liquid into a chamber of a nebulizer for a patient's breathing treatment. Often the liquid contains a bronchodilator, a mucolytic agent, or sterile saline solution for moisture.
- In the home, the patient may instill sprays via nasal spray bottles, vaporizers, or inhalers. Asthma patients rely on the use of inhalers to keep their bronchioles open by inhaling the mist of a bronchodilator. A mouthpiece, through which the patient inhales, is connected to a container of liquid drug.

Gas. Anesthetics, such as nitrous oxide, that are introduced via the respiratory route for general anesthesia.

Powder. Drug in powder form to reduce bronchial asthma attacks, to be inhaled through a special device called a Spinhaler. The powdered drug, cromolyn sodium (Intal), is inside a capsule that is inserted into the Spinhaler.

Supplies

Considering the variety of drug forms you may be administering, you must become familiar with various supplies to be used (Fig. 4.9):

Medicine cup. Two types of disposable cups are commonly used. Paper cups are used for dispensing tablets and capsules. Plastic 1-oz medicine cups with measurements (ml, tsp, tbsp, dr, or oz) marked on the side are used for dispensing oral liquid medications. (See Table 5.1 for a list of common abbreviations used in medication orders.)

Mortar. Glass cup in which tablets (excluding enteric-coated tablets) may be placed to be crushed. Various other pill-crushing devices are available.

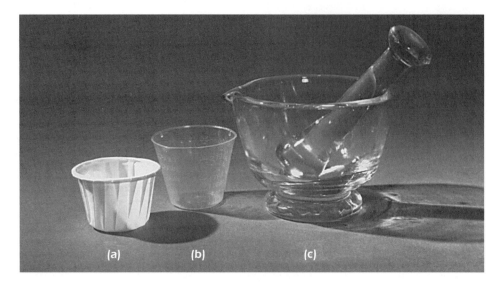

Figure 4.9 *Supplies for oral administration. (a) Tablets and capsules are usually administered in paper soufflé cups. (b) Liquids are measured in calibrated plastic cups. (c) A mortar and pestle are used when necessary to crush tablets.*

Note: In some areas a physician's order is required for pill crushing. Check the regulations in your area.

Pestle. Club-shaped glass tool used as the crushing device to pulverize tablets.

Finger cot. Rubber coverlet for one finger only, to be applied and lubricated before insertion of a rectal suppository (Fig. 4.10).

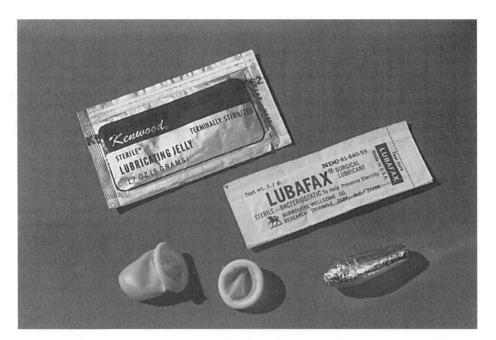

Figure 4.10 *Supplies for administration of rectal suppository. A finger cot and small packet of lubricant are required.*

Medication for injection is contained in an ampule or vial (Fig. 4.11):

Ampule. Small glass container that holds a single dose of sterile solution for injection. The ampule must be broken at the neck to obtain the solution.

Vial. Glass container sealed at the top by a rubber stopper to enhance sterility of the contents. Contents may be a solution or a powdered drug that needs to be reconstituted. Vials may be multiple dose or unit dose:

- Multiple-dose vials contain large quantities of solution (up to 50 cc) and may repeatedly be entered through the rubber stopper to remove a portion of the contents.
- Unit-dose vials contain small quantities of solution (1–2 cc) that are removed during a single use. Unit-dose vials are widely used today as a means of controlling abuse or removal of excess amounts of solution from a drug vial.

Needles. Needles for injections have two measurements that must be noted (Fig. 4.12):

- Length varies from short ($\frac{3}{8}$ inch) to medium (1–1$\frac{1}{2}$ inch) length for standard injections. Long needles (5 inch) may be used by the physician for intraspinal or intracardiac routes. Needles 2–5 inches long are used by the physician for intra-articular injections (into the joint).
- Gauge is a number that represents the diameter of the needle lumen. Needle gauges vary from 18 (largest) to 27 (smallest), with the higher gauge number representing the smaller lumen.

Syringes. The three most common disposable syringes for parenteral administration of drugs are the standard hypodermic syringe, the tuberculin (TB) syringe, and the insulin syringe (Fig. 4.13).

- The standard hypodermic syringe has a capacity of 2–3 cc. Most companies prepackage this type of syringe with a needle attached. Since you

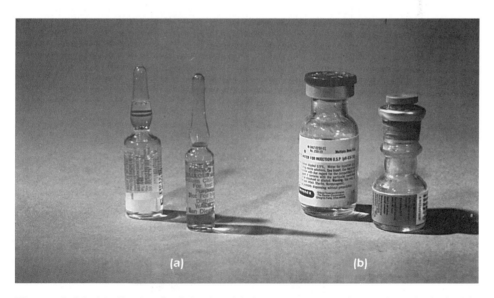

Figure 4.11 *Medication for injection. Various premeasured containers include (a) ampules and (b) vials.*

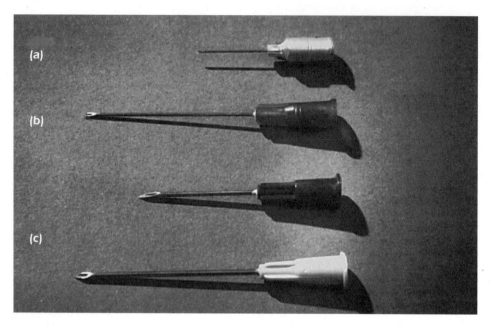

Figure 4.12 Needles commonly used for injections. Sizes vary in length and gauge. (a) 3/8 inch, 27 gauge; (b) 1 ½ inches, 21 gauge; (c) 1 inch and 1 ½ inches, 18 gauge.

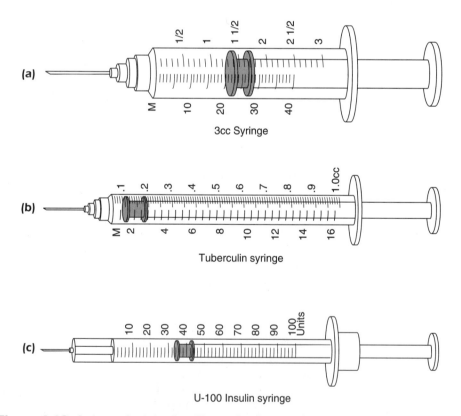

3cc Syringe

Tuberculin syringe

U-100 Insulin syringe

Figure 4.13 Syringes for injection. Type of syringe varies with type and quantity of medication. (a) 3 cc syringe, read at 1.4 cc or 23 minims; (b) tuberculin syringe, read at 0.05 cc; (c) insulin syringe, read at 32 units.

may use this type of syringe for either subcutaneous or intramuscular injections, you must choose the package with the needle length and gauge appropriate for the route and depth of injection you will give. All hypodermic syringes are marked with 10 calibrations per cc. Thus, each small line represents 0.1 cc. When preparing for an injection with this syringe, you must know the amount of solution needed to the nearest 0.1 cc (an additional scale on the syringe shows calibrations in minims, which is discussed later, in Chapter 9).

- The TB syringe is very narrow and is finely calibrated. The total capacity is only 1 cc. There are 100 fine calibration lines marking the capacity. Thus, each line represents 0.01 cc. Every tenth line is longer, to indicate 0.1-cc increments. Very precise small amounts of solution may be measured with the TB syringe. It is most commonly used for newborn and pediatric dosages and for intradermal skin tests. When preparing for an injection with this syringe, you must know the amount of solution needed to the nearest 0.01 cc.

- The insulin syringe is used strictly for administering insulin to diabetics. Like the TB syringe, it has only a 1-cc capacity. The 1-cc capacity is marked as 100 units (U) to represent a strength of 100 U of insulin when full. Each group of 10 U is further divided by 5 small lines on an even scale or 5 small lines on an odd scale. Thus, *each line represents 2 U*. A smaller insulin syringe, of only ½-cc capacity, may be used when less than 50 U (½ cc) of insulin is ordered. The smaller insulin syringe has 50 small calibration lines; thus, each represents 1 U of insulin.

It is extremely important that you can interpret the value of the calibrations on each of the syringes. Study the calibrations each time you prepare for an injection to prevent a medication error from negligent misinterpretation.

Oral Syringes.   Health care workers should be aware that some oral liquid medications are dispensed from the Pharmacy in disposable plastic syringes with rubber or plastic covers on the tip. These syringes are labeled "Not for injection" or "For oral use only".

Check your knowledge of this chapter before going any further.

Chapter Review Quiz

1. Which route of administration is used most often? Why?

   _____

   _____

Complete with the appropriate drug form:

2. A tablet placed under the tongue: _____

3. A tablet placed in the cheek pouch: _____

4. A tablet dissolved in the mouth for local action: _____

5. A coated tablet that dissolves in the intestines instead of in the stomach:

   _____

6. A capsule that has delayed action over a longer period of time:

   _____

7. A liquid drug form with an alcohol base: _____

8. A liquid medication that must be shaken before administration:

   _____

9. Drugs given by the rectal route include _____ _____.

10. The parenteral route refers to any route other than the gastrointestinal route. Name four parenteral routes:

    _____

    _____

    _____

    _____

Fill in the blanks:

11. Crushing tablets requires a _____ and _____ .

12. To administer a rectal suppository, you need a _____ and

    _____ .

13. Medicine for injection is contained in two types of glass containers:

    a. With rubber stopper on top: _____

    b. All glass to be broken at the neck: _____

14. Needles are selected according to two measurements: _____ and _____ .

15. The three most commonly used syringes for injections are: _____ , _____ , and _____ .

CHAPTER 5

Abbreviations and Systems of Measurement

OBJECTIVES

Upon completion of this chapter, the student should be able to:

1. Identify common abbreviations and symbols used for medication orders.
2. List the six parts of a medication order and the two additional items required on a prescription blank.
3. Describe the responsibilities of the health care worker regarding verbal and telephone orders for medications.
4. Interpret medication orders correctly.
5. Compare and contrast the three systems of measurement.
6. Convert dosages from one system to another by use of the table for metric, apothecary, and household equivalents.
7. Describe appropriate patient education for those who will be measuring and administering their own medications.

Abbreviations

Interpretation of the medication order is the first responsibility when preparing medication for administration. Knowledge of abbreviations and symbols is essential for accurate interpretation of the physician's order. The abbreviations and symbols in Table 5.1 must be memorized. You may see some abbreviations written with or without periods, and orders may vary in the use of capital versus lowercase letters. You may occasionally see other abbreviations not included in this list. *When in doubt, always question the meaning.*

TABLE 5.1. COMMON ABBREVIATIONS FOR MEDICATION ORDERS

Note: Abbreviations can be written with or without periods.

a	before	NS, N/S	normal saline (sodium chloride, 0.9%)
aa, a͞a	of each	OD	right eye; overdose
ac	before meals	OS	left eye
ad lib	as desired	os	mouth
AM, am	morning	OTC	over the counter
amp	ampule	OU	both eyes
amt	amount	oz, ℥	ounce
aq	water	p̄	after
bid	twice a day	pc	after meals
c̄	with	per	by means of
cap	capsule	PM, pm	afternoon
cc	cubic centimeter (equivalent to ml)	po, PO, per os	by mouth, orally
cm	centimeter	PRN, prn	whenever necessary
comp	compound	pt	pint
d	day	q̄	every
DC, disc, dc	discontinue	qd	every day
dil	dilute	qh	every hour
dr, ℨ	dram	q2h	every 2 hours
D/RL	dextrose, c̄ Ringer's lactate	q3h	every 3 hours
DS	double strength	qid	four times a day
DW	distilled water	QNS	quantity not sufficient
D5W	dextrose, 5% in water	qod	every other day
EC	enteric coated	qs	quantity sufficient
elix	elixir	qt	quart
et	and	R	rectal
ext	extract	RL, R/L	Ringer's lactate
fl, fld	fluid	Rx	take, prescription
gr	grain	s̄	without
g, Gm	gram	SC, subcu, subq	subcutaneous
gtt	drop	sig	label
h, hr	hour	SL	sublingual
hs, HS	at bedtime, at hour of sleep	sol	solution
IM	intramuscular	sos	once if necessary
inj	by injection	sp	spirits
IU	International Units	SR	sustained release
IV	intravenous	ss, s̄s̄	one-half
IVP	intravenous pyelogram	stat	immediately
IVPB	intravenous piggyback	supp	suppository
kg, Kg	kilogram	syr	syrup
KVO, TKO	keep vein open, to keep open	T	temperature
L	liter	tab	tablet
LA	long acting	tbsp, T, tbs	tablespoon
lb, #	pound	tid	three times a day
m, m̨ , min	minim	tinct, tr	tincture
mEq	milliequivalent	TO	telephone order
μg, mcg	microgram	TPR	temperature, pulse, respiration
mg	milligram	tsp, t	teaspoon
ml, mL	milliliter (equivalent to cc)	U, u	unit
mm	millimeter	ung	ointment
NaCl	sodium chloride	vag	vaginal
noc, noct, n	night	VO	verbal order
NPO, npo	nothing by mouth	×	times

Medication orders contain six parts.

1. Date.
2. Patient's name.
3. Medication name.
4. Dosage or amount of medication.
5. Route or manner of administration (if no route is specified, the oral route is usually the appropriate one). When in doubt, always check with the physician.
6. Time to be administered, or frequency.

Medication orders must always be written and signed by a physician. In an emergency the physician may give a verbal order (VO). It is the responsibility of the health care worker to repeat the order (i.e., medication and amount) before administration and to write down medication, amount, and time of administration as soon as it is given. The physician will sign the medication order after the emergency. Always determine the policy of the agency before taking a telephone order (TO). Most agencies require a registered nurse to take telephone orders. In some extended care facilities, licensed practical (vocational) nurses are allowed to take telephone orders. When taking a telephone order, always obtain the name of the person calling in the order and write the name of that person and the time the call was made next to the medication ordered, e.g., "TO Dr. A. Smith, per Mary Jones, CMA @ 1300." Also repeat all of the details regarding the medication, dosage, frequency, etc., as you write down the order. If you are the medical assistant, or nurse, calling in the prescription to the facility for the physician, be sure to repeat the name of the drug, dosage, frequency, and route to the physician as you write it on the patient's office record, adding the time the call was made and the name of the nurse receiving the call in the facility. This documentation is extremely important in preventing medication errors and legal complications. The physician must sign all verbal and telephone orders within 24 hours.

Note: Regulations vary from state to state regarding phone orders. Check the rules in your state regarding who can call in an order and who can receive a phone order.

Medication orders can be written on the patient's record in the physician's office, clinic, or institution, or on a prescription blank (Fig. 5.1). It is the responsibility of the health care worker to check the medication order for completeness by noting the six items—date, patient name, medication name, dosage, route, and frequency (plus additional items if using the prescription blank)—and to question any discrepancy, omission, or unusual order. The prescription blank contains two additional items: the physician's Drug Enforcement Administration registration number if the medication is a controlled substance, and the number of times that the prescription can be refilled. If there are to be no refills, write the word "NO," "NONE," or "Ø" after Refill. Never leave a blank space in that area on the prescription blank.

Systems of Measurement

In order to carry out a medication order accurately, the person administering medications must have an understanding of the different systems of measurement. The

---

COMMUNITY MEDICAL CLINIC

1700 South Tamiami Trail, Sarasota, FL 34239, (813) 952-2577

Patient Name: *Mary Chase* Date: *12-10-96*

Address:_____

R

Cephalexin 250 mg
28
I qid

Private Pay
Private Insurance
Medicaid
CMC

Refill: *0* Physician Signature: *J. Brown* M.D.

Physician Name (printed): J. Brown

Physician DEA#:_____

5371-1 11/92

Figure 5.1 Prescription blank. Check for completeness and accuracy, including date, patient's name, medication name, dosage, route, frequency or time, number of refills, and DEA number for controlled substances.

original system of weights and measures for writing medication orders was the *apothecary system*. An apothecary is a pharmacist or druggist. A few drugs are still ordered by the apothecary system. However, the *metric system* is the preferred system of measurement and is used more frequently at the present time. The third system of measurement is the *household system*, which is the least accurate. However, this system is more familiar to the layperson and is therefore used in prescribing medications for the patient at home. The health care worker must understand all three systems of measurement for accurate administration of medicines and for patient education as well. Medication orders are concerned with only two types of measurement: (1) measuring fluids, or liquid measure, and (2) measuring solids, or solid weight.

The apothecary system of liquid measurement includes the minim, fluid dram, fluid ounce, pint, quart, and gallon. The apothecary system for measuring solid weights includes the grain, dram, ounce, and pound (see Table 5.2).

Rules for writing dosages in the apothecary system are as follows:

1. Lowercase Roman numerals are used and *follow* the unit of measurement (e.g., gr iv means 4 grains; ℥ ii means 2 ounces).
2. The symbol ss may be used for one-half (e.g., gr iss means 1½ grains; gr viiss means 7½ grains).
3. All other fractions are written with Arabic numbers and may precede the unit of measurement (e.g., $1/150$ gr or $3¼$ gr).

The metric system was invented by the French in the late 18th century and is the international standard for weights and measures. The metric system of liquid measurement includes the liter and the milliliter, which is approximately equivalent to the cubic centimeter. The metric system for measuring solid weights includes the gram and the milligram as the measures most commonly used for medication prescriptions.

At times you will find it necessary to convert a dosage from the apothecary system to the metric or household system. It is important to memorize the few basic equivalents most commonly used. Table 5.3 lists commonly used approximate equivalents for liquid measurement. These figures are easily committed to memory. When conversions are necessary in the measurement of solids, you will find it useful to consult Table 5.4 for metric and apothecary equivalents.

Equipment most commonly used for measuring medications includes the medicine cup and various syringes calibrated in milliliters and/or minims.

TABLE 5.2. ABBREVIATIONS AND SYMBOLS FOR THE APOTHECARY SYSTEM

grain	gr
minim[a]	m, m̡ , min
drop[a]	gtt
dram	dr, ℥
ounce	oz, ℥
pint	pt
quart	qt

[a]A drop is approximately equivalent to 1 minim of water, but the type of solution may cause variation. When minims are ordered, they should always be measured with a minim glass or in a tuberculin syringe for accuracy. If the order specifies drops, they may be measured with a medicine dropper.

TABLE 5.3. COMMON APPROXIMATE EQUIVALENTS FOR LIQUID MEASUREMENT

Metric	Apothecary	Household
1 ml	15 m	
5 ml	1 dr	**1 tsp**
15 ml	4 dr	1 tbsp
30 ml	1 oz	2 tbsp
240 ml	8 oz	1 measuring cup (240 ml)
500 ml	1 pt (16 oz.)	1 pt
1,000 ml	1 qt (32 oz)	1 qt

Note: Memorize all equivalents above.

TABLE 5.4. METRIC AND APOTHECARY EQUIVALENTS FOR SOLID MEASUREMENT

Metric (Grams)	Metric (Milligrams)	Apothecary
1 g	**1,000 mg**	**gr xv**
0.6 g	600 mg	gr x
0.5 g	**500 mg**	gr viiss
0.3 g	300 mg	gr v
0.2g	200 mg	gr iii
0.1 g	100 mg	gr iss
0.06 g	**60 mg**	**gr i**
0.05 g	50 mg	gr ¾
0.03 g	**30 mg**	**gr ½ or gr ss**
0.02 g	20 mg	gr ⅓
0.015 g	15 mg	gr ¼
0.016 g	16 mg	gr ¼
0.010 g	10 mg	gr ⅙
0.008 g	8 mg	gr ⅛
0.006 g	6 mg	gr 1/10
0.005 g	5 mg	gr 1/12
0.003 g	3 mg	gr 1/20
0.002 g	2 mg	gr 1/30
0.001 g	1 mg	gr 1/60
	0.6 mg	gr 1/100
	0.5 mg	gr 1/120
	0.4 mg	gr 1/150
	0.3 mg	gr 1/200

Note: Memorize all equivalents in boldface.
Pounds–Kilograms (kg) Conversion
    1 pound = 0.453592 kg
    1 kg   = 2.2 pounds (lb)
To convert pounds to kg, divide number of pounds by 2.2.
Warning: Be very careful in calculating the weight in kilograms. The slightest error, especially in pediatric doses, could result in serious or fatal consequences.

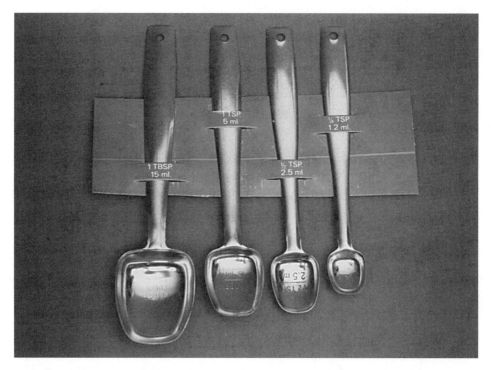

Figure 5.2 For accurate household measurement, standard measuring spoons are used.

PATIENT EDUCATION

When explaining dosage preparation, always speak directly to the patient and observe the patient for comprehension. Many elderly patients have difficulty hearing but are reluctant to admit lack of understanding. Ask them to repeat the directions.

Many elderly patients also have vision problems. Be sure the directions for dosage preparation are written clearly. If a family member will be assisting in preparation and administration of medications, include that person in the instruction. Be sure that any measuring equipment to be used is clearly marked.

Measuring spoons and clearly marked measuring cups should be used when available for household measurement. Such calibrated utensils are more accurate than tableware (Fig. 5.2). Teaspoons, tablespoons, teacups, and drinking glasses vary in size and capacity, and therefore measurements are inaccurate with such utensils.

Chapter Review Quiz

Interpret the following orders:

1. Keflex 250-mg cap PO q6h

2. Neosporin ophth sol gtt ii OS qid

3. Feosol 65 mg tab i qid pc and hs c̄ snack

4. Diuril 500 mg PO qAM

5. Dyazide 1 cap bid

6. Demerol 50 mg IM q4h prn for pain

7. Metamucil 1 tsp mixed c̄ 8 oz H_2O bid ac

8. Dulcolax supp hs qod prn for constipation

9. Actifed syr dr ii qid prn for cough

10. Nitrostat 1 tab SL prn for angina attack, may repeat q5min × 3

11. Compazine supp 25 mg sos for nausea

12. DC Phenergan 48h post-op

13. Tolinase 250 mg qd c̄ breakfast

14. Mandol 0.5 g IVPB q8h

_____

15. Potassium chloride 20 mEq in NS 1L ql2h

_____

16. NPH insulin 20 U SC qd ac breakfast

_____

17. ASA 5 gr supp R prn T > 101

_____

18. Vasocidin opth sol 1 gtt OD q3h

_____

19. Ceclor 20 mg/kg/qd in 2 equal doses ql2h

_____

20. Temazepam 15 mg cap hs prn, may repeat × 1 q noc

_____

Fill in the blanks:

21. Which is the oldest system of measurement for medication?

_____

22. Which system of drug measurement is used most frequently throughout the world?

_____

23. Which is the least accurate system for measuring medicine?

_____

24. Two different types of equipment used to measure drugs are _____ and _____ .

Use Table 5.3 to complete the following conversions, and place the correct answer in the blank:

25. gr V = _____ mg

26. 0.5 mg = gr _____

27. gr XV = _____ g

28. 16 mg = gr _____

29. 1 g = _____ mg

30. gr iss = _____ g

31. gr ⅓ = _____ mg

32. 0.5 g = _____ mg

33. 60 mg = gr _____

34. 1 g = gr _____

35. gr X = _____ mg

36. 1 mg = gr _____

37. 0.1 g = gr _____

38. 0.06 g = gr _____

39. 1 dr _____ = cc = _____ tsp

40. 1 oz _____ = _____ tbsp

41. 1 cc = _____ min

42. 1 oz = _____ dr

43. 1 kg = _____ pounds

44. 30 m = _____ ml

45. 5 gr = _____ mg

CHAPTER 6

Safe Dosage Preparation

OBJECTIVES

Upon completion of this chapter, the student should be able to:

1. Identify the three steps for calculation of the dosage ordered when it differs from the dose on hand.
2. Write the formula for each of the two methods of dosage calculation presented in this chapter.
3. Convert from one system of measurement to another using the ratio and proportion method.
4. Solve dosage problems using the basic calculation method.
5. Solve dosage problems using the ratio and proportion method.
6. List the cautions with the basic calculation method.
7. List the cautions with the ratio and proportion method.
8. Calculate safe dosages for infants and children.
9. List the variables when assessing geriatric patients for safe dosage.
10. List some steps to reduce medication errors.

"First, do no harm." Health care workers are dedicated to the principle of helping others, not harming them. Nowhere is this principle more important than in the calculation, preparation, and administration of safe dosages. One careless moment can lead to a catastrophe. It is the responsibility of the health care worker to be absolutely certain that the medication administered is exactly as prescribed by the physician, *and* is also an *appropriate* dose for that particular patient. Doses for children and the elderly can vary significantly from the average dose. Therefore, it may be necessary to compute a partial dose from the dose on hand for the average patient.

Many medications are dispensed by the pharmacist in unit dose form, in which each individual dose of medicine is prepackaged in a separate packet, vial, or prefilled syringe. Although much of the mixing and measuring of medications is now completed by the pharmacist, the person who is administering medications must understand the preparation of dosages in order to ensure accuracy. On occasion the dosage ordered differs from the dose on hand. Consequently, it may be necessary to calculate the correct dosage. Calculations can be a simple procedure if you follow the necessary steps in sequential order.

A working knowledge of basic arithmetic is required for accurate calculation of drug dosage. In order to understand the calculation of correct dosage, you must evaluate your basic arithmetic skills by completing the following mathematics pretest.

Basic Arithmetic Test

1. $6\frac{1}{4} + 3\frac{2}{3}$
2. $4\frac{2}{3} - 2\frac{1}{2}$
3. $2\frac{2}{3} \times 3\frac{2}{5}$
4. $\frac{2}{5} \div \frac{3}{4}$
5. $2\frac{2}{3} \div 5$
6. Write six and a third as a decimal.
7. $6.67 + .065 + 0.3$
8. $10.4 - .037$
9. $.223 \times .67$
10. $46.72 \div 6.4$
11. Write 8% as a fraction and reduce.
12. Change $\frac{2}{5}$ to a decimal.
13. Write .023 as a percent.
14. Express 12% as a decimal.
15. Express .4 as a fraction and reduce.
16. Change 3/5 to a percent.
17. Change $12\frac{1}{2}\%$ to a decimal.
18. What is 75% of 160?
19. What is 9.2% of 250?
20. What is $37\frac{1}{2}\%$ of 192?
21. Which fraction is the largest: $\frac{1}{2}$, $\frac{2}{5}$, or $\frac{3}{10}$?
22. Which is the largest: $\frac{1}{3}$, 0.4, or 60%?
23. Write the Roman numeral XXV as an Arabic numeral.
24. Write 154 as a Roman numeral.
25. The label on the bottle reads 0.5 g per tablet. The doctor orders 0.25 g. How many tablets should you give?

After completing the quiz, check your answers (see following). If there is an error, review mathematics for that area until all problems can be solved accurately and easily. A minimum score of 80% is recommended as indicating readiness for dosage calculations. Those not meeting this criterion should seek remedial assistance in review of basics before beginning calculations.

ANSWERS TO BASIC ARITHMETIC TEST

1. $9^{11}/_{12}$	8. 10.363	14. 0.12	20. 72
2. $2^1/_6$	9. 0.14941	15. $^2/_5$	21. $^1/_2$
3. $9^1/_{15}$	10. 7.3	16. 60%	22. 60%
4. $^8/_{15}$	11. $^2/_{25}$	17. 0.125	23. 25
5. $^8/_{15}$	12. 0.4	18. 120	24. CLIV
6. 6.333	13. 2.3%	19. 23	25. $^1/_2$
7. 7.035			

Calculation Guidelines

Remember, there is no margin of error in administration of medications. It is possible for a small error in arithmetic to seriously harm a patient. A misplaced decimal point could cause a fatality. Safe dosage preparation requires (1) a working knowledge of basic arithmetic and (2) meticulous care with all calculations.

Calculations can be as simple as 1, 2, 3. When the dosage ordered differs from the dosage on hand, the problem can be solved simply by completing three basic steps:

1. Check whether all measures are in the same system. Convert if necessary by using Tables 5.3 and 5.4 or use the ratio and proportion method.
2. Write the problem in equation form using the *appropriate formula and labeling all parts*, and complete the necessary calculations.
3. *Check the accuracy* of your answer for reasonableness, and have someone else verify your calculations.

There are several different methods of calculating dosage. Either of the methods presented in this book may be used, or both methods may be used to verify accuracy. The two methods presented here are *basic calculation* and *ratio and proportion*. Basic calculation requires only simple arithmetic, while ratio and proportion requires the ability to determine an unknown, X.

Method 1: Basic Calculation

Use the following formula:

$$\frac{\text{Desired dose}}{\text{On-hand dose}} \times \text{quantity of on-hand dose}$$

in short form:

$$\frac{D}{OH} \times Q$$

EXAMPLE 1

The physician orders aspirin gr 10 q4h PRN for fever over 101°. On hand are aspirin gr 5 tabs.

Step 1. Check to see if all measures are in the same system. No conversion is necessary. Both measures are in grains.

Step 2. Use the formula $\dfrac{D}{OH} \times Q$ and label all parts:

$$\frac{10 \text{ gr}}{5 \text{ gr}} \times 1 \text{ tab} = 10 \div 5 = 2$$

$$2 \times 1 = 2 \text{ tabs}$$

> *Note:* The labels of the desired and on-hand doses must be the same. The label of the answer must be the same as the quantity.

Step 3. Check for reasonableness. A dose of 2 tabs is within normal limits.

If the calculations resulted in an answer such as 1/4 tablet or 5 tablets, the answer is not reasonable and the calculations should be rechecked. If calculations are correct after recheck, any unusual dosage should be checked with the person in charge: the pharmacist or the physician. *When in doubt, always question.*

EXAMPLE 2

The order reads Ampicillin 0.5 g. The unit dose packet reads 250 mg/cap.

Step 1. Check to see if all measures are in the same system. Convert grams to milligrams:

$$1 \text{ g} = 1,000 \text{ mg}$$

$$0.5 \text{ g} = 0.5 \times 1,000 = 500 \text{ mg}$$

Step 2. Use the formula $\dfrac{D}{OH} \times Q$ and label all parts:

$$\frac{500 \text{ mg}}{250 \text{ mg}} \times 1 \text{ cap} =$$

Reduce fractions to lowest terms:

$$\frac{500}{250} = 50 \div 25 = 2$$

$$2 \times 1 = 2 \text{ caps}$$

Step 3. Check for reasonableness. A dose of 2 caps is within normal limits.

EXAMPLE 3

The narcotics drawer contains vials of meperidine (Demerol) labeled 75 mg in 1 ml. The preoperative order reads Demerol 60 mg IM on call.

Step 1. Check to see if all measures are in the same system. No conversion is necessary.

Step 2. Use the formula $\dfrac{D}{OH} \times Q$ and label all parts:

$$\frac{60 \text{ mg}}{75 \text{ mg}} \times 1 \text{ ml} =$$

Reduce fractions to lowest terms:

$$\frac{60}{75} = \frac{12}{15} = \frac{4}{5}$$

Convert fractions to decimals:

$$\frac{4}{5} = 5\overline{)4.0}^{\,0.8}$$

Multiply by quantity.

$$0.8 \times 1 \text{ ml} = 0.8 \text{ ml}$$

Note: Fractions must be converted to decimals and rounded off to one decimal place to coincide with the markings on the syringe.

Step 3. Check for reasonableness. A dose of 0.8 ml is within normal limits.

EXAMPLE 4

The physician orders Versed 3 mg IM preoperatively. On hand are vials labeled 5 mg per ml.

Step 1. Check to see if all measures are in the same system. No conversion is necessary.

Step 2. Use the formula $\dfrac{D}{OH} \times Q$ and label all parts:

$$\frac{3 \text{ mg}}{5 \text{ mg}} \times 1 \text{ ml} = 3 \div 5 = 5\overline{)3.0}^{\,0.6}$$

$$0.6 \times 1 \text{ ml} = 0.6 \text{ ml}$$

Step 3. Check for reasonableness. A dose of 0.6 ml is within normal limits.

EXAMPLE 5

The order reads atropine sulfate 0.6 mg IM on call to surgery. Available ampules are labeled atropine sulfate 0.4 mg/ml.

Step 1. Check to see if all measures are in the same system. No conversion is necessary

Step 2. Use the formula $\dfrac{D}{OH} \times Q$ and label all parts:

$$\frac{0.6\ mg}{0.4\ mg} \times 1\ ml = 0.6 \div 0.4 = 0.4\overline{)0.6}^{1.5}$$

$$1.5\ ml \times 1\ ml = 1.5\ ml$$

Step 3. Check for reasonableness. A dose of 1.5 ml is within normal limits.

CAUTIONS FOR THE BASIC CALCULATION METHOD

1. *Label* all parts of the formula.
2. Use the *same label* for desired and on-hand doses.
3. Use the *same label* for the quantity and the answer (the amount to be given).
4. *Reduce fractions* to lowest terms before dividing.
5. *Multiply by the quantity* after dividing.
6. Take *extra care* with *decimals*.
7. *Convert* fractions to decimals.
8. *Round off* decimals to one decimal place after computation is complete.
9. *Verify the accuracy* of calculations with an instructor.
10. Question the answer if not within normal limits (e.g., less than 1/2 tab, more than 2 tabs, or more than 2 ml for injection).

Method 2: Ratio and Proportion

A *ratio* describes a relationship between two numbers.

Example: 1 g : 15 gr

A *proportion* consists of two ratios that are equal.

Example: 1 g : 15 gr = 2g : 30 gr

Always label each term in the equation. The terms of each ratio must be in the same sequence. In the examples above, you will see that the first term of each ratio is labeled g and the second term of each ratio is labeled gr.

To solve a problem with the ratio and proportion method, set up the formula with the known terms on the left and the desired and unknown terms on the right. Use X to represent the unknown. Label all terms.

For example, we know that 1,000 mg is equal to 1 g (known). We need to administer 500 mg (desired) and do not know how many grams are equivalent (unknown = X). To convert a dosage from one system to another when a table of metric and apothecary equivalents (such as Table 5.4) is unavailable, set up the problem as a proportion:

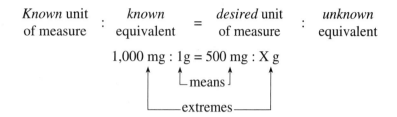

To solve the problem, multiply the two outer terms, or extremes, and then multiply the two inner terms, or means. Using our example:

$$1,000 \; X = 500 = 1,000 \overline{)500.0}^{\;0.5}$$

$$X = 0.5 \text{ g}$$

We now know that our desired dose, 500 mg, is equal to 0.5 g.

When the dose ordered differs from the dose on hand, the problem can be solved simply by completing three basic steps:

1. Verify that all measures are in the same system. Convert if necessary by using a table of metric and apothecary equivalents if available or by using the ratio and proportion method if the equivalent is unknown.
2. Set up the problem as a proportion, *label all terms*, and complete the calculations. Use the following formula:

$$\frac{\text{dose}}{\text{on hand}} : \frac{\text{known}}{\text{quantity}} = \frac{\text{dose}}{\text{desired}} : \frac{\text{unknown}}{\text{quantity}}$$

   Note: The answer should be stated as a whole number or a decimal. Convert fractions to decimals and round off to one decimal place.
3. Check the accuracy of your answer for reasonableness and also have someone else verify your calculations.

EXAMPLE 1

The preoperative order reads Demerol 60 mg IM on call. The narcotics locker contains ampules labeled meperidine (Demerol) 100 mg/2 ml.

Step 1. Verify that all measures are in the same system. No conversion is necessary.

Step 2. Set up the problem as a proportion and label all terms:

$$\frac{\text{dose}}{\text{on hand}} : \frac{\text{known}}{\text{quantity}} = \frac{\text{dose}}{\text{desired}} : \frac{\text{unknown}}{\text{quantity}}$$

$$100 \text{ mg} : 2 \text{ ml} = 60 \text{ mg} : X \text{ ml}$$

$$100 \text{ X} = 120 = 100\overline{)120.0}^{\,1.2}$$

$$X = 1.2 \text{ ml}$$

Step 3. Check for reasonableness. A dose of 1.2 ml is within normal limits.

EXAMPLE 2

The physician is treating a child weighing 44 pounds for epilepsy. The order reads phenobarbital elixir 3 mg/kg @ HS. Phenobarbital elixir is labeled 15 mg/5 ml. How many ml will the child receive?

Step 1. Verify that all measures are in the same system. Pounds must be converted to kilograms (kg). To convert lbs to kg, divide the number of pounds by 2.2.

The child weighs 20 kg.

The order reads 3mg/kg. Therefore 3 mg × 20 kg = 60 mg dose.

Step 2. Set up the problem as a proportion. Label all terms.

$$\frac{\text{dose}}{\text{on hand}} : \frac{\text{known}}{\text{quantity}} = \frac{\text{dose}}{\text{desired}} : \frac{\text{unknown}}{\text{quantity}}$$

$$15 \text{ mg} : 5 \text{ ml} = 60 \text{ mg} : X \text{ ml}$$

$$15 \text{ X} = 300 = 15\overline{)300}^{\,20}$$

$$X = 20 \text{ ml}$$

Step 3. Check for reasonableness. An oral dose of 20 ml is a large amount for a young child to take at one time. The physician might want to divide the daily dose. If so, the order would be written: phenobarbital 30 mg BID.

EXAMPLE 3

Meperidine Oral Solution is available as Demerol Syrup 50 mg/5 ml. The order reads Demerol liquid 150 mg PO q6h PRN.

Step 1. Verify that all measures are in the same system. No conversion necessary.

Step 2. Set up the problem as a proportion. Label all terms.

$$\frac{dose}{on\ hand} : \frac{known}{quantity} = \frac{dose}{desired} : \frac{unknown}{quantity}$$

$$50\ mg: 5\ ml = 150\ mg : X\ ml$$

$$50\ X = 750 = 50\overline{)750}^{\ 15}$$

$$X = 15\ ml$$

Step 3. Check for reasonableness. An oral dose of 15 ml is appropriate for an adult.

EXAMPLE 4
An 88-pound child with cancer has an order for pain medication that reads morphine liquid PO 0.2 mg/kg q 4 h PRN. Available Morphine Solution is labeled 20 mg/5 ml.

Step 1. Verify that all measures are in the same system. Pounds must be converted to kilograms (kg). To convert lb to kg, divide number of pounds by 2.2. The child weighs 40 kg.

The order reads 0.2 mg/kg. Therefore, 0.2 mg × 40 = 8-mg dose.

Step 2. Set up the problem as a proportion. Label all terms.

$$\frac{dose}{on\ hand} : \frac{known}{quantity} = \frac{dose}{desired} : \frac{unknown}{quantity}$$

$$20\ mg : 5\ ml = 8\ mg : X\ ml$$

$$20\ X = 40 = 20\overline{)40}^{\ 2}$$

$$X = 2\ ml$$

Step 3. Check for reasonableness. An oral dose of 2 ml is appropriate for a terminally ill child.

EXAMPLE 5
The physician orders Benadryl elixir 25 mg q12h. The bottle in the medicine cupboard is labeled 12.5 mg/5 ml.

Step 1. Verify that all measures are in the same system. No conversion is necessary.

Step 2. Write the problem as a proportion and label each term:

$$\frac{\text{dose}}{\text{on hand}} : \frac{\text{known}}{\text{quantity}} = \frac{\text{dose}}{\text{desired}} : \frac{\text{unknown}}{\text{quantity}}$$

$$12.5 \text{ mg}: 5 \text{ ml} = 25 \text{ mg} : X \text{ ml}$$

$$12.5 \text{ X} = 125 = 12.5\overline{)125.00} = 125\overline{)1250}^{\,10}$$

$$X = 10 \text{ ml}$$

Step 3. Check for reasonableness. The dose 10 ml is within normal limits for oral solution.

CAUTIONS FOR THE RATIO AND PROPORTION METHOD

1. *Label* all parts of the equation.
2. The ratio on the *left* contains the *known* quantity, and the ratio on the *right* contains the *desired* and *unknown* quantities.
3. Terms of the second ratio must be in the same sequence as those in the first ratio.
4. *Multiply* the *extremes first* and then the *means*.
5. Take *extra care* with *decimals*.
6. *Convert* fractions to decimals. *Round off* decimals to one decimal place.
7. *Label* the answer.
8. *Verify the accuracy* of calculations with an instructor.
9. *Question* any unusual dosage not within normal limits (e.g., less than ½ tab, more than 2 tabs, or more than 2 ml for injection).

Pediatric Dosage

Children are not miniature adults. You cannot merely take part of an adult dose and give it to a child. There are many other variables to consider. There are numerous formulas available for computing *approximate* child's dose based on either body surface area, weight, or age. However, other factors must be taken into consideration as well. In neonates, renal function and some enzyme systems needed for drug absorption and metabolism are not fully developed. The neonate's blood-brain barrier is more permeable and his total body water contributes a greater percentage of his body weight, also affecting drug absorption.

Appropriate dosage for children, as well as adults, must take into consideration variables such as age, weight, sex, and metabolic, pathologic, or psychologic conditions. Recommended pediatric drug dosages are derived from data obtained in clinical trials utilizing sick children. When preparing drug dosages for children, it is important to always refer to recommended dosages as listed in drug inserts, *Physician's Desk Reference (PDR),* or *AHFS Drug Information (Formulary).*

Recommended dosages of drugs are often expressed in the references as a number of milligrams per unit of body weight, per unit of time. For example, the recommended dose for a drug might be 6 mg/kg/24 hours. This information can then be used to:

1. Calculate the dose for the individual patient.
2. Check on the appropriateness of the prescribed dose, watching particularly for possible overdoses.

EXAMPLE 1

The recommended dose of meperidine (Demerol) is 6 mg/kg/24 h for pain, in divided doses every 4–6 hours, as necessary. Demerol is available in ampules or cartridges labeled 50 mg/ml. How much Demerol would be appropriate for a 33-pound child as a single dose every 6 hours?

Step 1. Convert pounds to kilograms (divide number of pounds by 2.2).

$$33 \text{ pounds} = 15 \text{ kg}$$

$$6 \text{ mg per kg in 24 hr is recommended}$$

$$6 \text{ mg} \times 15 \text{ kg} = 90 \text{ mg in 24 hr}$$

Step 2. Calculate the number of *milliliters needed in 24 hr*. Write the problem as a proportion and label each term.

$$\frac{\text{dose}}{\text{on hand}} : \frac{\text{known}}{\text{quantity}} = \frac{\text{dose}}{\text{desired}} : \frac{\text{unknown}}{\text{quantity}}$$

$$50 \text{ mg}: 1 \text{ ml} = 90 \text{ mg} : X \text{ ml}$$

$$50 \text{ X} = 90 = 50\overline{)90.0}^{\,1.8}$$

$$X = 1.8 \text{ ml in 24 hr}$$

Then, calculate the number of *milliliters needed in 6 hr*. Remember, the unknown quantity is always the last term in the equation.

$$24 \text{ hr}: 1.8 \text{ ml} = 6 \text{ hr} : X \text{ ml}$$

$$24 \text{ X} = 10.8 = 24\overline{)10.80}^{\,0.45}$$

$$X = 0.45 \text{ ml dose every 6 hr}$$

Step 3. The appropriateness of this dose can be checked by applying *Clark's Rule:*

$$\frac{\text{Child's weight in lbs}}{\text{Average adult wt}} \times \text{adult dose} = \text{child's } \textit{approximate} \text{ dose}$$

$$\frac{33}{150} \times 100 \text{ mg} = 22 \text{ mg approximate child's dose}$$

Demerol is available in ampules labeled 100 mg/2 ml

100 mg: 2 ml = 22 mg: X ml

$$100\ X = 44 = 100\overline{)44.00}$$
$$\underline{400}$$
$$400$$

X = 0.44 ml dose to be administered

Remember, this is a *general* rule and other variables must be considered when assessing for appropriateness of dosage.

Geriatric Dosage

Special consideration must be given to preparation and administration of safe dosage to older adults. As with children, the dose frequently needs to be reduced. Factors leading to possible dangerous cumulative effects can include slower metabolism, poor circulation, or impairment of liver, kidneys, lungs, or central nervous system. Any chronic disease, debility, dehydration, or electrolyte imbalance can affect assimilation of drugs and interfere with therapeutic effect. Many drugs can impair mental status of the elderly, leading to confusion. Any elderly person taking many drugs is also at risk for potentially lethal interactions. There is no formula to guide you in safe geriatric dosage. Careful assessment on an *individual* basis, constant monitoring, and reduction of dosage, whenever possible, are the rules to follow. Each individual reacts differently to drugs, and changes occur over time. You have the responsibility to question the appropriateness of any drug, and especially as the patient's condition changes.

Prevention of Medication Errors

Medication errors can occur for a number of reasons: administering the wrong drug, the wrong amount, at the wrong time, by the wrong route, or to the wrong patient. The Rights of Medication Administration will be discussed in the next chapter. However, we will consider here errors that can occur when the drug order is misinterpreted.

- Never leave the decimal point naked. Writing .2 instead of 0.2 could cause the decimal point to be missed and could result in an overdose. Always place a zero *before* a decimal point, for example, 0.2, 0.5.
- Never place a decimal point and zero after a whole number. The decimal point could be missed and the zero could be mininterpreted, for example, 5.0 mg could be read as 50 mg. The correct way is to write 5 mg.
- Avoid using decimals whenever whole numbers can be used as alternatives, for example, 0.5 g can be expressed as 500 mg.

- If you have difficulty interpreting the spelling of a drug or the number used for the dosage, or the dosage seems inappropriate, *always question* the order. This is not only your duty, but you have an ethical and legal responsibility to be sure that the drugs you administer are safe. If a medication error results in legal action, you could be held accountable, even though the order was written incorrectly. You are expected to recognize inappropriate dosage, to check reference books with unfamiliar drugs and to ask the physician or pharmacist about any questionable dosage.

Check your knowledge of this chapter before going any further.

Chapter Review Quiz

SECTION A

Use the preceding VISUAL IDENTIFICATION GUIDE to find the most appropriate available form to deliver the dosage ordered. Use only *one* form of each drug. Indicate the *amount* and *which drug form* you should give for the following orders. *Use the smallest number of tablets possible.*

Drug and Dose Ordered	*Amount to Administer*
1. Atenolol (Tenormin) 75 mg	_____ of _____ mg tab
2. Buspirone (Buspar) 25 mg	_____ of _____ mg tab
3. Alprazolam (Xanax) 0.75 mg	_____ of _____ mg tab
4. Bumetanide (Bumex) 2 mg	_____ of _____ mg tab
5. Cimetidine (Tagamet) 200 mg	_____ of _____ mg tab
6. Furosemide (Lasix) 60 mg	_____ of _____ mg tab
7. Levothyroxine (Synthroid) 0.3 mg	_____ of _____ mg tab
8. Propranolol (Inderal) 15 mg	_____ of _____ mg tab
9. Prednisone (Deltasone) 15 mg	_____ of _____ mg tab
10. Sertraline (Zoloft) 75 mg	_____ of _____ mg tab

SECTION B

Show your work. Label and circle your answer:

1. The physician orders procaine penicillin G 500,000 U. Available is Bicillin in a vial labeled penicillin G procaine 600,000 U/ml. How many ml would you administer?

2. The medication order reads Demerol 60 mg IM. The narcotic drawer contains vials labeled meperidine (Demerol) 75 mg/ml.

A. How many ml would you administer?_____

B. How many ml would you discard and mark as "wasted" on the narcotic record? _____

3. Lasix is available in 40-mg tablets. The order reads Lasix 60 mg PO qAM. How many tablets should you give?

4. Atropine 0.6 mg is ordered. Available vials of atropine are labeled 0.4 mg/ml. How many ml would you administer?

5. Acetaminophen elixir 650 mg is ordered. The container is labeled 325 mg/5 ml.

A. How many ml would you administer?_____

B. How many teaspoons per dose?_____

6. Morphine sulfate PO 30 mg liquid is ordered. Morphine oral solution is labeled 20 mg/ml. How many ml would you administer?

7. The medication order reads heparin 5,000 units. Vials available in the medication cupboard are labeled heparin 10,000 U/ml. How many milliliters should you draw into the syringe?

8. Digoxin elixir is available in 50 μg/ml. The physician orders 75 μg Lanoxin qd. How many milliliters should you give?

9. The physician orders prednisone 7.5 mg qd. Prednisone is available in 5-mg and 10-mg scored tablets, which can be broken in half. Which strength tablet and how many tablets should you give?

10. Amoxicillin suspension 750 mg q8h is ordered. Liquid medication available is labeled 250 mg/5 ml. How many milliliters should you give?

11. Calcium carbonate 1,000 mg qd is prescribed, to be given in divided doses bid. Available tablets contain calcium 250 mg/tab. How many tablets should be taken each time?

12. Robitussin A-C contains 10 mg of codeine in each teaspoon (5 ml). If 2 tsp Robitussin A-C is prescribed q4h, how much codeine would be contained in each dose?

13. The physician orders Mintezol tablets for a 110-pound child with creeping eruption. The recommended dose is 20 mg/kg. Mintezol tablets are labeled 500 mg. How many tablets should be given for each dose?

14. The physician orders Ceclor Suspension 200 mg q8h for a 44-pound child. Ceclor Suspension is available 250 mg/5 ml.

   A. How many ml should be administered each time? _____

   B. Recommended dosage of Ceclor is 30 mg/kg/daily. How many mg would be appropriate for this child daily? _____

15. List five variables to consider in determining a child's dose:

   _____ , _____ ,

   _____ , _____ ,

   and _____ .

16. List five factors that could lead to serious cumulative effects with medicines in the elderly:

   _____ , _____ ,

   _____ , _____ ,

   and _____ .

More questions and their answers are available in the Instructor's Guide.

CHAPTER 7

Responsibilities and Principles of Drug Administration

OBJECTIVES

Upon completion of this chapter, the student should be able to:

1. Describe four responsibilities of the health care provider in safe administration of medications.
2. List the six Rights of Medication Administration.
3. Explain moral, ethical, and legal responsibilities regarding medication errors.
4. Cite three instances of medication administration that require documentation.
5. Explain the rights of the health care worker to question or refuse to administer medications.

Responsible Drug Administration

The safe and accurate administration of medications requires knowledge, judgment, and skill. The *responsibilities* of the health care provider in this vital area include:

1. Adequate, up-to-date *information* about all medications to be administered, including purpose, potential side effects, cautions and contraindications, and possible interactions.
2. *Wisdom* and judgment to accurately *assess* the patient's needs for medications, to *evaluate* the response to medications, and to plan appropriate interventions as indicated.
3. *Skill in delivery* of the medication accurately, in the best interests of the patient, and with adequate documentation.
4. *Patient education* to provide the necessary information to the patient and family about why, how, and when medications are to be administered and potential side effects and precautions with administration by the layperson.

Responsibility for safe administration of medications requires that the health care worker be familiar with every medication before administration. Knowledge of the typical and most frequently used drugs of the systems (as described in Part II of this text) is imperative. However, this is only a framework upon which to build and add other knowledge of new drugs or new effects as changes in medicine become known. Unfamiliar drugs should never be administered. Resources such as the *PDR*, the *AHFS Drug Information*, the *USP/NF*, package inserts, and pharmacists must be consulted *before* administration in order to become familiar with the desired effect, potential side effects, precautions and contraindications, and possible interactions with other drugs or with foods.

Responsibility for safe administration of medications requires *complete planning* for patient care, including prior *assessment*, *interventions*, and *evaluations* of the results of drug therapy. Assessment involves taking a complete history, including all medical conditions (e.g., pregnancy or illness), allergies, and all other medications in use, including over-the-counter drugs. Assessment also involves careful observation of the patient's vital signs, posture, skin temperature and color, and facial expression before and after drug administration. Appropriate interventions require judgment in timing, discontinuing medicine if required, and taking steps to counteract adverse reactions, as well as knowing what and when to report to the physician. Evaluation and documentation of results also play a vital role for all health care providers, including the physician, in planning effective drug therapy.

The safe administration of medications necessitates training to develop skills in delivery of medications. The goal is to maximize the effectiveness of the drug with the least discomfort to the patient. Sensitivity to the unique needs of each patient is encouraged (e.g., awareness of difficulty swallowing or impaired movement that could affect administration of medications).

Patient education is an essential part of the safe administration of medicines. If the patient is to benefit from drug therapy, he or she must understand the importance of taking the medicine in the proper dosage, on time, and in the proper way. Information for patients should be in language they understand, with instruction both verbal and written, as well as demonstrations of techniques when indicated.

Administration of medication carries moral, ethical, and legal responsibilities. Some rules and regulations vary with the institution, agency, or office. When in doubt, consult those in authority—supervisors or administrators—and/or policy and procedure books. However, documentation on the patient's record is always required for all medicines given, as well as for patient education provided. In addition, controlled substances given must also be recorded in a narcotics record.

Meticulous care in preparation and administration of medications reduces the chances of error. However, if a mistake is made, it is of the utmost importance to report it immediately to the one in charge so that corrective action can be taken for the patient's welfare. The patient's record should reflect the corrective action taken for justification in case of legal proceedings. An incident report must also be completed as a legal requirement. Failure to report errors appropriately can jeopardize the patient's welfare, as well as increase the possibility of civil suits against the health care provider and/or the risk of loss of professional license or certificate. Honesty is not only the best policy, it is the *only* policy for moral, ethical, and legal reasons.

Principles of Administration

When preparing to administer medications, several basic principles should always be kept in mind:

1. *Cleanliness.* Essential to safe administration of medicines. Always wash hands before handling medicines and be sure preparation area is clean and neat.
2. *Organization.* Necessary for safe administration of medicines. Always be sure medications and supplies are in the appropriate area and in adequate supply. When stock drugs are used, they should be reordered immediately.
3. *Preparation area.* Should be well lighted and away from distracting influences.

Guidelines to review before giving medicines are called the six Rights of Medication Administration (Fig. 7.1):

1. Right medication
2. Right amount
3. Right time
4. Right route
5. Right patient
6. Right documentation

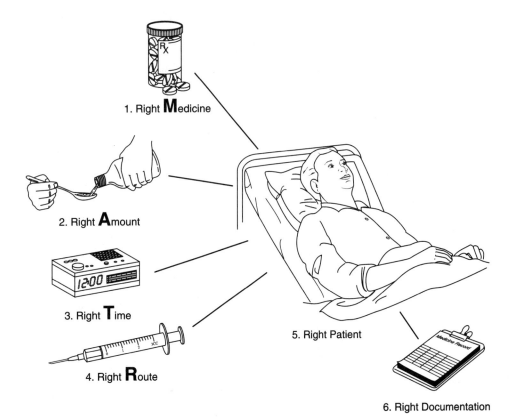

1. Right **M**edicine

2. Right **A**mount

3. Right **T**ime

4. Right **R**oute

5. Right Patient

6. Right Documentation

Figure 7.1 The Six Rights of Medication Administration. Using the acronym MATR, read down, saying, "It matters to the patient." Don't forget #6, the right documentation.

RIGHT MEDICATION

You can confirm that you have the right medication by carefully comparing the name of the drug prescribed (on the physician's order sheet, prescription blank, medication record, or medicine card) with the label on the package, bottle, or unit-dose packet (medications with each dose separately sealed in an individual paper, foil, plastic, or glass container). *Never* give medication in which the name of the medication is obscured in any way. Some drugs have names that sound or look similar (e.g., digoxin and digitoxin, or Inderal and Isuprel), and therefore it is essential to scrutinize every letter in the name when comparing the medicine ordered with the medicine on hand. Accuracy can be facilitated by placing the unit-dose packet next to the name of the drug ordered on the patient's record, while comparing the drug ordered with the drug on hand.

If there is any question about the drug order because of handwriting, misspelling, inappropriateness, allergies, or interactions, you have the *right* and *responsibility to question* the physician and/or the pharmacist.

Never give medications that someone else has prepared. *Never* leave medications at the bedside unless specifically ordered by the doctor (e.g., nitroglycerin tablets and contraceptives are frequently ordered to be left with the patient for self-administration). If the patient is unable to take a medication when you present it, the medication must be returned (in an unopened packet) to the patient's drawer in the medicine cart or medicine room. Never open the unit-dose packet until the patient is prepared to take the medicine.

RIGHT AMOUNT

Administering the right amount of drug is extremely important. Drug dosage ordered must be compared *very carefully* with the dose listed on the label of the package, bottle, or unit dose packet. Here again, accuracy can be facilitated by placing the unit-dose packet next to the written order on the patient's record while comparing the dose ordered with the dose on hand.

The three different systems of measurement (household, apothecary, and metric) were discussed in Chapter 5. It is important to consult a table of equivalents (Table 5.4), if necessary, to convert from one system to another. Directions for calculation of different drug doses were presented in Chapter 6. Drug calculations are infrequent with unit-dose packaging. However, if it is necessary to compute calculations, such calculations must be checked by another trained health care worker, pharmacist, or doctor to verify accuracy. Be especially careful when the dose is expressed in decimals or fractions. Always recheck the dose if less than one tablet or more than one tablet are required, or with less than 1 milliliter or more than 1 milliliter for injection. An unusual dosage should alert you to the possibility of error. Those who administer medications have the right, as well as the responsibility, to question any dosage that is unusual or seems inappropriate for the individual patient. Remember that drug action is influenced by the condition of the patient, metabolism, age, weight, sex, and psychological state (see Chapter 3). The health care worker has the responsibility of reporting the results of careful assessment and observations in order to assist the physician in prescribing the right dosage for each patient.

Directions for measurement and preparation of the right dose are described in Chapters 8 and 9. An important part of the patient education includes complete instructions about the importance of preparing and taking the right amount of medicine prescribed by the physician.

RIGHT TIME

The time for administration of medications is an important part of the drug *dosage*, which includes the amount, frequency, and number of doses of medication to be administered. For maximum effectiveness, drugs must be given on a prescribed schedule. The physician's order specifies the number of times per day the medicine is to be administered (e.g., bid, or twice a day). Some medications need to be maintained at a specific level in the blood and are therefore prescribed at regular intervals around the clock (e.g., q4h, or every 4 hours). Some medications, such as some antibiotics, are more effective on an empty stomach and are therefore prescribed ac (before meals). Medications that are irritating to the stomach are ordered pc (after meals). Drugs that cause sedation are more frequently prescribed at hs (hour of sleep). If the physician does not prescribe a specific time for administration of a drug, the health care worker arranges an appropriate schedule, taking into consideration the purpose, action, and side effects of the medication. Patient education includes instruction about the right time to take specific medicines and why.

RIGHT ROUTE

The route of administration is important because of its effect on degree of absorption, speed of drug action, and side effects. Many drugs can be administered in a variety of ways (see Chapter 4). The physician's order specifies the route of administration. If no route is specified, the oral route is used unless conditions warrant otherwise (e.g., nausea, vomiting, or difficulty swallowing). Those administering medications have the right and responsibility to question the appropriateness of a route based on assessment and observation of the patient. Change of route may be indicated because of the patient's condition. However, the route of administration may not be changed without the physician's order.

RIGHT PATIENT

The patient who is to receive the medication must be identified by use of certain techniques to reduce the chance of error. The patient's wrist identification band should be checked *first*, and then the patient should be called by name or asked to state his name, *before* administering the medication. If the patient questions the medication or the dosage, recheck the order and the medicine before giving it.

RIGHT DOCUMENTATION

Another essential duty is *documentation*. Every medication given must be recorded on the patient's record, along with *dose, time, route,* and *location* of injections. If the medication is given on a PRN (as necessary) basis (e.g., for pain), notation should also be made on the patient's record of the effectiveness of the medication. The person administering the medication must also sign or initial the record after administration (the policy of each facility determines the exact procedure to be followed). The accuracy of medication documentation is a very important legal responsibility. At times, patients' records are examined in court, and the accuracy of medication documentation can be a critical factor in some legal judgments.

Documentation also includes the recording of narcotics administered on the special controlled substances record kept with the narcotics. If narcotics are destroyed because of partial dosage, cancellation, or error, two health care workers must sign as witnesses of the disposal of the drug (the policy about documentation of narcotics may vary with the agency).

In summary, safe and effective administration of medications involves current drug information; technical and evaluation skills; and moral, ethical, and legal responsibilities. Guidelines include the six Rights of Medication Administration. In addition, the health care worker has the right and responsibility to question any medication order that is confusing or illegible or that seems inappropriate, and the right to refuse to administer any medication that is not in the best interests of the patient. The primary concern in administration of medications is the welfare of the patient.

MED WATCH

The Food and Drug Administration (FDA) issued a form in 1993 to assist health care professionals in reporting serious adverse events or product quality problems associated with medications, medical devices, or nutritional products regulated by the FDA, for example, dietary supplements or infant formulas. Even the large, well-designed clinical trials that precede FDA approval cannot uncover every problem that can come to light once a product is widely used. Or a drug could interact with other drugs in ways not revealed during clinical trials. Reports by health care professionals can help ensure the safety of drugs and other products regulated by the FDA.

In response to these voluntary reports from the health care community, the FDA has issued warnings, made labeling changes, required manufacturers to do postmarketing studies, and ordered the withdrawal of certain products from the market. Such actions can prevent injuries, suffering, disabilities, congenital deformities, and even deaths.

You are not expected to establish a connection, or even wait until the evidence seems overwhelming. The agency's regulations will protect your identity and the identities of your patient and your facility. With your cooperation, MED WATCH can help the FDA better monitor product safety, and when necessary, take swift action to protect your patients and you. MED WATCH encourages you to regard voluntary reporting as part of your professional responsibility. See Fig. 7.2 for a MED WATCH form, which can be reproduced, and for instructions for completing and submitting this form to the FDA.

Check your knowledge of this chapter before going any further.

ADVICE ABOUT VOLUNTARY REPORTING

Report experiences with:
- medications (drugs or biologics)
- medical devices (including in-vitro diagnostics)
- special nutritional products (dietary supplements, medical foods, infant formulas)
- other products regulated by FDA

Report SERIOUS adverse events. An event is serious when the patient outcome is:
- death
- life-threatening (real risk of dying)
- hospitalization (initial or prolonged)
- disability (significant, persistent or permanent)
- congenital anomaly
- required intervention to prevent permanent impairment or damage

Report even if:
- you're not certain the product caused the event
- you don't have all the details

Report product problems – quality, performance or safety concerns such as:
- suspected contamination
- questionable stability
- defective components
- poor packaging or labeling

How to report:
- just fill in the sections that apply to your report
- use section C for all products except medical devices
- attach additional blank pages if needed
- use a separate form for each patient
- report either to FDA or the manufacturer (or both)

Important numbers:
- 1-800-FDA-0178   to FAX report
- 1-800-FDA-7737   to report by modem
- 1-800-FDA-1088   for more information or to report quality problems
- 1-800-822-7967   for a VAERS form for vaccines

If your report involves a serious adverse event with a device and it occurred in a facility outside a doctor's office, that facility may be legally required to report to FDA and/or the manufacturer. Please notify the person in that facility who would handle such reporting.

Confidentiality: The patient's identity is held in strict confidence by FDA and protected to the fullest extent of the law. The reporter's identity may be shared with the manufacturer unless requested otherwise. However, FDA will not disclose the reporter's identity in response to a request from the public, pursuant to the Freedom of Information Act.

The public reporting burden for this collection of information has been estimated to average 30 minutes per response, including the time for reviewing instructions, searching existing data sources, gathering and maintaining the data needed, and completing and reviewing the collection of information. Send your comments regarding this burden estimate or any other aspect of this collection of information, including suggestions for reducing this burden to:

Reports Clearance Officer, PHS
Hubert H. Humphrey Building,
Room 721-B
200 Independence Avenue, S.W.
Washington, DC 20201
ATTN: PRA

and to:
Office of Management and
Budget
Paperwork Reduction Project
(0910-0291)
Washington, DC 20503

Please do NOT
return this form
to either of these
addresses.

U.S. DEPARTMENT OF HEALTH AND HUMAN SERVICES
Public Health Service • Food and Drug Administration

FDA Form 3500-back   **Please Use Address Provided Below – Just Fold In Thirds, Tape and Mail**

**Department of
Health and Human Services**
Public Health Service
Food and Drug Administration
Rockville, MD 20857

Official Business
Penalty for Private Use $300

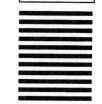

NO POSTAGE
NECESSARY
IF MAILED
IN THE
UNITED STATES
OR APO/FPO

BUSINESS REPLY MAIL
FIRST CLASS MAIL   PERMIT NO. 946   ROCKVILLE, MD

POSTAGE WILL BE PAID BY FOOD AND DRUG ADMINISTRATION

MEDWATCH
**The FDA Medical Products Reporting Program
Food and Drug Administration
5600 Fishers Lane
Rockville, MD 20852-9787**

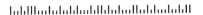

Figure 7.2 MED WATCH form. The FDA Medical Products Reporting Program for voluntary reporting by health professionals of adverse events and product problems.

(Continued)

MEDWATCH
THE FDA MEDICAL PRODUCTS REPORTING PROGRAM

For **VOLUNTARY** reporting
by health professionals of adverse
events and product problems

Form Approved: OMB No. 0910-0291 Expires: 12/31/94
See OMB statement on reverse

FDA Use Only (EPHO)

Triage unit
sequence #

Page ____ of ____

A. Patient information

1. Patient identifier	2. Age at time of event:	3. Sex	4. Weight
In confidence	or _____ Date of birth:	☐ female ☐ male	____ lbs or ____ kgs

B. Adverse event or product problem

1. ☐ Adverse event   and/or   ☐ Product problem (e.g., defects/malfunctions)

2. Outcomes attributed to adverse event (check all that apply)

☐ death _____ (mo/day/yr)
☐ life-threatening
☐ hospitalization – initial or prolonged
☐ disability
☐ congenital anomaly
☐ required intervention to prevent permanent impairment/damage
☐ other: _____

3. Date of event (mo/day/yr)	4. Date of this report (mo/day/yr)

5. Describe event or problem

6. Relevant tests/laboratory data, including dates

7. Other relevant history, including preexisting medical conditions (e.g., allergies, race, pregnancy, smoking and alcohol use, hepatic/renal dysfunction, etc.)

PLEASE TYPE OR USE BLACK INK

C. Suspect medication(s)

1. Name (give labeled strength & mfr/labeler, if known)

#1 _____

#2 _____

2. Dose, frequency & route used	3. Therapy dates (if unknown, give duration) from/to (or best estimate)
#1	#1
#2	#2

4. Diagnosis for use (indication)	5. Event abated after use stopped or dose reduced
#1	#1 ☐ yes ☐ no ☐ doesn't apply
#2	#2 ☐ yes ☐ no ☐ doesn't apply

6. Lot # (if known)	7. Exp. date (if known)	8. Event reappeared after reintroduction
#1	#1	#1 ☐ yes ☐ no ☐ doesn't apply
#2	#2	#2 ☐ yes ☐ no ☐ doesn't apply

9. NDC # (for product problems only)
_____ – _____

10. Concomitant medical products and therapy dates (exclude treatment of event)

D. Suspect medical device

1. Brand name

2. Type of device

3. Manufacturer name & address	4. Operator of device
	☐ health professional ☐ lay user/patient ☐ other: _____
6. model # _____ catalog # _____ serial # _____ lot # _____ other #	5. Expiration date (mo/day/yr) 7. If implanted, give date (mo/day/yr) 8. If explanted, give date (mo/day/yr)

9. Device available for evaluation?   (Do not send to FDA)
☐ yes   ☐ no   ☐ returned to manufacturer on _____ (mo/day/yr)

10. Concomitant medical products and therapy dates (exclude treatment of event)

E. Reporter (see confidentiality section on back)

1. Name, address & phone #

2. Health professional?	3. Occupation	4. Also reported to
☐ yes ☐ no		☐ manufacturer ☐ user facility ☐ distributor

5. If you do NOT want your identity disclosed to the manufacturer, place an " X " in this box. ☐

Mail to: MEDWATCH
5600 Fishers Lane
Rockville, MD 20852-9787

or FAX to:
1-800-FDA-0178

FDA Form 3500 (6/93)   Submission of a report does not constitute an admission that medical personnel or the product caused or contributed to the event.

Figure 7.2 (Continued)

Chapter Review Quiz

Complete the statements by filling in the blanks:

1. Before administering any medication, you should have the following information about the drug:

   _____   _____

   _____   _____

2. Before administering any medication, you should have the following three pieces of information about the patient:

   _____   _____

   other _____

3. Assessment of the patient's need for pain medication and reactions to drugs includes observation of the following four signs:

   _____   _____

   _____   _____

4. Patient education about medication should include the following four pieces of information:

   _____   _____

   _____   _____

5. When administering a controlled substance, documentation is necessary in two places:

   _____   _____

6. Documentation of an injection given for pain should include the following five pieces of information:

   _____   _____

   _____   _____

   _____

7. Name the six Rights of Drug Administration:

   _____

   _____

   _____

   _____

   _____

   _____

8. Medication errors must be reported immediately, and documentation includes recording the information in the following two areas:

_____   _____

CHAPTER 8

Administration by the Gastrointestinal Route

OBJECTIVES

Upon completion of this chapter, the student should be able to:

1. Describe the advantages and disadvantages of administering medications orally, by nasogastric tube, and rectally.
2. Explain appropriate action when patient is NPO, refuses medication, vomits medication, or has allergies.
3. List special precautions in preparation of timed-release spansules, enteric-coated tablets, and oral suspensions.
4. Demonstrate measurement of liquid medications with medicine cup and syringe.
5. Demonstrate proficiency in administering medications orally, by nasogastric tube, and rectally.
6. Satisfactorily complete all of the activities listed on the checklists.

Medications are administered by the gastrointestinal route more often than any other way. Gastrointestinal administration includes four categories: oral, nasogastric tube, gastric tube, and rectal.

Advantages of the oral route include:

- Convenience and patient comfort
- Safety, since medication can be retrieved in case of error or intentional overdose
- Economy, since there are few equipment costs

Disadvantages of the oral route include:

- Slower onset of absorption and action
- Rate and degree of absorption that vary with gastrointestinal contents and motility

- Some drugs (e.g., insulin and heparin) destroyed by digestive fluids and must be administered by injection
- Cannot be used with nausea or vomiting
- Dangerous to use if patient has difficulty swallowing (dysphagia), because of possible aspiration
- Cannot be used for unconscious patients
- Cannot be used if patient is NPO (e.g., before surgery or while fasting for a laboratory test or X-ray examination)

Administration of medications by nasogastric tube is sometimes ordered when the patient is unable to swallow for prolonged periods of time because of illness, trauma, surgery, or unconsciousness. Medications are usually administered intravenously when these conditions exist for short periods of time. *Advantages of the nasogastric tube* include:

- Ability to bypass the mouth and pharynx when necessary
- Elimination of numerous injections

The *disadvantage of the nasogastric tube* with a conscious patient is the discomfort of the tube in the nose and throat for prolonged periods of time.

When a patient is unable to take nourishment by mouth for a very extended period of time, the surgeon will sometimes insert a *gastric tube* through the skin of the abdomen, directly into the stomach. This G-tube, or peg tube, as it is sometimes called, is secured in place and can remain there for feeding purposes indefinitely. Medication can be administered via the G-tube, directly into the stomach.

Medications are sometimes administered by the rectal route when nausea or vomiting are present, or the patient is unconscious or unable to swallow. *Advantages of the rectal route* include:

- Bypassing the action of digestive enzymes
- Avoidance of irritation to the upper GI tract
- Useful with dysphagia

Disadvantages of the rectal route include:

- Many medications are unavailable in suppository form
- Some patients have difficulty retaining suppositories (e.g., the elderly and children)
- Prolonged use of some rectal suppositories can cause rectal irritation (e.g., aminophylline)
- Absorption may be irregular or incomplete if feces are present

Administration of Medications Orally

GUIDELINES FOR ADMINISTRATION OF ORAL MEDICATIONS

1. Wash your hands (Fig. 8.1)
2. Locate appropriate medication sheet and check for completeness of the order (i.e., date, patient's name, medication name, dosage, route, and time).
3. Check for special circumstances (e.g., allergies or NPO).
4. Be sure that you know the purpose of the drug, possible side effects, contraindications, cautions, interactions, and normal dosage range. If unfamiliar with the drug, consult a reference book for this information.
5. Select appropriate receptacle in which to place medication (i.e., paper medicine cup for tablets or capsules and plastic medicine cup for liquids).
6. Locate medication in medication cupboard or medication cart drawer and compare the label against the medication sheet for the five Rights of Medication Administration: right medicine, right amount, right time, right route, and right patient (Fig. 8.2).
7. If the dose ordered differs from the dose on hand, complete calculations on paper and check for accuracy with instructor or coworker in clinical setting.
8. Prepare the dosage as ordered. Do not open unit dose packages until you are with the patient (Fig. 8.3). If medication is liquid, see "Preparation of Liquid Medications" later in this section.
9. Take tray to patient and place it on table nearby.
10. Check patient's identification bracelet (Fig. 8.4).
11. Call patient by name and explain what you are doing. Answer any questions. Recheck medication order if patient expresses any doubts. Use this opportunity for patient education about the medication.
12. Monitor patient's vital signs if required for specific medication (e.g., blood pressure, apical pulse, or respiration).

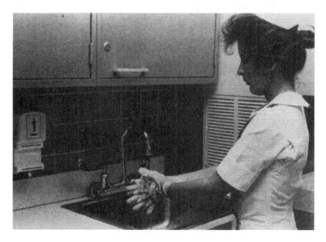

Figure 8.1 Medical asepsis handwash.

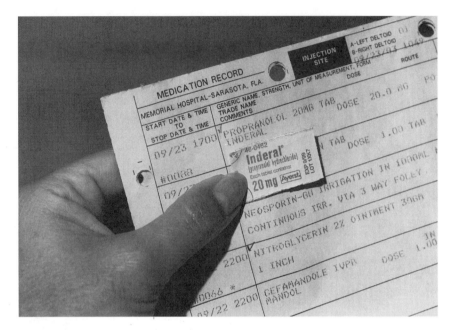

Figure 8.2 Compare name and dosage on medication package with the medication sheet.

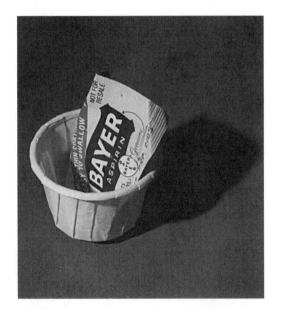

Figure 8.3 Keep the unit-dose packet intact until you are with the patient.

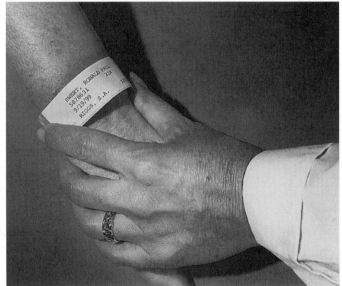

Figure 8.4 Check identification to be sure it is the right patient.

13. Open unit-dose package and place container in the patient's hand. Avoid touching the medication (Fig. 8.5).
14. Provide full glass of water and assist the patient as necessary (e.g., raise the head of the bed and provide drinking straw if required).
15. Stay with the patient until the medication has been swallowed. Make the patient comfortable before you leave the room.

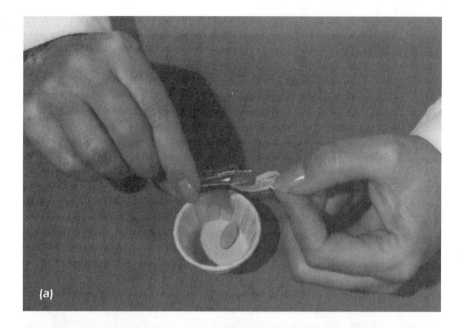

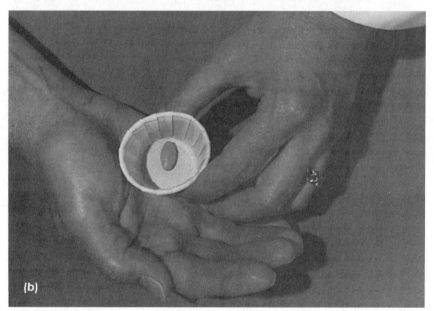

Figure 8.5 Do not touch medicine. (a) Open the unit dose packet and drop the tablet in a cup. (b) Place the cup containing the medicine in the patient's hand.

16. Discard used medicine cup and wrappers in wastebasket.
17. Return clean tray to medicine cart or medicine room.
18. Record the medication, dosage, time, and your signature or initials in the correct place on patient's record.
19. Document on patient's record and report if a medication is withheld or refused and the reason. Record *and report* any unusual circumstances associated with administration or any adverse side effects.

SPECIAL CONSIDERATIONS FOR ORAL ADMINISTRATION

1. If patient is NPO, check with the person in charge regarding appropriate procedure, based on reason for NPO. If patient is fasting for laboratory X-ray tests, medication can usually be given at a later time with possible modification of time schedule. If patient is NPO for surgery, nausea, or dysphagia, it may be necessary to consult the doctor regarding a change of route. Do not omit the medications completely without specific instructions to that effect. Abrupt withdrawal of some medications, for example, phenytoin (Dilantin) or diazepam (Valium), may lead to seizures.

2. Always check the patient's record for *allergies* and be aware of the components of combination products. Patients with a history of allergy should be watched carefully for possible drug reactions when any new medication is administered.

3. Give the most important medicine first.

4. Elevate the patient's head, if not contraindicated by the patient's condition, to aid in swallowing.

5. Stay with the patient until the medication is swallowed. *Do not* leave the medication at the bedside or in the patient's possession unless ordered by physician.

6. Administer oral medications with water, unless ordered otherwise. *Do not* give medicine with fruit juice, milk, or any other liquid unless indicated by specific directions. The absorption of many medicines (e.g., antibiotics) is inhibited by interaction with acid or alkaline products.

7. Medications whose action depends on contact with the mucous membranes of the mouth or throat (e.g., topical anesthetics or fungicides) *should not* be administered with any fluid or food.

8. *Do not* open or crush timed-release capsules or enteric-coated tablets.

9. If tablets must be divided, place on paper towel and cut with a knife on score marks only, for accuracy. *Do not* break by hand. If available, a pill-cutter may be used.

10. When removing tablets or capsules from a stock bottle, pour into lid and from there into medicine cup. *Do not* touch tablets or capsules.

11. *Do not* administer any medication that is discolored, has precipitated, is contaminated, or is outdated.

12. If a patient is NPO, refuses the medication, or vomits within 20–30 min. of taking the medication, always report this to the person in charge. A written order from the physician is required to change either the medication or the route of administration. Document on the patient's record the time of emesis and appearance of the emesis, for example, medication remained intact.

13. If the patient refuses a medication, determine the reason. Report the refusal and reason to the person in charge and record all information on patient's record.

14. Tablets (unless enteric coated) may be crushed with mortar and pestle. Capsules (except timed-release capsules) may be opened and the contents mixed with applesauce or ice cream to facilitate administration for patients with difficulty swallowing (e.g., children and the elderly). Check diet to be

sure these foods are allowed. Be sure that any equipment used to crush medication is wiped clean.

Note: In some areas a physician's order is required for pillcrushing. If available, ask for the medication to be ordered in liquid or powdered form.

PREPARATION OF LIQUID MEDICATIONS

Follow the "Guidelines for Administration of Oral Medications," at the beginning of this section. Preparation of *liquid medications* requires these additional steps:

1. Shake bottle if indicated. Remove cap and place cap upside down on table.
2. Hold medicine bottle with label side upward to prevent smearing of label while pouring (Fig. 8.6).
3. In other hand, hold medicine cup at eye level and place thumbnail on level to which medication will be poured (Fig. 8.6).
4. While holding the medicine cup straight at eye level, pour the prescribed amount of medication.
5. Replace cap on bottle.
6. Compare the information on the medication sheet against the label on the stock bottle and the quantity of drug in the cup.
7. Replace medication bottle in cupboard or medicine cart.

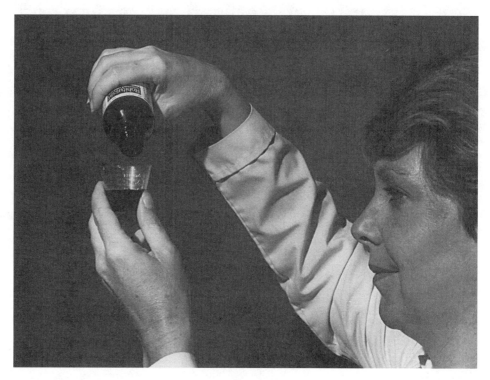

Figure 8.6 Hold the medicine bottle with label side up and medicine cup at eye level, with thumbnail marking measurement.

8. Recheck the five Rights of Medication Administration.*
9. Proceed with the "Guidelines for Administration of Oral Medications."

When administering liquid medication to someone who is unable to drink from a cup (e.g., infants and persons with wired jaws), a syringe may be used. Follow the "Guidelines for Administration of Oral Medications." Administration of *liquid medications orally via syringe* requires these additional steps:

1. Pour prescribed medication into medicine cup.
2. Withdraw prescribed amount with syringe.
3. Check medication and order using the five Rights of Medication Administration.
4. Identify the patient and elevate the patient's head.
5. Be sure the patient is alert and able to swallow.
6. Place the syringe tip in the pocket between the cheek and the gums. (When administering large amounts of liquid via syringe, it helps to fit a 2-inch length of latex tubing on the syringe tip to facilitate instillation of the medication into the cheek pocket.)
7. Instill the medication slowly to lessen chances of aspiration.
8. Be sure all medication is swallowed before leaving the patient.
9. Proceed with "Guidelines for the Administration of Oral Medications."
10. Remember the "sixth right" and document appropriately.

Administration of Medications by Nasogastric Tube

A nasogastric tube is not inserted solely for the purpose of administering medication. However, medications are sometimes ordered by this route when a nasogastric tube is in place for tube feeding or for suction. When medications are ordered by nasogastric tube, follow the "Guidelines for Administration of Oral Medications" and "Preparation of Liquid Medications."

Administration of medication by nasogastric tube requires these additional steps:

1. Check the medication order using the five Rights of Medication Administration.
2. Wash hands (Fig. 8.1). Wear gloves when handling tubes, if it is the policy at your facility.
3. Prepare the medication as ordered and take to the patient's room. Be sure the medication is at room temperature.
4. Check identification bracelet, call the patient by name, and explain the procedure. Elevate head of bed, if not contraindicated.
5. Hold the end of the tube up and remove the clamp, plug, or adapter.
6. Make sure that the tube is properly placed in the stomach by using at least two tests (Fig. 8.7):

*Remember the "sixth right" and document appropriately.

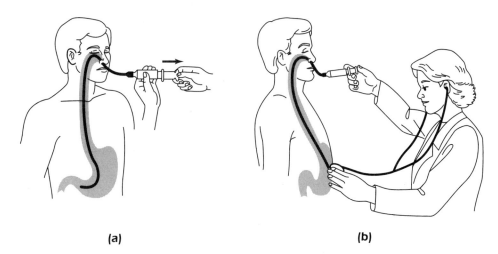

Figure 8.7 Test for correct placement of nasogastric tube. (a) Aspirate with syringe. (b) Listen with stethoscope as you inject 15 cc of air.

    a. Aspirate with bulb or piston syringe for stomach contents to verify correct placement. Then flush tube with normal saline solution.

    b. Place a stethoscope over the patient's stomach, attach the syringe to the tube, and inject about 15 cc of air. If you hear a swooshing sound, air has entered the stomach, verifying correct placement.

7. Clamp the tube with your fingers by bending it over upon itself or by pinching it. While tube is closed, remove plunger or bulb from syringe, leaving syringe attached firmly to tubing (Fig. 8.8a).

8. Pour medication into syringe. Release or unclamp the tubing and let medication flow through by gravity. Never force fluids down a nasogastric tube (Fig. 8.8b). Watch the patient during the procedure and stop immediately at any sign of discomfort by pinching the tube. Holding the syringe too high causes fluid to run in too quickly, possibly causing nausea and vomiting.

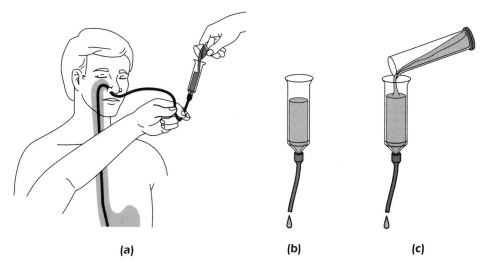

Figure 8.8 (a) Close tube before filling syringe. (b) Let fluid flow in by gravity. Hold syringe at level of patient's shoulder. (c) Flush tube with water.

9. Before the syringe empties completely, flush the tube by adding 30–50 ml of water to the syringe (Fig. 8.8c). If the patient's input and output are being monitored, be sure to add this amount to the patient's record.

10. After the water has run in, pinch the tube, remove the syringe, and clamp or plug the tube. If the patient is on suction, be sure to leave suction turned *off* for at least 30 min until medication is absorbed.

11. Position patient on right side and/or elevate head of bed to encourage the stomach to empty. Make the patient comfortable.

12. Proceed with "Guidelines for the Administration of Oral Medications" for documentation.

Administration of Medications by Gastric Tube

If a patient has a gastric tube in place in the abdomen, medications can be administered per order in this way. Directions for "Administration of Medications by Nasogastric Tube" can be followed, only omitting number 6. No test for placement of tube is necessary. The rest of the directions regarding flushing the tube afterward and positioning the patient, etc., should be followed carefully. Remember to document appropriately.

Administration of Medications Rectally

Medications are sometimes ordered to be administered by rectal route. The medicine may be in suppository form or in liquid form to be administered as a retention enema. This treatment is more effective with the patient's cooperation. Tact and consideration are required for successful administration of rectal medications. Remember to respect the patient's dignity and privacy by closing the door and curtains completely. Do not expose the patient unnecessarily.

The retention enema is administered in the same way as a cleansing enema. However, the retention enema must be retained approximately 30 min or more for absorption of the medication. Therefore, the patient is instructed to lie quietly on either side to aid in retention. If the patient is uncooperative, unconscious, or has poor sphincter control, the buttocks can be taped together with 2-inch paper adhesive for 30 min. Do not use this method unless absolutely necessary. Remember to treat the patient with dignity. Always explain everything you are doing and why. Even if patients are unconscious or unable to speak, they may be able to hear and cooperate in some way if they understand.

ADMINISTRATION OF RECTAL SUPPOSITORY

1. Wash hands (Fig. 8.1)
2. Check the medication order using the five rights of Medication Administration.

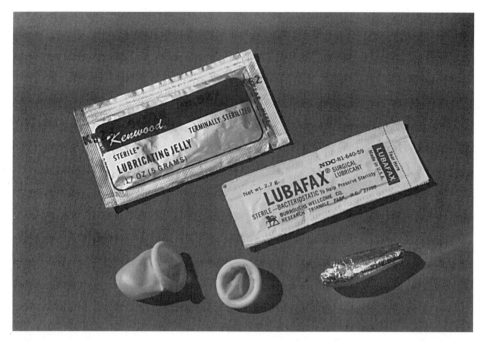

Figure 8.9 *Supplies for administration of rectal suppository. A finger cot and a small packet of lubricant are required.*

3. Identify medication (purpose, side effects, contraindications, cautions, and normal dose range). Research information if necessary.
4. Assemble supplies (finger cot or disposable glove and water-soluble lubricant (Fig. 8.9).
5. Select the medication as ordered, checking medication name and dosage again. Some suppositories are stored in a refrigerator, and some may be stored at room temperature, according to manufacturer's instructions.
6. Check patient's identification bracelet, call the patient by name, and explain the procedure. Answer any questions.
7. Close door and curtain completely.
8. Lower the head of the bed if necessary and position the patient on side with upper knee bent. Keep patient covered, exposing only the rectal area (Fig. 8.10).
9. Put on disposable glove, or finger cot on index finger. With infants, use little finger.
10. Remove suppository from wrapper and lubricate the tapered end with water-soluble lubricant.
11. With ungloved hand, separate the patient's buttocks gently so you can see anus.
12. Ask patient to take a deep breath. Insert the lubricated suppository gently into the rectum and push gently with gloved index finger until the suppository has passed the internal sphincter (Fig. 8.11).
13. Urge the patient to retain the suppository for at least 20 min. If patient is unable to cooperate, hold the buttocks together as required.

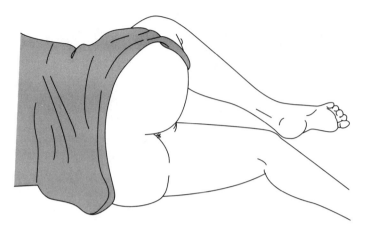

Figure 8.10 Drape and position patient on side with upper knee bent.

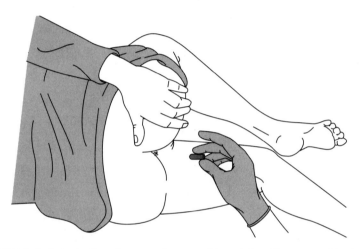

Figure 8.11 Lubricate tip of suppository and insert it with covered index finger.

14. Remove and dispose of glove or finger cot, turning it inside out as you remove it.
15. Be sure the patient is comfortable, with covers and bed adjusted appropriately.
16. Wash hands.
17. Record the medication in the appropriate place (the sixth right).

 Check your knowledge of this chapter before going any further.

Chapter Review Quiz

1. Name six disadvantages of oral administration compared with administration by injection.

   _____

   _____

   _____

   _____

   _____

   _____

Match the column on left with the appropriate action on the right. Actions may be used more than once:

2. ____	To facilitate swallowing	a.	Watch closely for drug reactions
3. ____	If NPO for lab tests	b.	Crush tablet, mix with applesauce
4. ____	Patient vomits 15 min after medication	c.	Administer first
		d.	Cannot be opened
5. ____	Most medications		
6. ____	Patient is allergic to penicillin	e.	Elevate patient's head
		f.	Notify person in charge
7. ____	Most important medicine	g.	Modify schedule, give medicine later
8. ____	Tablet cannot be swallowed		
9. ____	Timed-release capsules	h.	Administer with water
10. ____	Dilantin ordered PO, patient NPO for surgery	i.	Leave medication at bedside

Complete the following statements by filling in the blanks:

When pouring liquid medicine:

11. The bottle should be held _____

12. The medicine cup should be held _____

13. The bottle cap should be placed _____

14. If medication is in suspension, the bottle should first be

_____

When administering medication by nasogastric tube:

15. Check tube placement first with two tests:

_____

_____

Check the appropriate answer:

16. _____ a. Medication should be pushed through the nasogastric tube by pressure on barrel of syringe.

_____ b. Medication should flow through the nasogastric tube by gravity.

17. _____ a. Medication should be cold.

_____ b. Medication should be at room temperature.

18. _____ a. Patient's head should be elevated.

_____ b. Patient should be placed in Trendelenburg position.

19. Name four steps in administration of a rectal suppository that are different from PO administration.

_____

_____

_____

_____

20. Medication documentation should include:

_____

_____

_____

_____

CHECKLIST FOR ADMINISTRATION OF ORAL MEDICATIONS

Activity   *Rating*
                                                                                     S / U

1. Washed hands.   ____ ____

2. Checked medication sheet for date, dosage, time, route, and   ____ ____
   allergies.

3. Identified medication: purpose, side effects, contraindications,   ____ ____
   cautions, interaction, and normal dosage range.

4. Selected appropriate medicine cup and placed on tray.   ____ ____

5. Selected correct medication and checked label against med-   ____ ____
   ication sheet for five Rights of Medication Administration.

6. Calculated correct dosage on paper if necessary.   ____ ____

7. Placed medication as ordered in cup without opening packet   ____ ____
   or touching medication. Prepared liquid medication by shak-
   ing if necessary, pouring away from label and measuring at
   eye level.

8. Identified patient by checking bracelet and calling the patient   ____ ____
   by name.

9. Explained procedure to patient and answered any questions   ____ ____
   about medication.

10. Checked patient's vital signs if necessary for specific medi-   ____ ____
    cine.

11. Opened unit dose packages and offered medication in con-   ____ ____
    tainer to patient.

12. Provided drinking water and assisted patient as necessary.   ____ ____

13. Made patient comfortable and left unit in order.   ____ ____

14. Recorded medication, dosage, time, and signature or initials   ____ ____
    on patient's record (the sixth right).

Note: S, satisfactory; U, unsatisfactory.

CHECKLIST FOR ADMINISTRATION OF RECTAL SUPPOSITORY

Activity	*Rating* *S / U*
1. Washed hands.	____ ____
2. Checked the medication order for date, dosage, time, route, and allergies.	____ ____
3. Identified medication: purpose, side effects, contraindications, cautions, and normal dosage range.	____ ____
4. Assembled supplies: finger cot or glove and lubricant.	____ ____
5. Selected correct medication and checked label with medication order for five Rights of Medication Administration.	____ ____
6. Identified patient by checking bracelet and calling patient by name.	____ ____
7. Explained procedure to patient and answered any questions about medication.	____ ____
8. Closed door and curtain.	____ ____
9. Positioned patient on side with upper knee bent and only rectal area exposed.	____ ____
10. Put on disposable glove, or finger cot on index finger.	____ ____
11. Removed wrapping from suppository and lubricated tapered end.	____ ____
12. With ungloved hand, separated buttocks gently.	____ ____
13. Instructed patient to take a deep breath and inserted suppository gently, pushing it past the sphincter.	____ ____
14. Instructed patient about retaining the suppository.	____ ____
15. Removed glove or finger cot correctly and disposed of it appropriately.	____ ____
16. Made patient comfortable and left unit in order.	____ ____
17. Washed hands.	____ ____
18. Recorded medication, dosage, time, and signature or initials on patient's record.	____ ____

Note: S, satisfactory; U, unsatisfactory.

CHAPTER **9**

Administration by the Parenteral Route

OBJECTIVES

Upon completion of this chapter, the student should be able to:

1. Define parenteral, systemic, local, topical, and transcutaneous delivery systems, and IPPB therapy.
2. Name four parenteral routes with systemic effects.
3. Explain administration via the sublingual and buccal routes, including instructions to the patient.
4. Demonstrate application of nitroglycerin ointment and the transdermal patch.
5. Identify three conditions treated with transcutaneous delivery systems.
6. Compare and contrast advantages and disadvantages of inhalation therapy.
7. Describe patient education for those receiving inhalation therapy with hand-held nebulizers.
8. List cautions when administering IPPB therapy.
9. Identify the three parts of the syringe and the three parts of the needle.
10. Select appropriate-length and correct-gauge needles for various types of injections.
11. List three types of syringes and a purpose for each.
12. Demonstrate drawing up medications from a vial and an ampule.
13. Describe and demonstrate an intradermal injection.
14. Describe and demonstrate a subcutaneous injection.
15. Describe five sites for intramuscular injection and demonstrate intramuscular injection.
16. Give purpose and demonstration of Z-track injection.
17. List four types of administration for local effects.

Parenteral routes include any route other than the gastrointestinal tract. The most common form of parenteral administration is injection. However, other routes must be considered as well: the skin, mucous membranes, eyes, ears, and respiratory tract.

Parenteral administration can be understood more easily if the purpose of administration or the effects desired are considered as two categories: systemic and local.

Systemic effects are those affecting the body as a whole, the entire system. The goal of administering drugs for systemic effects is to distribute the medication through the circulatory system to the area requiring treatment. Parenteral routes with systemic effects include (1) sublingual or buccal, (2) transcutaneous (transdermal), (3) inhalations, and (4) injections.

Local effects are those limited to one particular part (location) of the body, with very little, if any, effect on the rest of the body. Medications in this category include:

1. Medications applied to the skin for skin conditions, sometimes called *topical* medications
2. Drugs applied to the mucous membranes to treat that specific tissue
3. Medication instilled in the eyes
4. Medication instilled in the ears

Sublingual and Buccal Administration

With sublingual administration, the medication is placed under the tongue. The drug is absorbed directly into the circulation through the numerous blood vessels located in the mucosa of this area. With buccal administration, the medication is placed in the pouch between the cheek and the gum at the back of the mouth. The sublingual route is used more commonly than the buccal. Medications absorbed in this way are unaffected by the stomach, intestines, or liver. Absorption via this route is quite rapid, and therefore this method is used frequently when quick response is required (e.g., with nitroglycerin to treat acute angina pectoris). The constricted coronary blood vessels are usually dilated within a few minutes, bringing quick relief from pain.

PATIENT EDUCATION

For the sublingual or buccal route, include the following instructions:
1. Hold the tablet in place with mouth closed until medication is absorbed.
2. Do not swallow the medication.
3. Do not drink or take food until medication is completely absorbed.

Transcutaneous Drug Delivery System

Transcutaneous, or transdermal, systems deliver the medication to the body by absorption through the skin. Nitroglycerin ointment, for example, is applied to the skin in prescribed amounts every few hours for prevention of angina pectoris. The absorption is slower, and therefore this method is not effective in the treatment of acute angina attacks. Other transcutaneous delivery systems utilize a patch impregnated with a particular medication, applied to the skin, and left in place for continuous absorption. Examples of transcutaneous drug delivery systems include nitroglycerin, (Transderm-Nitro), in which the patch is usually left in place for 24 hours in prophylactic treatment of chronic angina; scopolamine, (Transderm-Scop), in which the patch is placed behind the ear and left in place up to 72 h, as necessary, to prevent motion sickness; and fentanyl (Duragesic), applied every 72 h in the management of chronic pain in patients requiring opiate analgesia. (See Analgesics, Chapter 19.) Absorption by this method is slower, but the action is more prolonged than with other methods of administration.

PATIENT EDUCATION

For those applying transcutaneous systems of administration, include the following instructions. With nitroglycerin ointment (Fig. 9.1):

1. Squeeze the prescribed amount of ointment onto Appli-Ruler paper. When the ointment reaches the correct marking, give the tube a slight twist to cut off the ointment and recap the tube.
2. *Do not* touch the ointment! Absorption of ointment through the skin of the fingers can cause a severe headache.
3. Carefully fold the Appli-ruler paper lengthwise with the ointment inside.
4. Flatten the folded paper carefully to spread the ointment inside. *Do not* allow the ointment to reach the edges of the paper. Keep paper folded.
5. Rotate sites for application. Appropriate areas include chest, back, upper arms, and upper legs. *Do not* shave the area. Be sure the area is clean, dry, and free of irritation, rash, and abrasion.
6. After the area for application is exposed, open the paper carefully and apply paper to the skin, ointment side down. *Do not* touch ointment. Fasten paper in place with paper tape.
7. Remove previous paper carefully, without touching the inside, and discard in trash container. Cleanse area and inspect skin for any sign of irritation. Report and record any skin changes.
8. Wash hands immediately.
9. Report and record any skin changes.

With transdermal sealed drug delivery systems (Fig. 9.2):

1. Select site for administration, rotating areas. Be sure the skin is clean, dry, and free of irritation.
2. Open the packet carefully, pulling the two sides apart *without touching the inside*.
3. Apply the side containing the medication to the skin. Press the adhesive edges down firmly all around. If for any reason the adhesive edges do not stick, fasten in place with paper tape. This is usually unnecessary.
4. Remove previous patch carefully, without touching the inside, and discard in trash container. Cleanse area and inspect skin for irritation.
5. Wash hands immediately.

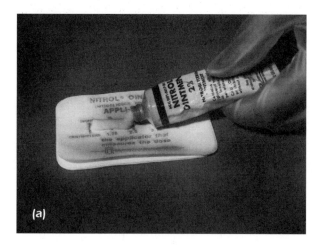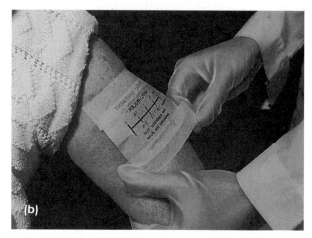

Figure 9.1 Transdermal administration of nitroglycerin ointment. (a) Ointment is measured on Appli-Ruler paper. (b) Paper containing ointment is applied to the skin.

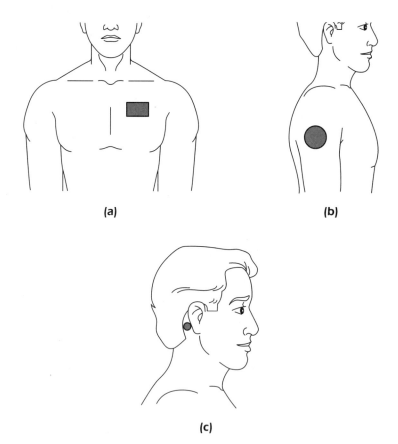

Figure 9.2 Transdermal drug delivery. Dermal patches vary in size and shape. (a, b) For prevention of angina pectoris; (c) For prevention of motion sickness. Analgesic patches are also available.

Inhalation Therapy

Medications are frequently administered by inhalation method, especially to those with chronic pulmonary conditions, such as asthma. Patients may self-administer the medication with a metered-dose inhaler (MDI) or small-volume nebulizer, or the physician may prescribe intermittent positive pressure breathing (IPPB) therapy, to be administered by trained personnel.

Advantages of inhalation therapy include:

1. Rapid action of the drug, with local effects within the respiratory tract.
2. Potent drugs may be given in small amounts, minimizing the side effects.
3. Convenience and comfort of the patient.

Disadvantages of inhalation therapy include:

1. Requires cooperation of the patient in proper breathing techniques for effectiveness.
2. Adverse systemic side effects may result rapidly because of extensive absorption capacity of the lungs.
3. Improperly administered, or too frequently administered, inhalations can lead to irritation of the trachea or bronchi, or bronchospasm.
4. Asthmatic and COPD (chronic obstructive pulmonary disease) patients sometimes become dependent on a small-volume nebulizer or MDI.
5. If not cleaned properly, the small-volume nebulizer can be a source of infection.

METERED-DOSE INHALER (MDI)

Metered-dose inhalers (Fig. 9–3) have become more popular in recent years. MDIs are portable, easy to use, and recently more drugs have become available in the inhaler form. Proper administration by the patient is essential for drug effectiveness. Elderly patients may have difficulty coordinating the depression of the canister and inhaling at the same time. A *spacer* may be added to act as a reservoir for the aerosol, allowing the patient to first depress the canister and then inhale. Many spacers have an audible horn or whistle to signal the patient if inspiration is too rapid. One type of spacer device, InspirEase, is described in Figure 9.4 with instructions for use. MDIs may be used in pediatric patients with a mouthpiece or a mask. A full MDI canister provides approximately 200 puffs of medication.

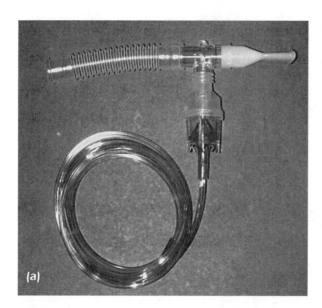
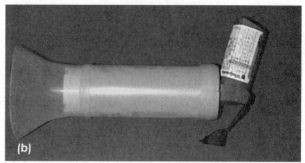
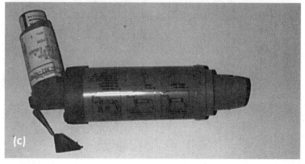

Figure 9.3 (a) Metered dose inhaler (MDI) with spacer. (b) MDI, spacer, and mask (pediatric patients). (c) Small volume nebulizer.

PATIENT EDUCATION

How to Use a Metered-Dose Inhaler (MDI)

1. Sit upright or stand.
2. Assemble inhaler and shake for 10 seconds.
3. Place the mouthpiece between the lips, forming a seal, or use a spacer prescribed by your physician.
4. Exhale slowly and completely.
5. Push down on the inhaler while breathing in slowly and deeply.
6. Hold your breath for at least 5–10 seconds.
7. Exhale slowly.

If your prescription is for more than 1 puff, rest for 1 or 2 minutes before the second dose.

Important: If using an inhaled steroid (such as Azmacort, Aerobid, Beclovent, or Vanceril), rinse your mouth out with tap water after using the inhaler.

SMALL-VOLUME NEBULIZERS (MINI-NEBS, MED-NEBS)

Many drugs for the respiratory system may be delivered in aerosol form via a small-volume nebulizer. The nebulizer is powered by a gas source, usually a small air compressor in the home care setting. For optimal drug deposition in the lung, proper breathing techniques must be used by the patient. The patient should be

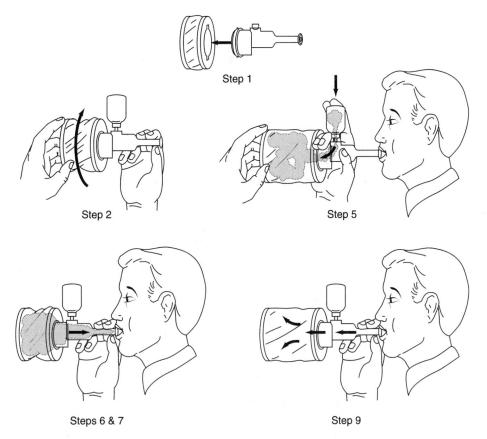

Step 1

Step 2

Step 5

Steps 6 & 7

Step 9

1. Connect the mouthpiece which fits your inhaler, to the reservoir bag by lining up the locking tabs with the openings in the reservoir. Push in the tabs, and twist to lock the mouthpiece.
2. Gently untwist the reservoir bag to extend it to its full size.
3. Shake the medication canister before placing its stem firmly in the area designated for it in the mouthpiece.
4. Place the mouthpiece in your mouth and close your lips tightly around it.
5. Press down on the medication canister to release a dose of medication into the reservoir bag.
6. Breathe in slowly through the mouthpiece. If you hear a whistling sound, breathe more slowly until the sound stops.
7. Breathe in the entire contents of the bag, that is, until the bag collapses completely.
8. Hold your breath while slowly counting to five.
9. Breathe out slowly through the mouthpiece.
10. Repeat steps 6 through 9.
11. Remove the mouthpiece from your mouth. Take the medication canister off the mouthpiece. Unlock the mouthpiece from the bag by untwisting it and pulling it free. Clean and store the equipment.

Figure 9.4 Instructions for use of the InspirEase extender device. (Courtesy of Key Pharmaceuticals, Inc.)

instructed to inhale slowly and deeply, perform a short breath, hold, and exhale slowly. In addition to the side effects of the drugs themselves (see Chapter 26), patients should be cautioned that dizziness may occur if they hyperventilate (breathing too rapidly). Proper cleaning of equipment on a daily basis is essential to avoid infection.

PATIENT EDUCATION

Proper Home Cleaning of Small-Volume Nebulizer

1. Dissemble the pieces of the nebulizer. Wash in mild soapy water and rinse thoroughly.
2. Place in a solution of 1 part vinegar to 2 parts water. Soak for 20–30 minutes.
3. Wash your hands with soap and water.
4. Remove the nebulizer parts from vinegar solution and rinse with warm tap water.
5. Allow to dry completely.
6. Reassemble pieces for next use.

PATIENT EDUCATION

With use of an inhaler or nebulizer, include the following instructions:

1. Name of the medication, dosage, and how often it is to be administered.
2. Desired effects and possible adverse side effects (e.g., palpitations, tremor, nervousness, dizziness, headache, nausea, dry mouth, irritated throat, hoarseness, or coughing).
3. Notify the physician if any adverse side effects occur or if the medication seems ineffective. The doctor may want to change the dosage or the medication.
4. Caution *not* to take any other medication, including over-the-counter drugs, without doctor's permission. Many drugs and alcohol can interact with these drugs causing serious side effects.
5. Rising slowly from a reclining position will help prevent dizziness.
6. Rinsing the mouth after inhalation will counteract dry mouth or unpleasant taste.
7. Step-by-step demonstration with the patient, answering all questions.
8. Rinsing equipment after use and storage of medication as indicated on the package.
9. Importance of not smoking.
10. Importance of handwashing before treatments.

INTERMITTENT POSITIVE PRESSURE BREATHING (IPPB)

Intermittent positive pressure breathing treatments may be ordered by the physician. IPPB combines administration of an aerosol with a mechanical breather to assist patients who are unable to take a deep breath on their own. Health care personnel, such as respiratory therapists or nurses, are specifically trained in the use of this equipment.

Cautions with IPPB therapy include:

1. Monitor vital signs closely, watching for a sudden drop in blood pressure, tachycardia, and decreased or shallow respirations.
2. Observe for nausea or distended abdomen.
3. Watch for tremors or dizziness.
4. Assure the patient that coughing after the treatment is to be expected. The goal of the treatment is to aid in coughing up the loosened secretions.
5. Record effectiveness of therapy and any side effects observed or reported by the patient.

Injections

To administer injections, you must be familiar with equipment.

SYRINGES

The syringe has three parts (Fig. 9.5):

1. *Barrel.* The outer, hollow cylinder that holds the medication. It contains the calibrations for measuring the quantity of medication.
2. *Plunger.* The inner, solid rod that fits snugly into the cylinder. Pulling back on the plunger allows solution to be drawn into the syringe. Pushing forward on the plunger ejects solution or air from the syringe.
3. *Tip.* The portion that holds the needle. Most tips are plain. Some larger syringes contain a metal attachment at the tip, called a Luer-Lok, which locks the needle in place.

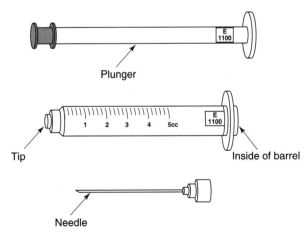

Figure 9.5 *Parts of a syringe and needle that must remain sterile during preparation and administration of medication.*

Most syringes are plastic and disposable after one use. Some syringes for special procedures are glass and must be resterilized after use.

NEEDLES

The needle has three parts (Fig. 9.6):

1. *Hub.* The flared end that fits on the tip of the syringe.
2. *Shaft.* The long, hollow tube embedded in the hub. Needles have shafts with different lengths. Shorter needles (½, ⅜, and ⅝ inches) are used for intradermal (into the skin) or subcutaneous (into the tissue just below the skin) injections. Longer needles (1½ and 2 inches) are used for intramuscular (into the muscle) injections. The length of the needle depends on the type of injection and the size of the patient (i.e., shorter needles for children and thin adults and longer needles for larger adults). The gauge is the size of the lumen, or hole, through the needle, or the diameter of the shaft. The gauge is numbered in reverse order (i.e., the thinner needle with the smaller diameter has the larger number, e.g., 25 gauge for subcutaneous injections and 19–21 gauge, a thicker needle with a larger opening for IM or IV injections. The size of the gauge is determined by the site of the injection and the viscosity of the solution (e.g., blood and oil require a thicker-gauge needle, e.g., 15–18).
3. *Tip.* The tip is the pointed end with a beveled edge.

Three main types of syringes are used for injections. The type used is determined by the medication and the dosage. The three types are:

1. *Standard syringe.* Used most frequently for subcutaneous or intramuscular injections, calibrated or marked in cubic centimeters (cc) or milliliters (ml) and minims (m) (Fig. 9.7). The most commonly used size is 3 cc or 2½ cc. Larger sizes of 5–50 cc are available for other purposes (e.g., irrigations, withdrawing fluids from the body, and intravenous injections).
2. *Tuberculin (TB) syringe.* Used for intradermal injections of very small amounts of a substance (e.g., testing for tuberculosis or for allergies). The TB syringe is also used for subcutaneous injections when a small amount of medication, less than 1 cc, is ordered (e.g., in pediatrics). The TB syringe is calibrated in tenths of a cubic centimeter and in minims and holds only a total of 1 cc, or 1 ml (Fig. 9.8).

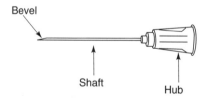

Bevel

Shaft

Hub

Figure 9.6 *Needle showing the hub, the shaft, and the tip (bevel).*

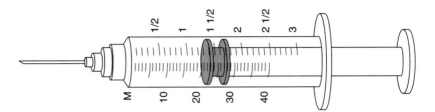

Figure 9.7 3-cc syringe.

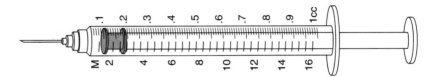

Figure 9.8 Tuberculin syringe.

3. *Insulin syringe.* Used only for injection of insulin and is calibrated in units. The size in common use today is U-100, in which 100 units of insulin is equal to 1 cc (Fig. 9.9). Formerly insulin and insulin syringes were also available in U-40 and U-80 sizes, and the insulin had to conform to the syringe size. However, these forms are obsolete, and you will be using the U-100 insulin and syringe.

Prefilled cartridges are also available, in which a premeasured amount of a medication is contained in a disposable cartridge with a needle attached. These prefilled units are made ready for injection by placing the cartridge and needle unit in a holder. An example of such a unit is the Carpuject, produced by SANOFI Winthrop Pharmaceuticals, New York (Fig. 9.10). A different type of unit, the Tubex, is produced by Wyeth Laboratories, Philadelphia, PA. Follow the manufacturer's directions regarding assembly of the different cartridge units.

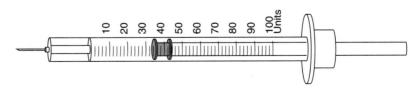

Figure 9.9 U-100 insulin syringe.

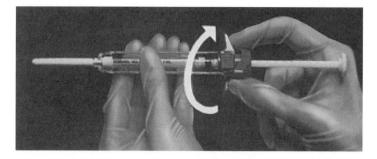

Place cartridge, needle end first, into open end of holder. Twist blue lock to close.

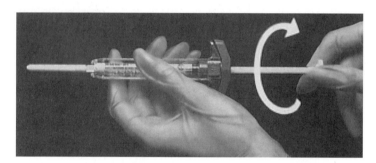

To engage, turn plunger rod clockwise. Proceed with injection in normal manner, leaving needle guard on until just before use.

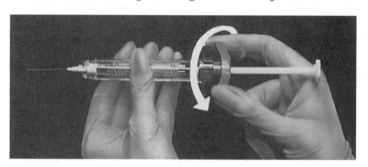

To disengage, turn plunger rod counterclockwise. Pull back plunger fully. Twist blue lock open to release.

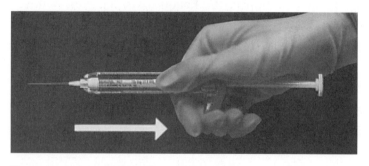

Place thumb on cartridge and slide back.

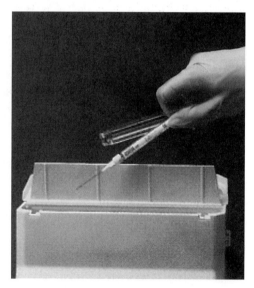

Invert holder and release used cartridge-needle unit into disposal bin.
Do not recap!
Holder autoclavable if sterility is desired.

Figure 9.10 Carpuject prefilled cartridge. (Reprinted with permission from SANOFI Winthrop Pharmaceuticals, New York.)

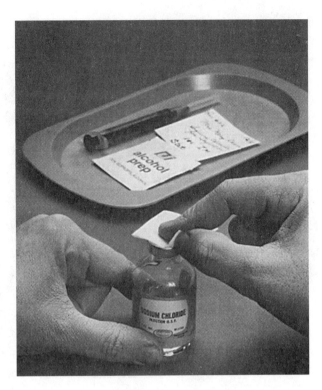

Figure 9.11 Preparing to withdraw medication from a vial.

DRAWING UP MEDICATIONS

1. Wash hands.
2. Assemble equipment (i.e., syringe, needle, packaged alcohol wipes, and medication ampule or vial) on a tray.
3. Check the order using the five Rights of Medication Administration.
4. If medication is contained in a vial, first remove the protective cap. If the vial has been opened previously, wipe the rubber diaphragm on top with an alcohol wipe. Check vial for date and discoloration of contents (Fig. 9.11).
5. Seat the needle securely on the syringe by pressing firmly downward on the top of the needle cover. Pull the needle cover straight off. **Note:** Luer-Loks require a half-turn to lock the needle in place.
6. Draw air into the syringe equal to the amount of solution you will be withdrawing from the vial. Insert needle into center of rubber diaphragm and inject air into vial (Fig. 9.12). Invert vial and withdraw prescribed dosage (Fig. 9.13). Be sure syringe is filled to proper level with solution and no bubbles are present. Withdraw needle from vial. For intramuscular injections, a small bubble (0.2 ml) of air may now be added to the correct dose of medicine already in the syringe.
7. The needle must now be recapped *carefully* to maintain sterility and prevent needle sticks. Hold the filled syringe, *without moving it,* in a vertical position with the needle upright, in your dominant hand. Hold the sterile cap in your

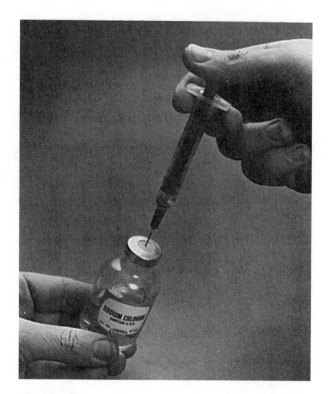

Figure 9.12 Injection of air into vial.

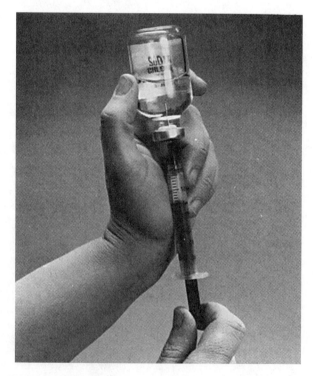

Figure 9.13 Withdrawal of prescribed amount of medication.

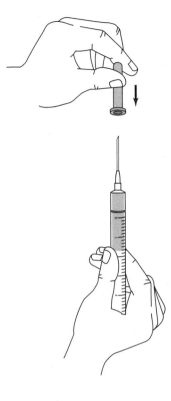

Figure 9.14 Recapping **sterile** needle. The syringe is held steady while the cap is **moved down carefully** to cover the sterile needle. Contaminated needles are **never** recapped but are discarded **uncapped** in sharps container.

nondominant hand and, slowly and *carefully,* place the cap over the needle snugly. *Do not contaminate the needle* by touching it to the outside of the cap. Remember, *only sterile needles are to be recapped* (Fig. 9.14).

An alternate method would be to remove the needle from the syringe carefully and discard the needle in the sharps container, replacing it with a sterile, capped needle.

8. If medication is contained in an ampule, hold tip with alcohol wipe to protect your fingers and break open along the scored marking at the neck. Tip vial and withdraw prescribed amount of medication. Recap needle carefully according to previous directions (Fig 9.14).

9. Place filled syringe with needle covered on tray with alcohol wipes and patient's name card.

If two drugs are to be combined in a syringe, you must first check for compatibility of the drugs.

ADMINISTRATION BY INJECTION

Intradermal injections are usually administered into the skin on the inner surface of the lower arm. For allergy testing, the upper chest and upper back areas may also be used. A small amount (0.1–0.2 ml) is injected so close to the surface that a wheal, or bubble, is formed by the skin expanding (Fig. 9.15).

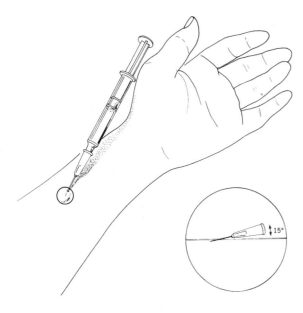

Figure 9.15 Intradermal injection.

Technique for intradermal injection is as follows:

1. Wash hands.
2. Assemble equipment (i.e., TB syringe, 26 or 27 gauge, ⅜-inch needle, alcohol wipes, and medication).
3. Check the order using the five Rights of Medication Administration and draw up medication.
4. Identify patient and explain procedure. Arm should be supported on flat surface.
5. Put on gloves.
6. Cleanse skin with alcohol wipe on inner surface of the forearm (or other area if ordered by the physician). Allow the skin to dry thoroughly. (If you inject before the skin is dry, you might introduce alcohol into the skin and interfere with test results). Avoid areas with hair or blemishes.
7. Hold the patient's arm in your nondominant hand and stretch the skin taut.
8. Hold the syringe so that the bevel is up and the needle is almost flat against the patient's arm. Insert the needle slowly only far enough to cover the lumen or opening in the needle. The point of the needle should be visible through the skin.
9. Inject the medication *very slowly.* You should see a small white bubble in the skin forming immediately. If no bubble forms, withdraw the needle slightly; it may be too deep. If solution leaks out as you inject, the needle is not deep enough.
10. After correct amount of medication is injected, withdraw needle and apply gentle pressure with alcohol wipe. *Do not* massage the area or you may interfere with test results.
11. Discard syringe with needle *uncapped* into sharps container immediately without touching needle. Remove gloves. Wash hands.
12. Note drug name, dosage, time, date, and site of injection on patient's record (Sixth Right–Documentation).

13. Instruct the patient not to scrub, scratch, or rub the area. Provide written instructions regarding time to return for reading. Tell the patient to contact the physician immediately or report to an emergency facility if breathing difficulty, hives, or a rash appears.

Note: Since intradermal injections are practically bloodless, some facilities omit gloves for this procedure. Follow the policy at your facility.

> **Caution:** Do not start allergy testing unless emergency equipment is available nearby and personnel are trained in emergency care in case of anaphylactic response. Patients receiving allergy testing should remain in office or clinical facility for 30 minutes after injection to be observed for possible anaphylactic reaction.

Subcutaneous injections are administered into the fatty tissues on the upper outer arm, front of the thigh, abdomen, or upper back (Fig. 9.16). A 2½–3-cc syringe is usually used with a 24–26-gauge, ⅜–⅝-inch needle. No more than 2 cc of medication may be administered subcutaneously.

Technique for subcutaneous injection is as follows:

1. Wash hands.
2. Assemble equipment (correct-size syringe and needle, alcohol wipes, and medication).
3. Check the order with the five Rights of Medication Administration and draw up medication.
4. Identify patient and explain procedure.
5. If patient is receiving frequent injections, be sure to rotate injection sites.
6. Put on gloves.
7. Cleanse skin with alcohol wipe.
8. Pinch the skin into a fat fold of at least 1 inch (Fig. 9.16).
9. Insert the needle at a 45-degree angle. Then release skin fold.
10. Pull back on the plunger (aspirate). If any blood appears in the syringe, withdraw the needle. Place pressure with alcohol swab over injection site until bleeding stops. Discard the syringe with needle *uncapped* into sharps container immediately. You will then have to draw up fresh solution with another sterile syringe and needle.
11. Inject the medication *slowly*, pushing the plunger all the way. Too rapid injection may cause pain.
12. Place alcohol wipe over the entry site, applying pressure with it, as you withdraw the needle.
13. Massage the site gently with the alcohol wipe to speed absorption. (*Do not* massage with heparin injection.) Be sure there is no bleeding.
14. Discard syringe with needle *uncapped* into sharps container immediately.
15. Remove gloves and discard.
16. Wash hands.

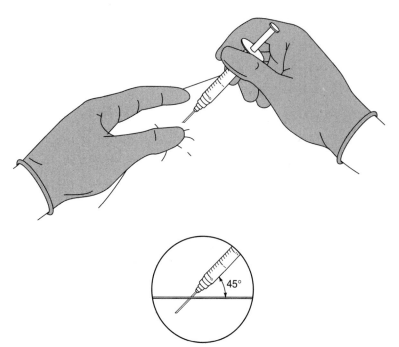

Figure 9.16 Subcutaneous injection. The tissue is pinched, and the needle is held at a 45-degree angle.

17. Note the medication, dosage, time, date, site of injection, and your signature on the patient's record (Sixth Right–Documentation).
18. Observe the patient for effects and record observations.

Intramuscular injections are administered deep into large muscles (Fig. 9.17). There are five recommended sites.

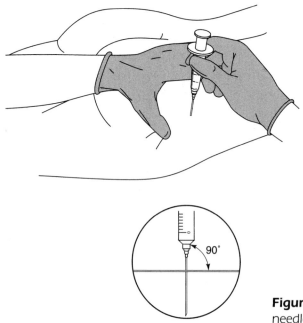

Figure 9.17 Intramuscular injection. The skin is held taut, with the needle at a 90-degree angle.

1. *Dorsogluteal.* Upper outer quadrant of the buttock (preferred site for adults).
2. *Ventrogluteal.* Above and to the outside of the buttock area, on the hip.
3. *Deltoid.* Upper outer arm above the axilla.
4. *Vastus lateralis.* Front of the thigh toward the outside of the leg.
5. *Rectus femoris.* Front of the thigh toward the midline of the leg.

The intramuscular route has two advantages over the subcutaneous route:

1. A larger amount of solution can be administered (up to 3 cc, or a maximum of 1 cc in children).
2. Absorption is more rapid because the muscle tissue is more vascular (i.e., contains many blood vessels).

The needle must be long enough to go through the subcutaneous tissue into the muscle. The length of the needle varies with the size of the patient. With a child or very thin, emaciated adult, a 1-inch needle is usually adequate. For most adults, a $1\frac{1}{2}$-inch needle is appropriate. However, for an obese person, a 2-inch needle might be required. The needle is inserted at a 90-degree angle with the skin spread taut (Fig. 9.17).

Because there are more large blood vessels and nerves in this deeper tissue, the site for injection must be chosen more precisely. Using the illustrations as a guide, follow these steps in selecting the site:

1. *Dorsogluteal site.* Most commonly used for adults, but not for children under 3 years old (Fig. 9.18). Position the patient flat on the stomach (prone) with the toes pointed inward or on the side with the upper leg flexed. Identify the site by drawing an imaginary line from the posterior superior iliac spine to the greater trochanter of the femur. These two bony prominences can be palpated with the thumb and forefinger. The injection is given above and to the outside of this line. Note that this site is high enough to avoid the sciatic nerve and the major blood vessels.

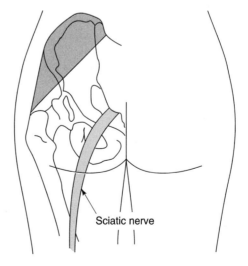

Figure 9.18 Dorsogluteal site for IM injection.

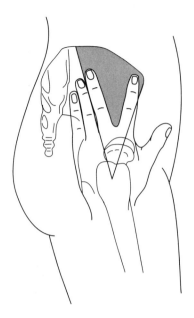

Figure 9.19 Ventrogluteal site for IM injection.

2. *Ventrogulteal site.* Can be used for all patients. Position the patient on the back or side (Fig. 9.19). Identify the site by placing the palm of your hand on the patient's greater trochanter. Place the index finger on the anterior superior iliac spine and the middle finger on the iliac crest. The injection is made into the center of the V formed between the index and middle fingers.

3. *Deltoid site.* Seldom used because the muscle is smaller and is close to the radial nerve (Fig. 9.20). The maximum solution that can be used is 1 cc; and a shorter needle, 1 inch, is used. Caution must be exercised to avoid the clavicle, humerus, acromium, brachial vein and artery, and radial nerve. Identify the site by drawing an imaginary line across the arm at the level of the armpit.

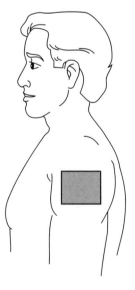

Figure 9.20 Deltoid site for IM injection.

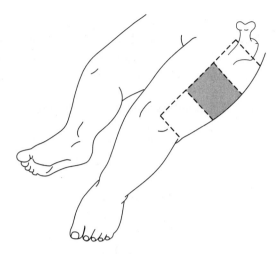

Figure 9.21 Vastus lateralis site for IM injection, preferred for infants.

The injection is made above this line and below the acromium on the outer aspect of the arm.

4. *Vastus lateralis.* Located on the anterior lateral thigh, the preferred site for infants, since these muscles are the most developed for children under the age of 3 years (Fig. 9.21). In the elderly, nonambulatory, and emaciated adult, this muscle may be wasted and insufficient for injection. Identify the midportion on the side of the thigh by measuring one hand breadth above the knee and one hand breadth below the great trochanter. The area between is the site for injection.

5. *Rectus femoris.* Located just medial to the vastus lateralis, but does not cross the midline (Fig. 9.22). It is the preferred site for self-injection because of its

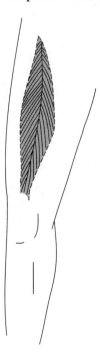

Figure 9.22 Rectus femoris site for IM injection.

accessibility. It is located in the same way as the vastus lateralis. **Caution:** Do not get too close to the midline, which is adjacent to the sciatic nerve and major blood vessels. If the muscle is not well developed, injections in this site may be painful.

Technique for intramuscular injection is as follows:

1. Wash hands.
2. Assemble equipment (i.e., correct-size syringe, needle, alcohol wipes, and medication).
3. Check the order with the five Rights of Medication Administration and draw up the medication, or insert appropriate prefilled cartridge into Tubex or Carpuject holder.
4. After measuring correct amount of medication in syringe, draw 0.2 cc air into syringe to clear needle. Recap carefully using method illustrated in Fig. 9.14.
5. Identify the patient and explain procedure.
6. If patient is receiving frequent injections, be sure to rotate sites.
7. Put on gloves.
8. Position the patient and expose area to be used for injection.
9. Cleanse skin with alcohol wipe.
10. With your nondominant hand, stretch the skin taut at the injection site.
11. Insert the needle at a 90-degree angle with a quick dartlike motion of your dominant hand.
12. Pull back on the plunger (aspirate), and follow previous guidelines if blood appears.
13. Inject the medication at a slow, even rate.
14. Withdraw the needle rapidly, holding alcohol swab over the site.
15. Apply pressure and massage area gently with alcohol wipe.
16. Discard syringe with needle *uncapped* into sharps container immediately.
17. Discard gloves and wash hands.
18. Note the medication, dosage, time, date, site of injection, and your signature on the patient's record (Sixth Right–Documentation).
19. Observe the patient for effects and record observations.

The *Z-track method* (Fig. 9.23) is used for injections that are irritating to the tissue, such as iron dextran, hydroxyzine, or cephazolin. The dorsogluteal is the site for this type of intramuscular injection.

Technique for the Z-track method is as follows:

1. Draw up the medication and then add 0.3–0.5 cc of air to the syringe. Then replace the needle with a sterile one 2–3 inches long.
2. Stretch the skin as far as you can to the outer side and hold it there.
3. After cleansing the site, insert the needle with a dartlike motion, aspirate, and then inject the medication *slowly*. Wait 10 sec before withdrawing the needle.

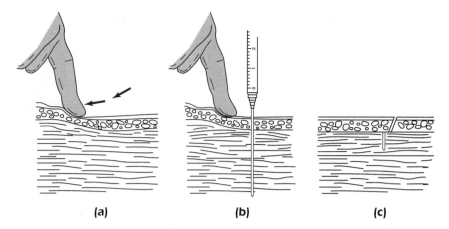

Figure 9.23 Z-track method of IM injection of iron preparations. (a) Skin and subcutaneous tissue pulled to one side and held there. (b) Needle is placed in muscle. (c) Z-track sealed when tissue released.

4. Withdraw the needle and allow the skin to return to normal position. This seals off the needle track.

5. Press firmly on injection site with alcohol swab. Do *not* massage the site, as this could spread the medication to the subcutaneous tissue, causing irritation.

6. Advise the patient that walking will aid absorption and to avoid tight garments, such as girdles, that cause pressure on the site.

Skin Medications

Topical medications for the skin are prescribed for a great variety of conditions and are available in a variety of forms: ointments, lotions, creams, solutions, soaks, and baths. Administration of topical medications requires knowledge of the condition being treated and the purpose of the treatment, and strict adherence to directions as prescribed by the doctor or provided by the pharmacist, or to instructions on the medication container or in a package insert. *When in doubt regarding administration techniques, always ask* a qualified person for advice. Some specific principles for skin medications are outlined in Chapter 12. In addition, good judgment is also required.

Several suggestions for applying topical medications include:

1. For burns, use sterile gloves to apply, and cover with sterile dressings because of the danger of infection. Use gentle, light touch because of pain.

2. For skin conditions in which there is irritation or itching, use cotton or snug-fitting gloves to apply. *Never* use gauze, which can cause additional irritation and discomfort.

3. Follow physician's order regarding covering or leaving open to the air.

4. Wash old medication off before applying new, unless specifically directed to do otherwise.

Application to the Mucous Membranes

Medications applied to the mucous membranes also come in a variety of forms: suppositories, ointments, solutions, sprays, gargles, and so on. Always follow the specific directions that accompany the individual medication, unless directed to do otherwise by the physician. When in doubt, always ask questions.

Eye Medications

Technique for instillation of eye medications is as follows:

1. Wash hands (Fig. 8.1).
2. Assemble eye medication (ophthalmic solution or ointment).
3. Check the order with the five Rights of Medication Administration. Pay particular attention to *percentage* on medication label and to *which eye* is to be treated (*OD* right eye, *OS* left eye, or *OU* both eyes).
4. Identify patient and explain procedure.
5. Position patient flat on back or upright with head back. Ask the patient to look up.
6. Carefully instill the ophthalmic solution, correct number of drops, or ointment into the lower conjunctival sac, using caution to avoid contamination of the tip of the dropper or ointment tube (Fig. 9.24). Do not let solution run from one eye to the other.
7. Tell the patient to close the eye gently so as not to squeeze out the solution.
8. Press gently on the inner canthus following administration of eyedrops

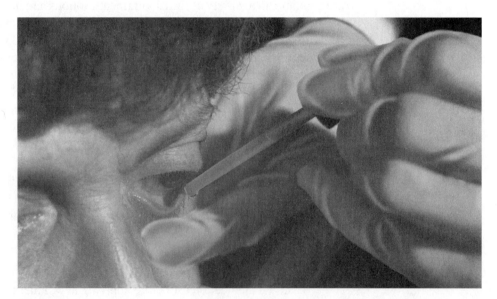

Figure 9.24 Instilling eye medication. Ophthalmic solution is dropped inside lower eyelid.

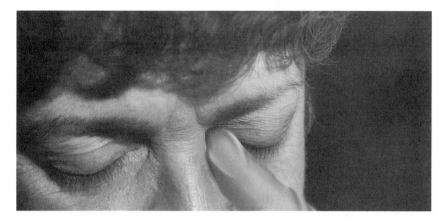

Figure 9.25 *Gentle pressure on the inner canthus following administration of ophthalmic medications. Systemic absorption is thus minimized with medications such as corticosteriods, miotics, and mydriatics.*

(Fig. 9.25). Systemic absorption is thus minimized with medications such as corticosteroids, miotics, and mydriatics.

9. Wash hands. Replace medication in appropriate place.

10. Record the medication, dosage, time, date, and which eye was treated, on the patient's record (Sixth Right–Documentation).

When in doubt about administration of any medication, always ask a qualified person for advice. Never guess! Remember that the patient who is receiving the medication could be you or your loved one. By thinking of yourself in the patient's place you will have the proper attitude to administer medications with competence, good judgment, and compassion.

Check your knowledge of this chapter before going any further.

CHECKLIST FOR INTRADERMAL INJECTION

Activity	*Rating* *S / U*
1. Washed hands.	____ ____
2. Checked medication order for date, dosage, time, route, and allergies.	____ ____
3. Identified medication: purpose, side effects, cautions, and normal dosage range.	____ ____
4. Assembled supplies: TB syringe, 27-gauge, $\frac{3}{8}$-inch needle, alcohol wipes, and medication.	____ ____
5. Checked medication vial against medication sheet using the five Rights of Medication Administration.	____ ____
6. Withdrew correct dose from vial *after* cleansing top with alcohol and injecting equivalent amount of air into vial.	____ ____
7. Recapped needle using sterile technique. See Figure 9.14 for technique.	____ ____
8. Identified patient by checking bracelet and calling patient by name.	____ ____
9. Explained procedure to patient and answered any questions regarding procedure.	____ ____
10. Positioned patient with inner forearm exposed and supported on a flat surface.	____ ____
11. Put on gloves.	____ ____
12. Selected area without hair or blemish, cleansed skin with alcohol wipe, and allowed skin to dry.	____ ____
13. Held patient's arm with nondominant hand, stretching the skin taut.	____ ____
14. Expelled any air bubbles from syringe.	____ ____
15. Inserted needle point slowly, bevel side up, only enough to cover needle opening. Point of needle visible through skin.	____ ____
16. Injected medication very slowly with immediate formation of small bubble.	____ ____
17. Withdrew needle and applied gentle pressure to injection site with alcohol wipe (no massage).	____ ____
18. Discarded syringe with needle *uncapped* into sharps container.	____ ____
19. Removed gloves.	____ ____
20. Washed hands.	____ ____
21. Recorded drug name, dosage, time, date, and site of injection on patient's record and signed or initialed entry (Sixth Right–Documentation).	____ ____
22. Observed patient for 30 min. for possible anaphylactic reaction. Identified location of emergency equipment and medication if required.	____ ____
23. Provided written instructions regarding time to return for reading. Instructed patient to avoid scrubbing, scratching, or rubbing the area and to report to emergency facility with dyspnea, hives, or rash.	____ ____

Note: S, satisfactory; U, unsatisfactory

CHECKLIST FOR SUBCUTANEOUS INJECTION

Activity	*Rating* S / U
1. Washed hands.	___ ___
2. Checked medication order for date, dosage, time, route, and allergies.	___ ___
3. Identified medication: purpose, side effects, contraindications, interactions, and normal dosage range.	___ ___
4. Assembled supplies: 2½–3-cc, TB or insulin syringe; 24–26-gauge, ⅜–⅝ inch needle; alcohol wipes; and medication vial or ampule.	___ ___
5. Checked medication against medication sheet using the five Rights of Medication Administration. Also checked drug for date and discoloration.	___ ___
6. Calculated correct dosage on paper if necessary and checked calculations with instructor.	___ ___
7. If drug contained in *vial*, withdrew correct amount after cleansing top with alcohol wipe and injecting equivalent amount of air into vial. If drug contained in *ampule*, held tip with alcohol wipe while breaking it at neck. Withdrew correct amount of drug without bubbles in syringe.	___ ___
8. Recapped needle using proper sterile technique.	___ ___
9. Identified patient by checking identification bracelet and calling patient by name.	___ ___
10. Explained procedure to patient and answered any questions.	___ ___
11. Selected appropriate site, using rotation if frequent injections.	___ ___
12. Put on gloves.	___ ___
13. Cleansed skin with alcohol wipe.	___ ___
14. Pinched skin into fold with nondominant hand.	___ ___
15. Expelled any air bubbles from syringe.	___ ___
16. Inserted needle at a 45-degree angle and released skin fold.	___ ___
17. While holding needle hub with nondominant hand, aspirated for blood (used new site if necessary).	___ ___
18. Injected medication slowly.	___ ___
19. Placed alcohol wipe over entry site, and applied pressure as needle was withdrawn. Massaged site gently (with heparin, pressure only, no massage).	___ ___
20. Disposed of syringe and needle *uncapped* in sharps container.	___ ___
21. Removed and discarded gloves.	___ ___
22. Washed hands.	___ ___
23. Recorded drug name, dosage, time, date, site of injection, and signature on patient's record. Also recorded effects after appropriate time (Sixth Right–Documentation).	___ ___

Note: S, satisfactory; U, unsatisfactory.

CHECKLIST FOR INTRAMUSCULAR INJECTION

Activity	*Rating* S / U

1. Washed hands. ____ ____

2. Checked medication order for date, dosage, time, route, and allergies. ____ ____

3. Identified medication: purpose, side effects, cautions, and normal dosage range. ____ ____

4. Assembled supplies: 2½, 3-cc, Tubex, or Carpuject syringe; 1½ inch needle, usually 21 ____ ____
   gauge; alcohol wipes; and medication.

5. Checked medication against medication sheet using the five Rights of Medication ____ ____
   Administration. If PRN medication, checked time of last dose.

6. If narcotic, signed, and checked time of last dose, on controlled substance sheet. ____ ____
   Calculated correct dosage on paper if necessary.

7. If drug contained in *vial,* withdrew correct amount after cleansing top with alcohol wipe ____ ____
   and injecting equivalent amount of air into vial. If drug contained in *ampule,* held tip
   with alcohol wipe while breaking it at neck. Withdrew correct amount of drug without
   bubbles in syringe. If drug contained in cartridge, assembled correctly in holder with
   drug at right level for dosage and no bubbles in syringe.

8. *After* drug measured accurately in syringe, drew 0.2 cc air into syringe. ____ ____

9. Recapped needle using sterile technique, See Figure 9.14 for techniques. ____ ____

10. Identified patient by checking bracelet and calling patient by name. ____ ____

11. Explained procedure to patient and answered any questions. ____ ____

12. Closed door to room and/or curtain around bed. ____ ____

13. Selected appropriate site, using rotation if frequent injections. ____ ____

14. Put on gloves. ____ ____

15. Positioned patient appropriately, exposing only the area for injection. ____ ____

16. Cleansed skin with alcohol wipe. ____ ____

17. With forefinger and thumb of nondominant hand, spread the skin taut at injection site. ____ ____

18. Inserted needle at a 90-degree angle with a quick, dartlike motion of dominant hand. ____ ____

19. Aspirated for blood (used new site if necessary). ____ ____

20. Injected medication at a slow, even rate. ____ ____

21. Applied pressure with alcohol wipe over entry site as needle was withdrawn rapidly. ____ ____
    Massaged site gently with alcohol wipe unless medication irritating (with Ancef,
    Vistaril, or iron dextran, pressure only, no massage).

22. Made sure there was no bleeding before covering patient and making patient comfort- ____ ____
    able.

23. Disposed of syringe and needle *uncapped* in sharps container. ____ ____

24. Discarded gloves appropriately. Washed hands. ____ ____

25. Recorded drug, name, dosage, time, date, site of injection, and signature on patient's _____
    record (Sixth Right–Documentation).

Note: S, satisfactory; U, unsatisfactory

CHECKLIST FOR INSTILLATION OF EYE MEDICATIONS

Activity	*Rating* *S / U*
1. Washed hands.	____ ____
2. Checked the order with the five Rights of Medication Administration. Noted percent, which eye, and allergies.	____ ____
3. Identified medication: purpose, side effects, and cautions.	____ ____
4. Identified patient by checking bracelet and calling patient by name.	____ ____
5. Explained procedure to patient and answered any questions regarding procedure.	____ ____
6. Positioned patient on back or upright with head back.	____ ____
7. Asked the patient to look up.	____ ____
8. Used aseptic technique to instill correct number of drops or ointment dosage into lower conjunctival sac.	____ ____
9. Gently closed the eyelid and applied pressure to the inner canthus, (eye drops only).	____ ____
10. Washed hands and replaced medication in appropriate place.	____ ____
11. Recorded medication, dosage, time, date, and which eye was treated, on patient's record (Sixth Right–Documentation).	____ ____

Chapter Review Quiz

Fill in the blanks:

1. Parenteral includes any routes other than_____ .

2. Systemic effects are those affecting _____ .

3. The four parenteral routes with systemic effects include

    _____   _____

    _____   _____

Label the routes according to their action. Use R for rapid and S for slow. Match each route with the appropriate definition:

Action		*Definition*	
4. ____	Sublingual	____ a.	Given with a needle
5. ____	Transcutaneous	____ b.	Nebulizer or IPPB
6. ____	Inhalation	____ c.	Under the tongue
7. ____	Injection	____ d.	Skin patch

8. What precautions should be observed when applying transcutaneous systems?

    _____ .

9. IPPB refers to _____ .

Select the correct needle for the purpose. Needle size may be used for more than one purpose.

Purpose		*Needle*	
10. ____	Subcutaneous injection	a.	21 gauge, $1\frac{1}{2}$ inch
11. ____	Intravenous injection	b.	25 gauge, $\frac{5}{8}$ inch
12. ____	Allergy testing	c.	18 gauge
13. ____	Intramuscular injection	d.	27 gauge, $\frac{3}{8}$ inch

14. What are the two purposes of the tuberculin syringe?

    _____

    _____

15. The insulin syringe is calibrated in _____,
and 1 cc is equal to _____ in an insulin syringe.

16. Disposable cartridges containing a premeasured amount of medication are
used with a plastic holder called a _____
or _____.

Match the injection with the proper technique:

Injection	**Technique**
17. _____ Intramuscular	a. Needle 45-degree angle, skin pinched up
18. _____ Subcutaneous	b. Needle flat, bevel up, skin taut
19. _____ Intradermal	c. Needle 90-degree angle, skin taut

20. List the five sites for intramuscular injections and when each is used.

_____

_____

_____

_____

_____

21. Why is the Z-track method used? _____

Describe Z-track administration. _____

_____

_____

22. Define local effects. _____

_____

List four areas to administer medication for local effects.

_____   _____

_____   _____

CHAPTER 10

Poison Control

OBJECTIVES

Upon completion of this chapter, the student should be able to:

1. Define poison, overdose, emetic, antidote, and ingestion.
2. Identify four routes by which poisons may be taken into the body.
3. List five conditions in which an emetic would not be given to induce vomiting, and describe substitute therapy.
4. Describe medication, dosage, and procedure for administration of the most common emetic.
5. Explain the purpose of activated charcoal and when it is given.
6. Name three clinical procedures required when caring for patients who have been poisoned.
7. Describe appropriate therapy for poisoning by inhalation, external poison, insect sting, and snakebite.
8. Identify two groups of people at risk for poisoning.
9. List 10 recommendations for patient education to help prevent poisoning.

A poison is a substance taken into the body by ingestion, inhalation, injection or absorption that interferes with normal physiological functions. In some cases, only a small amount of a substance can cause severe tissue damage directly (e.g., corrosives). In other cases, the substance can be beneficial in small amounts, but lethal in excessive amounts (e.g., overdose of medication).

In a case of suspected poisoning, the best policy is to contact a Poison Control Center directly, or through an emergency care facility. Instructions can then be given by phone for appropriate emergency treatment based on the type of poison and the patient's condition, age, and size.

Poisoning by Ingestion

The most common type of poisoning is by ingestion, or swallowing. An emetic, such as ipecac syrup, is usually administered to induce vomiting. However, there are some important exceptions to this therapy. *Do not* induce vomiting under these conditions:

1. Ingestion of corrosive substances such as mineral acids or caustic alkalis (e.g., carbolic acid, ammonia, drain cleaners, oven cleaners, dishwasher detergent, and lye). Check also for burns around or in the mouth. Vomiting can cause additional tissue damage.
2. Ingestion of volatile petroleum products (e.g., gasoline, kerosene, lighter fluid, and benzene). Vomiting can cause aspiration and/or asphyxiation.
3. Ingestion of convulsants (e.g., strychnine or iodine). Vomiting can precipitate seizures.
4. If patient is semiconscious, severely inebriated, in shock, convulsing, or has no gag reflex. Vomiting could cause choking, aspiration, and/or asphyxiation.
5. If patient is less than 1 year old.

Caution must be taken with the use of ipecac in patients with cardiac or vascular disease. Vomiting can increase blood pressure and precipitate a stroke, cardiac arrhythmias, or atrioventricular block.

If any of the above mentioned conditions exist, the patient should be transported *immediately* to an emergency care facility. Trained personnel can remove the stomach contents by gastric lavage and administer appropriate antidotes as indicated.

Antidotes, such as CNS (central nervous system) stimulants and/or CPR (cardiopulmonary resuscitation), may be required in poisoning with CNS depressants. Gastric lavage is *not* used in patients who have ingested corrosives, because of the danger of perforating the damaged tissue of the esophagus. If perforation exists, surgery is required. Observation is required in an acute care facility.

If none of the above mentioned conditions exist and the patient is 1–10 years old, and able to swallow, 1 tablespoon (15 ml, $\frac{1}{2}$ ounce) of ipecac syrup is administered PO and followed immediately with several glasses (8–16 oz) of water. Other liquids may be substituted for water. However, milk may slow emesis and carbonated drinks may cause distention; these liquids should therefore be avoided. If emesis does not occur within 20 min, the initial dose of 15 ml of ipecac syrup may be repeated. Never give more than 2 tablespoons. If there is no emesis within 30 min, gastric lavage is required.

If the person is over 10 years of age, give 2 tablespoons of ipecac with 8–16 oz of fluid. If vomiting has not occurred in 20 min, call the Poison Control Center.

Sometimes a substance such as activated charcoal is administered to minimize systemic absorption of the ingested poison. However, activated charcoal is given *only after* emesis or gastric lavage. If given before the ipecac, it will absorb the ipecac and prevent emesis.

Personnel caring for poisoning victims should observe the following cautions:

• *Be sure to save emesis.* It may be necessary to send it to a laboratory to determine the type of poison. If there is doubt about the poison, the doctor may also order urine and blood tests for toxicology.

- Closely monitor the vital signs of patients who have taken poison of any kind.
- Observe closely for possible confusion, tremors, convulsions, visual disturbances, loss of consciousness, respiratory distress, or cardiac arrhythmias.

Poisoning by Inhalation

Poisoning by inhalation requires symptomatic treatment: fresh air, oxygen, and CPR if indicated. Inhaling insect spray may require administration of an antidote.

External Poisoning of Skin or Eyes

External poisons should be flushed from the skin or eyes with a continuous stream of water for at least 15 minutes. The patient should then be transported to an emergency care facility for further treatment as required. Systemic absorption of poisons through the skin may require administration of an antidote.

Poisoning by Sting and Snakebite

Poisoning by insect sting (e.g., bee, wasp, scorpion, or fire ant) should be treated with a paste made of bicarbonate of soda and water, after removing the stinger of a bee or wasp, and an ice pack should be applied to the site of the sting. If the patient is allergic, watch closely for possible anaphylactic reaction. CPR and administration of adrenalin and corticosteroids may be required. Transport the patient to an emergency care facility immediately if indicated. Some allergic persons carry a kit with medication prescribed by their doctor (e.g., antihistamine and Isuprel SL to be self-administered if stung, or epinephrine for self-injection or injection by someone else).

A stingray, found in warm ocean and bay waters, can cause a wound and inject a poison. Immediate treatment includes submerging injured extremity in hot water at as high a temperature as patient can tolerate without injury for 30–90 minutes. Further treatment may be necessary in an emergency room including possible tetanus immunization.

The jellyfish, also found in warm ocean water, has a poisonous sting that can cause severe reactions, especially in those who are allergic. Immediate treatment consists of applying vinegar, ammonia, or alcohol to the sting site, then applying a paste of nonseasoned meat tenderizer. Topical hydrocortisone cream will also help counteract the effects of the poison. Always seek medical attention if there is a severe reaction.

Do not apply ice or a tourniquet to a snakebite. Venom is very irritating, and may cause sloughing of the tissues. Keep the patient quiet in order to slow circulation, and transport the patient, lying down, to an emergency care facility for antivenom injections. If possible, take the snake along, in a closed container, for identification purposes. It may be nonpoisonous.

People at Risk

Poisonings are the leading cause of health emergencies for children in the nation., and a major cause of death among young children because of their natural curiosity and active lifestyle. The danger is particularly great with flavored medications, such as aspirin or iron tablets. Great care must be taken to prevent poisoning of young children. The child between the ages of 1 and 5 years old is most at risk.

The Food and Drug Administration (FDA) reports that iron pills are the leading cause of poisoning deaths in children under 6. Although iron supplements have been sold in bottles with child-resistant caps, in the last decade more than 110,000 children were poisoned by eating adult iron pills and at least 33 have died. Therefore, in 1994 the FDA proposed requiring iron supplements to be sold in special "blister packs."

The health care worker can play a major role in reducing the number of accidental poisonings in children by stressing preventive measures to parents. One educational program teaches the child to stay away from dangerous products by labeling them with a "Mr. Yuk" sticker. Fig. 10.1 (Mr. Yuk says "No!") is a warning label for children who cannot read. These stickers are available from many poison information centers throughout the United States.

Another group at risk for poisoning is the elderly. Overdoses of medication can result in toxicity, with symptoms of confusion, dizziness, weakness, lethargy, ataxia, tremors, or cardiac irregularities. *Toxic reactions* from medications taken by the elderly can possibly result from:

1. Slower metabolism, impaired circulation, and decreased excretion, causing medication to remain in the body longer and build up to dangerous levels.
2. Wrong dosage due to impaired vision or poor memory (patients may forget that they have taken medicine and take a double dose).

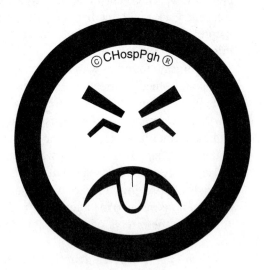

Figure 10.1 Mr. Yuk and similar stickers may be obtained from many Poison Control Centers throughout the United States. The number of the nearest Poison Control Center is frequently printed on these stickers. (Permission to reproduce Mr. Yuk has been granted by Children's Hospital of Pittsburgh.)

3. Interactions when many different medications are taken and over-the-counter medications are self-administered with inadequate medical supervision.
4. Medical conditions affecting absorption.

Many medicines and common household products resemble candy or food. Children may be attracted to the unique shapes and bright colors used in packaging. Impaired vision may contribute to mistakes by adults, especially the elderly. It is important to keep medicines and dangerous chemicals in an area separate from food and medicines. Don't be fooled by look-alikes (Fig. 10.2).

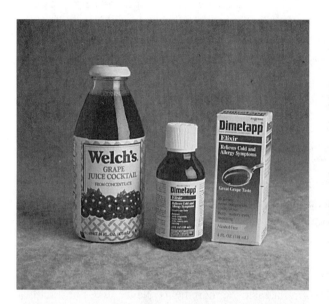
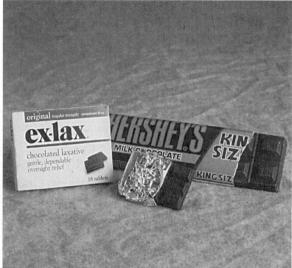
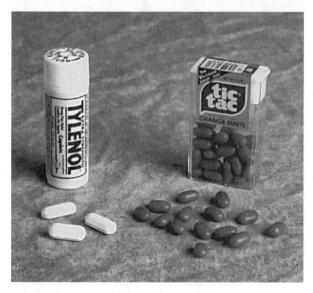
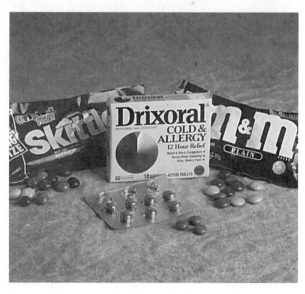

Figure 10.2 Look-alikes: Don't be fooled! Many common household products and medicines resemble candy or food. Keep these products in separate areas. "The compared products are chosen for illustration purposes only. The manufacturers do not intend any misuse of their products." (Permission to reproduce Look-alikes has been granted by the Florida Poison Control Center, Jacksonville, Florida.)

PATIENT EDUCATION CONCERNING POISONS

Public education is of paramount importance in preventing poisoning. The general public must be instructed in precautions with medications, and it is especially important to inform the parents and caretakers of young children and the elderly. It is the responsibility of all health care workers to provide the necessary information to help prevent poisoning.

To prevent poisoning, the American Medical Association recommends the following precautions:

1. Keep all medicines, household chemicals, cleaning supplies, and pesticides in a locked cupboard. There is no place that is "out of reach of children."
2. Never transfer poisonous substances to unlabeled containers or to food containers such as milk or soda bottles or cereal boxes. Keep in original labeled container.
3. Never store poisonous substances in the same area with food. Confusion could be fatal.
4. Never reuse containers of chemical products.
5. When discarding medication, always flush down the toilet. Never discard it in a wastebasket.
6. Do not give or take medications in the dark.
7. Never leave medications on a bedside stand. Confusion while a person is sleepy could result in a fatal overdose.
8. Always read the label before taking any medication or pouring any solution for ingestion.
9. Never tell children the medicine you are giving them is candy.
10. When preparing a baby's formula, taste the ingredients. Never store boric acid, salt, or talcum near the formula ingredients.
11. Never give or take any medication that is discolored, has a strange odor, or is outdated.
12. Don't take medicine in front of children.
13. Keep pocketbooks, purses, and pillboxes out of reach of children.
14. Rinse out containers thoroughly before disposing of them.

If you have small children who live or visit in your home, purchase 1 ounce of ipecac syrup at any pharmacy and keep it for emergency use in poisoning. Check with Poison Control Center before administering.

Obtain the number of your nearest Poison Control Center (Fig. 10.3) and place it on or near your telephone. There are more than 100 Poison Control Centers throughout the United States and Canada with computerized data to give you the latest information about poisons. Remember, *the wrong treatment is often more dangerous than none.* You can obtain the number of the Poison Control Center in your area by calling the nearest emergency care facility, or check the emergency numbers in your phone book. The Poison Control Center is also a good source of information regarding poisonous plants, insects, snakes, and reptiles.

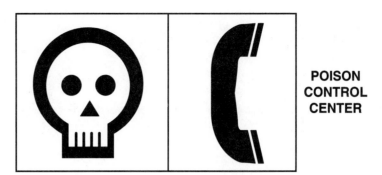

Figure 10.3 Obtain the number of your nearest Poison Control Center and place it near or on your telephone. (Permission to reproduce Poison Control Center logo has been granted by the America Association of Poison Control Centers, Inc., Washington D.C.)

 Check your knowledge of this chapter before going any further.

Chapter Review Quiz

Complete the statements by filling in the blanks:

1. Poisons can be taken into the body in four different ways:

   _____

   _____

   _____

   _____

2. In cases of poison ingestion, emetics are contraindicated under the following five conditions:

   _____

   _____

   _____

   _____

   _____

3. Gastric lavage is contraindicated when a patient has ingested what type of substance?

   _____

4. When is activated charcoal administered?

   _____

5. Why are gastric contents saved after emesis or gastric lavage?

   _____

6. What is the treatment for poisons that contact skin or eyes?

   _____

   _____

7. What two groups of people are most at risk for poisoning?

   _____

   _____

8. Name four conditions that may lead to toxic medication reactions in the elderly.

   _____

   _____

   _____

9. What is the leading cause of poisoning deaths in children under 6 years of age?

_____

_____

Note: A **Comprehensive Review Exam** for Part I can be found at the end of the text on page 493.

Answers to this comprehensive exam are available in the Instructor's Guide.

VISUAL IDENTIFICATION GUIDE

Use this section to quickly verify the identity of a capsule, tablet, or other solid oral medication. More than 200 leading products are shown in actual size and color, organized alphabetically by generic name. Each product is labeled with its brand name, if applicable, as well as its strength and the name of its supplier.

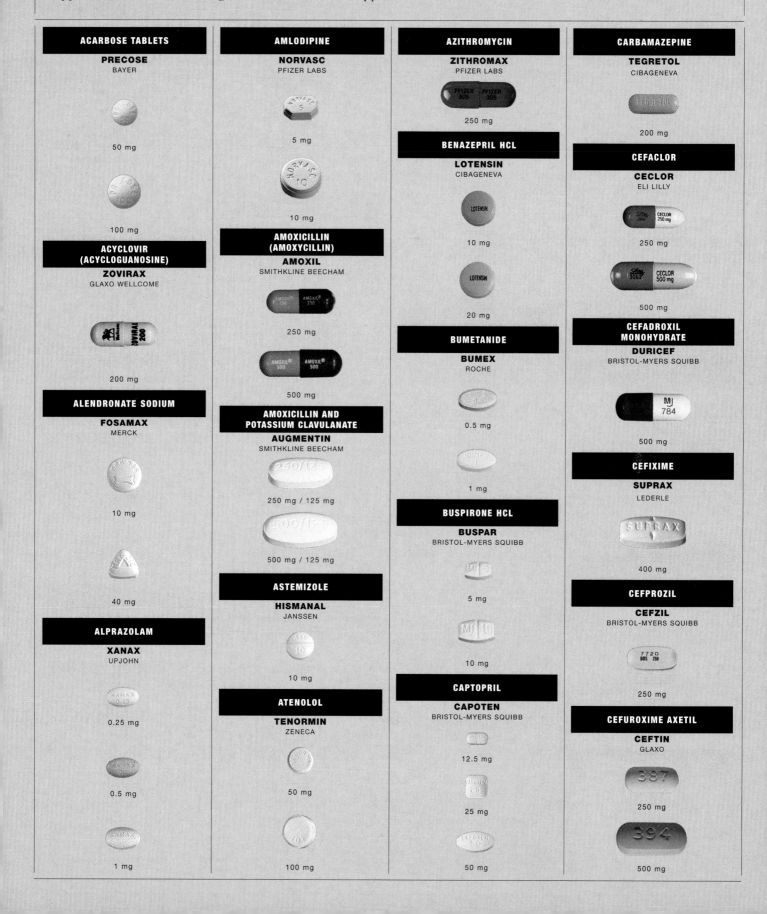

ACARBOSE TABLETS

PRECOSE
BAYER

50 mg

100 mg

ACYCLOVIR (ACYCLOGUANOSINE)

ZOVIRAX
GLAXO WELLCOME

200 mg

ALENDRONATE SODIUM

FOSAMAX
MERCK

10 mg

40 mg

ALPRAZOLAM

XANAX
UPJOHN

0.25 mg

0.5 mg

1 mg

AMLODIPINE

NORVASC
PFIZER LABS

5 mg

10 mg

AMOXICILLIN (AMOXYCILLIN)

AMOXIL
SMITHKLINE BEECHAM

250 mg

500 mg

AMOXICILLIN AND POTASSIUM CLAVULANATE

AUGMENTIN
SMITHKLINE BEECHAM

250 mg / 125 mg

500 mg / 125 mg

ASTEMIZOLE

HISMANAL
JANSSEN

10 mg

ATENOLOL

TENORMIN
ZENECA

50 mg

100 mg

AZITHROMYCIN

ZITHROMAX
PFIZER LABS

250 mg

BENAZEPRIL HCL

LOTENSIN
CIBAGENEVA

10 mg

20 mg

BUMETANIDE

BUMEX
ROCHE

0.5 mg

1 mg

BUSPIRONE HCL

BUSPAR
BRISTOL-MYERS SQUIBB

5 mg

10 mg

CAPTOPRIL

CAPOTEN
BRISTOL-MYERS SQUIBB

12.5 mg

25 mg

50 mg

CARBAMAZEPINE

TEGRETOL
CIBAGENEVA

200 mg

CEFACLOR

CECLOR
ELI LILLY

250 mg

500 mg

CEFADROXIL MONOHYDRATE

DURICEF
BRISTOL-MYERS SQUIBB

500 mg

CEFIXIME

SUPRAX
LEDERLE

400 mg

CEFPROZIL

CEFZIL
BRISTOL-MYERS SQUIBB

250 mg

CEFUROXIME AXETIL

CEFTIN
GLAXO

250 mg

500 mg

CIMETIDINE

TAGAMET
SMITHKLINE BEECHAM

300 mg

400 mg

CIPROFLOXACIN HCL

CIPRO
BAYER

250 mg

500 mg

CLARITHROMYCIN

BIAXIN
ABBOTT

250 mg

500 mg

CLONAZEPAM

KLONOPIN
ROCHE

0.5 mg

1 mg

CYCLOBENZAPRINE HCL

FLEXERIL
MERCK

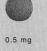

10 mg

DARVOCET-N 100

ACETAMINOPHEN AND PROPOXYPHENE NAPSYLATE
ELI LILLY

650 mg / 100 mg

DIAZEPAM

VALIUM
ROCHE

2 mg

5 mg

10 mg

DICLOFENAC SODIUM

VOLTAREN
CIBAGENEVA

50 mg

75 mg

DICYCLOMINE HCL

BENTYL
HOECHST MARION ROUSSEL

10 mg

20 mg

DIGOXIN

LANOXIN
BURROUGHS WELLCOME

0.125 mg

0.25 mg

DILTIAZEM HCL

CARDIZEM CD
HOECHST MARION ROUSSEL

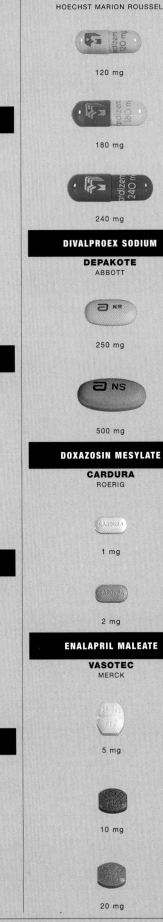

120 mg

180 mg

240 mg

DIVALPROEX SODIUM

DEPAKOTE
ABBOTT

250 mg

500 mg

DOXAZOSIN MESYLATE

CARDURA
ROERIG

1 mg

2 mg

ENALAPRIL MALEATE

VASOTEC
MERCK

5 mg

10 mg

20 mg

ERYTHROMYCIN BASE

ERY-TAB
ABBOTT

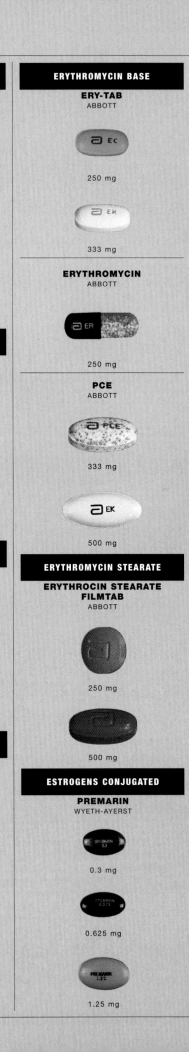

250 mg

333 mg

ERYTHROMYCIN
ABBOTT

250 mg

PCE
ABBOTT

333 mg

500 mg

ERYTHROMYCIN STEARATE

ERYTHROCIN STEARATE FILMTAB
ABBOTT

250 mg

500 mg

ESTROGENS CONJUGATED

PREMARIN
WYETH-AYERST

0.3 mg

0.625 mg

1.25 mg

ESTROPIPATE
(PIPERAZINE ESTRONE SULFATE)
OGEN
UPJOHN

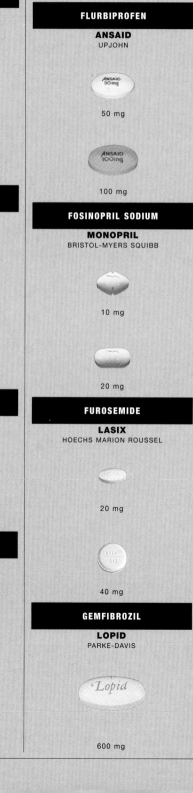

0.625 mg

1.25 mg

ETODOLAC
LODINE
WYETH-AYERST

300 mg

400 mg

FAMOTIDINE
PEPCID
MERCK

20 mg

40 mg

FINASTERIDE
PROSCAR
MERCK

5 mg

FIORINAL
BUTALBITAL AND ASPIRIN
AND CAFFEINE
SANDOZ

50 mg / 325 mg / 40 mg

50 mg / 325 mg / 40 mg

FLUOXETINE HCL
PROZAC
DISTA

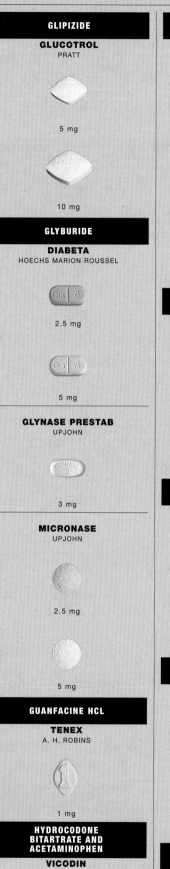

10 mg

20 mg

FLURBIPROFEN
ANSAID
UPJOHN

50 mg

100 mg

FOSINOPRIL SODIUM
MONOPRIL
BRISTOL-MYERS SQUIBB

10 mg

20 mg

FUROSEMIDE
LASIX
HOECHS MARION ROUSSEL

20 mg

40 mg

GEMFIBROZIL
LOPID
PARKE-DAVIS

600 mg

GLIPIZIDE
GLUCOTROL
PRATT

5 mg

10 mg

GLYBURIDE
DIABETA
HOECHS MARION ROUSSEL

2.5 mg

5 mg

GLYNASE PRESTAB
UPJOHN

3 mg

MICRONASE
UPJOHN

2.5 mg

5 mg

GUANFACINE HCL
TENEX
A. H. ROBINS

1 mg

HYDROCODONE
BITARTRATE AND
ACETAMINOPHEN
VICODIN
KNOLL

5 mg / 500 mg

IBUPROFEN
MOTRIN
UPJOHN

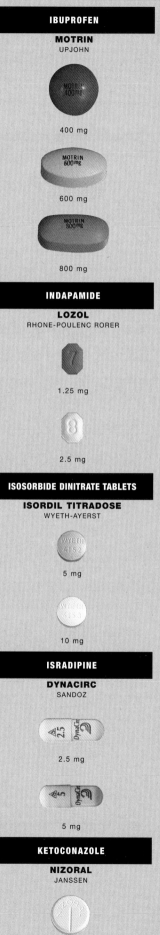

400 mg

600 mg

800 mg

INDAPAMIDE
LOZOL
RHONE-POULENC RORER

1.25 mg

2.5 mg

ISOSORBIDE DINITRATE TABLETS
ISORDIL TITRADOSE
WYETH-AYERST

5 mg

10 mg

ISRADIPINE
DYNACIRC
SANDOZ

2.5 mg

5 mg

KETOCONAZOLE
NIZORAL
JANSSEN

200 mg

KETOROLAC TROMETHAMINE	LORATADINE	METFORMIN HCL	NABUMETONE

KETOROLAC TROMETHAMINE

TORADOL
SYNTEX

10 mg

LEVOTHYROXINE SODIUM

SYNTHROID
KNOLL

0.05 mg

0.1 mg

0.15 mg

LISINOPRIL

PRINIVIL
MERCK

10 mg

20 mg

LISINOPRIL

ZESTRIL
STUART

5 mg

10 mg

20 mg

LORACARBEF

LORABID
ELI LILLY

200 mg

LORATADINE

CLARITIN
SCHERING

10 mg

LORAZEPAM

ATIVAN
WYETH-AYERST

0.5 mg

1 mg

LOSARTAN POTASSIUM

COZAAR
MERCK

25 mg

50 mg

LOVASTATIN (MEVINOLIN)

MEVACOR
MERCK

10 mg

20 mg

MEDROXYPROGESTERONE ACETATE

PROVERA
UPJOHN

2.5 mg

10 mg

METFORMIN HCL

GLUCOPHAGE
BRISTOL-MYERS SQUIBB

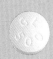

500 mg

850 mg

METHYLPHENIDATE HCL

RITALIN
CIBAGENEVA

5 mg

10 mg

METHYLPREDNISOLONE

MEDROL
UPJOHN

4 mg

METOPROLOL TARTRATE

LOPRESSOR
CIBAGENEVA

50 mg

100 mg

MISOPROSTOL

CYTOTEC
G. D. SEARLE

100 mcg

200 mcg

NABUMETONE

RELAFEN
SMITHKLINE BEECHAM

500 mg

NADOLOL

CORGARD
BRISTOL-MYERS SQUIBB

40 mg

80 mg

NAPROXEN

NAPROSYN
ROCHE

375 mg

500 mg

NAPROXEN SODIUM

ANAPROX
ROCHE

275 mg

ANAPROX DS
ROCHE

550 mg

NEFAZODONE HCL

SERZONE
BRISTOL-MYERS SQUIBB

100 mg

200 mg

NIFEDIPINE

PROCARDIA XL
PRATT

30 mg

60 mg

90 mg

NIZATIDINE

AXID
ELI LILLY

150 mg

NORTRIPTYLINE HCL

PAMELOR
SANDOZ

25 mg

50 mg

OFLOXACIN

FLOXIN
MCNEIL

300 mg

OMEPRAZOLE

PRILOSEC
ASTRA MERCK

20 mg

OXAPROZIN

DAYPRO
G. D. SEARLE

600 mg

OXYCODONE AND ACETAMINOPHEN

PERCOCET
DUPONT

5 mg / 325 mg

PAROXETINE HCL

PAXIL
SMITHKLINE BEECHAM

20 mg

PENICILLIN V POTASSIUM (PHENOXYMETHYL PENICILLIN POTASSIUM)

PEN-VEE K
WYETH-AYERST

250 mg

500 mg

PENTOXIFYLLINE

TRENTAL
HOECHST MARION ROUSSEL

400 mg

PHENYTOIN SODIUM, EXTENDED

DILANTIN KAPSEALS
PARKE-DAVIS

100 mg

POTASSIUM CHLORIDE

K-DUR
KEY

10 mEq

20 mEq

KLOR-CON 10
UPSHER-SMITH

10 mEq

MICRO-K 10 EXTENCAPS
A. H. ROBINS

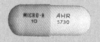

10 mEq

PRAVASTATIN SODIUM

PRAVACHOL
BRISTOL-MYERS SQUIBB

20 mg

PREDNISONE

DELTASONE
UPJOHN

5 mg

10 mg

20 mg

PROPRANOLOL HCL

INDERAL
WYETH-AYERST

10 mg

20 mg

40 mg

INDERAL LA
WYETH-AYERST

80 mg

QUINAPRIL HCL

ACCUPRIL
PARKE-DAVIS

10 mg

20 mg

RAMIPRIL

ALTACE
HOECHST MARION ROUSSEL

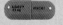

2.5 mg

5 mg

RANITIDINE HCL

ZANTAC
GLAXO

150 mg

300 mg

SERTRALINE HCL

ZOLOFT
ROERIG

50 mg

100 mg

SIMVASTATIN

ZOCOR
MERCK

10 mg

20 mg

SUCRALFATE

CARAFATE
HOECHST MARION ROUSSEL

1 gm

TAMOXIFEN

NOLVADEX
ZENECA

10 mg

TEMAZEPAM

RESTORIL
SANDOZ

15 mg

30 mg

TERAZOSIN

HYTRIN
ABBOTT

2 mg

5 mg

TERFENADINE

SELDANE
HOECHST MARION ROUSSEL

60 mg

TERFENADINE AND PSEUDOEPHEDRINE HCL

SELDANE-D
HOECHST MARION ROUSSEL

60 mg / 120 mg

THEOPHYLLINE

THEO-DUR
KEY

200 mg

300 mg

TRIAMTERENE AND HYDROCHLOROTHIAZIDE TABLETS

MAXZIDE
LEDERLE

37.5 mg/25 mg

75 mg/50 mg

TRIAMTERENE AND HYDROCHLOROTHIAZIDE CAPSULES

DYAZIDE
SMITHKLINE BEECHAM

37.5 mg / 25 mg

TRIAZOLAM

HALCION
UPJOHN

0.125 mg

0.25 mg

TRIMETHOPRIM AND SULFAMETHOXAZOLE

BACTRIM DS
ROCHE

160 mg / 800 mg

TYLENOL WITH CODEINE TABLETS

ACETAMINOPHEN AND CODEINE PHOSPHATE
MCNEIL

300 mg / 30 mg

VERAPAMIL

CALAN SR
G. D. SEARLE

240 mg

WARFARIN SODIUM

COUMADIN
DUPONT PHARMA

2 mg

2.5 mg

5 mg

PART II

Drug Classifications

CHAPTER 11

Vitamins and Minerals

OBJECTIVES

Upon completion of this chapter, the student should be able to:

1. Categorize vitamins as water soluble or fat soluble.
2. List vitamins and their sources, function, signs of deficiency, and symptoms of overdose if known.
3. Identify vitamins by name as well as letter.
4. List minerals and their sources, function, and signs of deficiency.
5. Identify the chemical symbol for each mineral.
6. Describe conditions that may require vitamin and/or mineral supplements.
7. Explain the role of antioxidants in nutrition therapy.

The National Academy of Sciences and the National Research Council of the Food and Nutrition Board have listed U.S. Recommended Dietary Allowances (U.S. RDA) of vitamins and minerals necessary for maintenance of good nutrition in the average healthy adult under normal living conditions in the United States. This information was published by the National Academy of Sciences, Washington, D.C., in 1980 and revised in 1989.

Under special circumstances, vitamin and mineral supplements are required for optimal function and health. *Indications for vitamin and mineral supplements include:*

Inadequate diet. Due to anorexia, weight reduction or other special diets, illness, alcoholism, or poor eating habits.

Malabsorption syndromes. Chronic gastrointestinal disorders or surgery that result in chronic diarrhea.

Increased need for certain nutrients. As in pregnancy and lactation (especially iron and calcium), infants under 1 year of age, adolescence, debilitation, illness, unusual physical activity, postmenopausal women (calcium).

Deficiency due to medication interactions. For example, potassium deficiency with diuretic use.

Nutrients function in groups or teams. Therefore, if diet supplementation is warranted, it is likely that both vitamins and some additional minerals are needed. An example of this teamwork is bone growth, development, and strength, which depends on calcium, magnesium, vitamin A, vitamin D, and several other nutrients (fluoride, etc.) However, patients should be advised to avoid self-medication with large doses of vitamins or minerals, which may not be indicated if the diet is well balanced and the individual is in good health. Overdoses of some vitamins, especially A and D, and some minerals, for example, iron, can be injurious to health. A need or deficiency should be established by a physician's diagnosis or blood test before exceeding Recommended Dietary Allowances (RDA). Supplementary (prophylactic) multivitamin preparations may reasonably contain 50–150% of the RDA of vitamins (except the amount of vitamins A and D and folic acid should not exceed the RDA). Combination vitamin preparations containing iron should not be used unless a deficiency has been established with a blood test or physician's diagnosis.

It is important to differentiate between water-soluble and fat-soluble vitamins in order to avoid build-up in the body with possible symptoms of overdose. Megadoses of vitamins (more than the RDA) should be taken only if prescribed by a physician and/or approved by the FDA. *Remember, the RDA includes the amount from foods you eat as well as supplements.* Research reports have indicated a possibility of damage to tissues with large quantities of vitamins (above RDA), especially those stored in the fat cells of the body.

The Recommended Dietary Allowances listed on the following pages are established for average, normal, healthy adults. Larger amounts are required with certain conditions (e.g., *pregnancy, lactation, and some illnesses*). Larger amounts are required for males than females. The RDAs on the following pages show the amount required for females first, with the amount for males afterward. Smaller amounts are required for children (consult references). However, megadoses should *never* be taken except under the direct supervision of a physician.

Fat-Soluble Vitamins

The fat-soluble vitamins are A, D, E, and K.

VITAMIN A (RETINOL, RETINAL, BETA CAROTENE)

Vitamin A is processed in the body from the carotene of plants, especially yellow-orange and dark-green leafy vegetables, fruits, oily saltwater fish, dairy products, and eggs (RDA 800–1,000 U/day). Beta carotene is an antioxidant. (See Antioxidants later in this chapter.)

Necessary for:

Resistance to infection
Proper visual function at night.

Normal growth and development of bones and soft tissue, and maintaining healthy epithelial tissue

Healing of wounds (sometimes prescribed for acne)

Possible connection to reproduction

Deficiencies may result from:

Malabsorption of fats or diarrhea

Obstruction of bile

Presence of mineral oil in the intestines

Overcooking of vegetables in an open container (heat and air cause oxidation)

Prolonged infection or fever

Signs of deficiency include:

Night blindness

Slow growth, anorexia, weight loss, bone and teeth deformities

Dry eyes and skin, pruritus, and photosensitivity

Impaired healing

Supplements of vitamin A (e.g., Aquasol A) may be necessary for:

Infants fed unfortified skim milk or mild-substitute formulas

Those with prolonged infection or fever

Diabetes or hypothyroidism

Liver disease

Vitamin A has been used as a screening test for fat absorption

Some dermatologic disorders, for example, psoriasis, are being treated investigationally with retinoids (synthetic vitamin A products). A retinoid product, Accutane, is prescribed for severe acne. This product can cause fetal abnormalities and is therefore contraindicated in pregnancy. Accutane has also caused increased intracranial pressure and other adverse side effects associated with hypervitaminosis A.

Symptoms of overdose (hypervitaminosis A) include:

Irritability and psychiatric symptoms

Fatigue and lethargy

Headache, insomnia, and myalgia

Brittle nails, dry skin with peeling, pruritus, hair loss, cracked lips

Anorexia, nausea, diarrhea, vomiting, abdominal discomfort

Yellow or orange skin pigmentation, jaundice, liver abnormalities

Acute toxicity with increased intracranial pressure, vertigo, coma

Joint pain, bone deformities, stunted growth

Caution should be used with kidney or liver problems or diabetes.

Long-term use of large doses of vitamin A is contraindicated for women who are, or may become, pregnant. Fetal malformations have been reported following maternal ingestion of large doses of vitamin A, either before or during pregnancy.

VITAMIN D (CALCIFEROL, CHOLECALCIFEROL, ERGOCALCIFEROL)

Vitamin D is synthesized in the body through the action of sunlight on the skin. Other sources include fish oils and food products fortified with vitamin D, such as milk and cereals (RDA 400 u/day).

Necessary for:

Maintenance of normal nerves and muscles

Regulating the absorption and metabolism of calcium and phosphorus for healthy bones and teeth

Pregnancy and lactation, when it is especially important

Signs of deficiency include:

Poor tooth and bone structure (rickets)

Skeletal deformities

Osteoporosis, osteomalacia

Tetany

Vitamin D supplements are prescribed as calcifediol, calcitriol, or ergocalciferol to prevent or treat rickets or osteomalacia and to manage hypocalcemia in cases of parathyroid malfunction. The difference between therapeutic dosage and that causing hypercalcemia is very small and dosage must be carefully regulated and monitored.

Symptoms of vitamin D overdose and toxicity include:

GI distress, weakness, headache

Cardiac arrhythmias

Vertigo, tinnitus

Muscle and/or bone pain

Kidney damage and kidney stone

Hypercalcemia and convulsions, calcium deposits in soft tissues

Fetal disorders

Caution not to exceed the RDA of vitamin D especially with:

Cardiovascular disorders

Kidney diseases

Pregnancy (possible fetal malformations or mental retardation)

Lactation

Interactions (overdose may antagonize) with:

Digitalis

Thiazide diuretics

Mineral oil may interfere with intestinal absorption of vitamin D

VITAMIN E (TOCOPHEROL)

Vitamin E is abundant in nature, found especially in cereals, wheat germ, seeds, nuts, vegetable oils, eggs, meat, and poultry (RDA 12–15 U/day). The main function of vitamin E is as an antioxidant (see Antioxidants later in this chapter).

Necessary for:

Normal metabolism
Protection of tissues of the eyes, skin, liver, breast, and muscles
Regulating use and storage of vitamin A
Protecting red blood cells (RBCs) from damage
Decreasing platelet clumping

Deficiencies are found in those with:

Alcohol abuse
Malabsorption syndromes, for example, celiac disease, sprue, cystic fibrosis
Pathologic conditions of liver and pancreas
Sickle-cell anemia
Also found in premature infants or low-birth weight neonates

Signs of deficiency are not firmly established. Premature infants may show irritability, edema, or anemia. Deficient adults may show muscle weakness and some abnormal lab values.

Symptoms of overdose are not clinically proven. However, since vitamin E is fat soluble, the potential for overdose exists, and caution is urged with megadoses of this and other fat-soluble vitamins.

Interactions: Excessive use of mineral oil may decrease the absorption of vitamin E.

VITAMIN K (PHYTONADIONE)

Vitamin K is found in green or leafy vegetables, vegetable oils, milk, eggs, and tomatoes, and is absorbed in the small intestine in the presence of bile salts (RDA 60–80 µg/day)

Necessary for blood clotting.

Deficiencies may result from reduced prothrombin in the blood due to:

Insufficient clotting factors in the newborn
Malabsorption syndromes, ulcerative colitis, prolonged diarrhea
Coumarin overdose
Prolonged use of salicylates, quinine, and some antibiotics

Signs of deficiency include:

Increased clotting time
Petechiae and bruising
Blood in the urine (hematuria)
Blood in the stool (melena)

Vitamin K is usually prescribed as phytonadione (Mephyton tabs or Aqua-mephyton IM or SC). Vitamin K is only effective for bleeding disorders due to low concentrations of prothrombin in the blood. It is not effective for bleeding from other causes such as heparin overdose. The American Academy of Pediatrics recommends that vitamin K (phytonadione) be routinely administered to infants at birth to prevent hemorrhagic disease of the newborn. Some state regulations currently require this prophylaxis.

Adverse effects are rare but hypersensitivity reactions have occurred with IV injections. Toxicity in infants can cause jaundice and possible brain degeneration.

Water-Soluble Vitamins

The *water-soluble vitamins* include the B-complex vitamins and vitamin C.

VITAMIN B₁ (THIAMINE)

Vitamin B₁ is a coenzyme utilized for carbohydrate, protein and fat metabolism. It is found in whole grains, wheat germ, peas, beans, nuts, yeast, meat, especially pork and organ meats, oysters, collard greens, oranges, and enriched cereals (RDA 1–1.5 mg/day).

Necessary for normal function of the nervous and cardiovascular systems.

Deficiencies in the United States may be due to:

Chronic alcoholism
Malabsorption

Signs of deficiency (beriberi; symptoms sometimes vague) include:

Anorexia and constipation, GI upset, nausea, emaciation
Neuritis, pain, tingling in extremities, loss of reflexes
Muscle weakness, fatigue, ataxia
Mental depression, memory loss, confusion
Hypersensitivity reactions have occurred mainly following repeated IV administration of the drug

VITAMIN B$_2$ (RIBOFLAVIN)

Vitamin B$_2$ is a coenzyme utilized in the metabolism of all cells. It is found in milk, eggs, nuts, meats, especially liver, yeast, enriched bread, and green leafy vegetables (RDA, 1.3–1.8 mg/day).

Necessary for cell growth and metabolism with release of energy from carbohydrates, protein, and fat in food. Also functions to regulate certain hormones and in formation of RBCs.

Deficiencies of vitamin B$_2$ in the United States may be due to:

Chronic alcoholism
Poor diet
Medications such as probenecid

Signs of deficiency include:

Glossitis (inflammation of the tongue)
Cheilosis (cracking at corners of mouth)
Dermatitis, photophobia, vision loss, burning or itching eyes

VITAMIN B$_6$ (PYRIDOXINE)

Vitamin B$_6$ is a coenzyme utilized in the metabolism of carbohydrates, fats, protein, and amino acids. It is found in meats, eggs, potatoes, legumes, peanuts, soybeans, wheat germ, yeast, and whole-grain cereals (RDA 1.6–2 mg/day). There is significant loss of B$_6$ when foods are frozen.

Deficiencies may be due to:

Chronic alcoholism
Drug interactions with isoniazid, other antitubercular drugs, oral contraceptives
Cirrhosis
Malabsorption syndromes

Signs of deficiency include:

In infants, seizure activity
In adults, peripheral neuropathy, oral sores, dermatitis, nausea, vomiting, and depression

Caution: Overdose in pregnant woman may result in newborns with seizures who have developed a need for greater than normal amounts of pyridoxine.

PATIENT EDUCATION

Patients taking levodopa alone (not combined with carbidopa) should be instructed not to take vitamin B6 supplement because it antagonizes the action of levodopa.

VITAMIN B$_{12}$ (COBALAMIN, CYANOCOBALAMIN)

Vitamin B$_{12}$ is found in meats (especially organ meats) and poultry, fish, and shell-fish, milk, cheese, and eggs. Absorption of vitamin B$_{12}$ depends on an intrinsic factor normally present in the gastric juice of humans. Absence of this factor leads to vitamin B$_{12}$ deficiency and pernicious anemia (RDA 2 μg/day).

Necessary for maturation of red blood cells and maintenance of the nervous system.

Deficiencies can be associated with:

Vegetarian diets
Gastrectomy or intestinal resections
Malabsorption syndromes
Pernicious anemia, megaloblastic (macrocytic) anemia

Signs of deficiency include:

Anemia and weakness first symptoms of clinical deficiency
Poor muscle coordination
Numbness of hands and feet
Mental confusion and irritability

Treatment for pernicious anemia consists of vitamin B$_{12}$, cyanocobalamin (Betalin 12 or Rubramin), 100–1,000 μg IM monthly for life to prevent neurologic damage.

Side effects include:

Transient diarrhea
Itching and urticaria
Anaphylaxis (rare)

Interactions may occur (decreased absorption of B$_{12}$) with:

Aminoglycoside antibiotics
Anticonvulsants
Slow-release potassium and colchicine

> **PATIENT EDUCATION**
>
> Patients should avoid taking large doses of vitamin B_{12} without confirmed deficiency, as megadoses may mask symptoms of folic acid deficiency or cause complications in those with cardiac or gout conditions.

FOLIC ACID (FOLACIN)

Folic acid is a vitamin included in the B-complex group and is found in leafy and green vegetables (broccoli), avocado, beets, orange juice, yeast, and organ meats (RDA 400 μg/day). Folic acid is lost with overcooking and reheating.

Necessary for protein synthesis, production of red blood cells, cell division, and normal growth and maintenance of all cells.

Deficiencies can be associated with:

Improper diet
Chronic alcoholism
Liver pathology
Intestinal obstruction
Megaloblastic and macrocytic anemia
Malabsorption syndromes, malnutrition
Renal dialysis or prolonged use of some medicines (listed below)

Signs of deficiency include:

Diarrhea, anorexia, weight loss, weakness
Sore mouth
Irritability, behavior disorders

Caution: Folic acid (Folvite) *should not be given to anyone with undiagnosed anemia*, since it may mask the diagnosis of pernicious anemia.

Interactions may occur with:

Phenytoin (Dilantin)
Estrogen (oral contraceptives)
Barbiturates, or nitrofurantoin

When these drugs are used, folic acid supplements may be required.

> **PATIENT EDUCATION**
>
> Patient should avoid taking folic acid supplements without consulting a physician first.

NIACIN (NICOTINIC ACID, NIACINAMIDE)

Niacin is a vitamin included in the B-complex group and is found in meat, chicken, milk, eggs, fish, green vegetables, cooked dried beans and peas, soybeans, nuts, peanut butter, and yeast (RDA 15–19 mg/day).

Necessary for lipid metabolism and nerve functioning, especially in circulation and maintenance of all cells.

Deficiency results in pellagra.

Signs of niacin deficiency include:

Peripheral vascular insufficiency
Dermatitis and varicose ulcers
Diarrhea
Dementia (mental problems)
Mouth sores
Lethargy, weakness, anorexia, indigestion

Niacin is used primarily to prevent and treat pellagra. Other treatment indications (usually as an adjunct with other medications) include:

Many vascular disorders (e.g., vascular spasm, arteriosclerosis, Raynaud's disease, angina, and varicose and decubital ulcers)
Circulatory disturbances of the inner ear, Meniere's syndrome
To lower blood lipid levels (see Chapter 25)
Daily doses of up to 1,000 mg appear to be safe.

Side effects of niacin, especially over 1,000 mg daily, can include:

Postural hypotension
Jaundice
Nausea, diarrhea, vomiting
Increased blood sugar and uric acid
Headache, flushing, and burning sensations of face, neck, and chest

Caution for patients with liver disease, gallbladder disease, gout, or diabetes.

PATIENT EDUCATION

Patients taking niacin should be instructed regarding possible side effects, especially flushing and a burning sensation, and should be cautioned to rise slowly from a reclining position. They should be told that the flushing usually resolves within 2 weeks. Taking niacin in divided doses, or extended-release products, can sometimes lessen this effect.

VITAMIN C (ASCORBIC ACID)

Vitamin C is a water-soluble vitamin found in fresh fruits and vegetables, especially citrus fruits, cantaloupe, tomatoes, cabbage, green peppers, and broccoli. It is unstable when exposed to heat or air or combined with alkaline compounds (e.g., antacids). Adding baking soda to vegetables for color retention destroys vitamin C. (RDA 60 mg/day).

Necessary for cellular metabolism and intracellular substances (collagen), and for normal teeth, gums, and bones. Also required for iron absorption. Vitamin C is considered an antioxidant. (See Antioxidants later in this chapter). Also promotes healing of wounds and bone fractures.

Deficiencies are associated with:

Pregnancy and lactation
Diet lacking fresh fruit and vegetables
Alcoholism, infections, trauma, and stress
GI disease
Smoking

Signs of vitamin C deficiency (scurvy) include:

Muscle weakness, and cramping, lethargy, anorexia, depression
Sore and bleeding mouth and gums
Capillary fragility (petechiae or bruising), dry, scaly skin
Degenerative changes in bone and connective tissue
Poor healing

Supplements of ascorbic acid are available in capsule, tablets (extended-release), or solution, chewables, or injection form. They are indicated for:

Treatment of scurvy (adults 100–250 mg BID, children 100–300 mg/day divided doses)
Hemodialysis patients (100–200 mg daily)
Infants beginning at 2–4 weeks of age (20–50 mg/day)
Prevention or treatment of the common cold (1–2 grams/day)

Dosages larger than that recommended are to be avoided because of the potential for side effects. In addition, since ascorbic acid is water soluble, more than 50% of the dose is excreted in the urine of normal subjects. Excretion of less than 20% of the dose over 24 hours suggests vitamin C deficiency.

Side effects of large doses of vitamin C, more than RDA, can include:

Heartburn, abdominal cramps, nausea, vomiting, and diarrhea
Increased uric acid levels, may precipitate gouty arthritis
Increased urinary calcium, may precipitate kidney stone formation
Scurvy in neonates following large amounts during pregnancy

Interactions may occur with:

Aspirin, causing elevated blood levels of aspirin
Barbiturates, tetracyclines, estrogens, oral contraceptives, which may increase requirements for vitamin C
Alcohol and smoking, which may decrease vitamin C level

PATIENT EDUCATION

Patients should be given the following information concerning vitamin C:

Vitamin C is destroyed by heat and air; therefore, raw fresh fruits and vegetables are best.
Large quantities of supplemental vitamin C are to be avoided, unless prescribed by a doctor, because of potential side effects, such as gastric irritation, increased uric acid, and urinary calcium.
Antacids should not be taken at the same time as vitamin C supplements because the alkaline compound neutralizes the ascorbic acid.
Megadoses of vitamin C taken during pregnancy may cause the newborn to require larger than average amounts of ascorbic acid.

See Table 11.1 for a summary of water- and fat-soluble vitamins.

TABLE 11.1. SUMMARY OF WATER- AND FAT-SOLUBLE VITAMINS

Name	Food Sources	Functions	Deficiency/Toxicity

Vitamin A (retinol, beta carotene)	Animal
	  Oily saltwater fish
	  Whole milk
	  Butter
	  Cream
	  Cod liver oil
	Plants
	  Dark green leafy vegetables
	  Deep yellow or orange fruit
	  Fortified margarine
		Dim light vision
		Maintenance of mucous membranes
		Growth and development of bones
		Healing of wounds
		Resistance to infection
		Beta carotene is an antioxidant
			Deficiency
			  Night blindness
			  Xerophthalmia
			  Bone growth ceases
			Toxicity
			  Irritability, lethargy
			  Joint pain, myalgia, headache
			  Stunted growth, fetal malformations
			  Jaundice, nausea, diarrhea
			  Dry skin and hair

Vitamin D (Cholecalciferol)	Animal
	  Fish oils
	  Salmon, herring, mackerel, sardines
	  Fortified milk
	Plants
	  Fortified cereals
		Healthy bones and teeth
		Muscle function
			Deficiency
			  Rickets
			  Osteomalacia
			  Poorly developed teeth
			  Muscle spasms
			Toxicity–(Hypercalcemia)
			  Kidney stones, kidney damage
			  Muscle/bone pain
			  GI distress

Vitamin E (tocopherol)	Animal
	  Meat, poultry, eggs
	Plant
	  Vegetable oils
	  Seeds, nuts
		Antioxidant	Deficiency
			  Destruction of RBCs, muscle weakness
			Toxicity
			  Prolonged bleeding time

Vitamin K (phytonadione)	Animal
	  Egg yolk
	  Milk
	Plant
	  Vegetable oil
	  Green leafy vegetables
	  Cabbage, broccoli
		Blood clotting	Deficiency
			  Prolonged blood clotting time
			Toxicity
			  Jaundice in infants

Vitamin B$_1$ (Thiamine)	Animal
	  Pork, beef, liver
	  Oysters
	  Eggs
	  Fish
	Plants
	  Yeast
	  Whole and enriched grains, wheat germ
	  Legumes, collard greens, nuts
		Coenzyme carbohydrate metabolism
		Normal nervous and cardiovascular systems
			Deficiency
			  GI upset
			  Neuritis, mental disturbance
			  Cardiovascular problems
			  Muscle weakness, fatigue
			Toxicity
			  None

(Continued)

TABLE 11.1. (Continued)

Name	Food Sources	Functions	Deficiency/Toxicity

Vitamin B_2 (Riboflavin)	Animal
	  Milk
	  Meat, liver
	Plants
	  Green vegetables
	  Cereals
	  Enriched bread
	  Yeast
		Aids release of energy from food	Deficiency
			  Cheilosis
			  Glossitis
			  Photophobia, vision problems
			  Dermatitis
			Toxicity
			  None

Vitamin B_6 (Pyridoxine)	Animal
	  Pork
	  Eggs
	Plants
	  Whole grain cereals, wheat germ
	  Legumes, peanuts, soybeans
	  Potatoes
		Synthesis of amino acids
		Antibody production
			Deficiency
			  Cheilosis, glossitis, dermatitis
			  Neuritis, depression
			Toxicity
			  Seizures in newborn

Vitamin B_{12} (cyanocobalamin)	Animal
	  Seafood/shellfish
	  Meat, poultry, liver
	  Eggs
	  Milk, cheese
	Plants
	  None
		Synthesis of RBCs
		Maintenance of nervous system
			Deficiency
			  Nerve, muscle, mental problems
			  Pernicious anemia
			Toxicity
			  None

Niacin (nicotinic acid)	Animal
	  Milk
	  Eggs
	  Fish
	  Poultry
	Plants:
	  Legumes, nuts
		Lipid metabolism
		Nerve functioning
			Deficiency
			  Pellagra
			Toxicity
			  Vasodilation of blood vessels

Folacin (folic acid)	Animal
	  Organ meats
	Plants
	  Green leafy vegetables
	  Avocado, beets
	  Broccoli
	  Orange juice
		Synthesis of RBCs	Deficiency
			  Glossitis
			  Macrocytic anemia
			  Irritability, behavior disorders
			Toxicity
			  None

Vitamin C (ascorbic acid)	Fruits
	  All citrus
	Plants
	  Broccoli
	  Tomatoes
	  Brussel sprouts
	  Cabbage
	  Green peppers
		Prevention of scurvy
		Formation of collagen
		Healing of wounds
		Absorption of iron
		Antioxidant
			Deficiency
			  Scurvy
			  Poor healing
			  Muscle cramps/weakness
			  Ulcerated gums/mouth
			  Capillary fragility
			Toxicity
			  Raise uric acid level
			  GI distress
			  Kidney stones
			  Rebound scurvy in neonates

Minerals

Minerals are chemical elements occurring in nature and in body fluids. The correct balance of each is required for maintenance of health. Minerals dissolved in the body fluids are called *electrolytes* because they carry positive or negative electrical charges required for body activities, such as conduction of nerve impulses, beating of the heart, skeletal muscle contraction, absorption of nutrients from the gastrointestinal tract, protein synthesis, energy production, blood formation and many other body processes.

Necessary for homeostasis (body balance), the correct ratio of fluids to electrolytes must be maintained for normal functioning of the body. Fluids and minerals are excreted daily and must be replaced with fluid and food intake.

The principal minerals in the body and their chemical symbols are sodium (Na), chloride (Cl), potassium (K), calcium (Ca), and iron (Fe).

SODIUM AND CHLORIDE

Sodium and chloride are the principal minerals in the intracellular body fluids. Blood contains approximately 0.9% sodium chloride. The best source of sodium and chloride is table salt (NaCl).

Deficiencies of sodium and chloride are associated with:

Excessive fluid loss: bleeding, diarrhea, vomiting, or excessive perspiration
Insufficient oral intake (starvation or extended fasting)
Alkalosis (chloride deficiency)

Treatment consists of intravenous therapy with sodium chloride (NaCl) according to needs:

Normal saline solution (0.9% sodium chloride)
Half-normal saline solution (0.45% sodium chloride)
Quarter-normal saline solution (0.2% sodium chloride)

Sometimes other minerals are required and are also added to the intravenous fluids.

POTASSIUM (K)

Potassium is another of the principal minerals within cells. Natural sources of potassium include citrus, bananas, tomatoes, potato skin, cantaloupe, avocadoes, apricots, dried and fresh fruits, cooked dried beans, and peas.

Necessary for:

Acid-base and fluid balance
Normal muscular irritability (heartbeat regulation)

Deficiencies are associated with:

Insufficient oral intake due to surgery, anorexia, or weight-reduction diets

Diarrhea or vomiting

Diabetic ketoacidosis

Diaphoresis (excessive perspiration)

Diuretic use, especially thiazides and furosemide

Digitalis toxicity

Long-term use of corticosteroids or long-term use of laxatives

Kidney disease

Signs of deficiency include:

Muscular weakness, paralysis

Cardiac arrhythmias

Lethargy and fatigue, mental apathy and confusion

Treatment consists of:

IV KCL given postoperatively or for severe dehydration (diluted according to directions)

One of the numerous oral products available, usually in effervescent tablet or powder form to be dissolved in water or juice and taken after meals (e.g., K-Lyte 50–100 mEq qd), or capsules to be swallowed (e.g., Micro-K), extended-release tablets (e.g. K-Dur, or Slow-K), or oral liquid preparations (e.g., Kaochlor)

Side effects can include:

Nausea, vomiting, or diarrhea

GI bleeding, or abdominal pain

Pain at the injection site or phlebitis may occur during IV administration of solutions containing 30 mEq or more potassium per liter. IV solutions containing potassium should always be run at a slow rate to prevent pain or hyperkalemia.

Hyperkalemia (excessive potassium in the blood) is not likely to result from oral administration, except in the case of severe renal impairment. Care must be taken when adding potassium to IV solutions that the dilute solution is thoroughly mixed, inverted and agitated, before the solution is hung for administration. Never add potassium to hanging IV solution.

Symptoms of potassium overdosage can include:

Listlessness

Confusion

Weakness or paralysis of extremities

Fall in the blood pressure and/or cardiac arrhythmias with possible heart block.

Cautions with use of potassium in the following conditions:

Cardiac disease

Renal impairment

Gastric or intestinal ulcers (extended-release products contraindicated)

Mental confusion (unable to follow directions properly)

PATIENT EDUCATION

Patients taking potassium should be instructed regarding:

Natural sources of potassium-rich foods.

Conditions requiring potassium supplements.

Directions for taking potassium supplements with or after meals to avoid GI distress and following directions on package carefully.

The importance of *dissolving* the tablet in at least 4 to 8 oz of water *completely* before taking it and *never* holding the tablet in the mouth or swallowing the tablet whole.

Notifying a doctor immediately of any side effects.

CALCIUM (CA)

Calcium is a mineral component of bones and teeth. It is absorbed in the small intestine with the help of vitamin D. Natural sources include milk and dairy products (RDA 1,000–1,200 mg/day). In postmenopausal women not receiving estrogen therapy, the RDA is about 1,500 mg/day. Those who are lactose intolerant (unable to take milk) should include dark green leafy vegetables, broccoli, canned fish with the bones, and dried peas and beans.

Necessary for:

Strong bones and teeth

Contraction of cardiac, smooth, and skeletal muscles

Nerve conduction

Blood coagulation, capillary permeability, and normal blood pressure

Renal function

The balance between calcium and magnesium is important in the prevention of heart disease

Deficiencies (supplements required) are associated with:

Pregnancy and lactation

Postmenopausal women (or those with estrogen deficiency)

Hypoparathyroidism

Long-term use of corticosteroids, some diuretics or anticonvulsants

Chronic diarrhea, pancreatitis, renal failure

Signs of deficiency may include:

Osteoporosis, or osteomalacia, including frequent fractures, especially in the elderly

Rickets in children

Muscle pathology, including cardiac myopathy or tetany and leg cramps

Increased clotting time

Treatment consists of calcium supplements 400–600 mg daily PO (e.g., Os-Cal or Tums E-X). Many products and combinations are available including calcium gluconate, calcium carbonate, or calcium lactate. Of these three, calcium carbonate delivers the highest amount of elemental calcium per tablet.

Adding vitamin D for calcium metabolism may be necessary without exposure to sunlight (See Vitamin D).

Side effects of calcium salts can include:

Constipation from oral products

Tissue irritation from IV products

When injected IV, calcium salts should be administered *very slowly* to prevent tissue necrosis or cardiac arrhythmias

Caution: Calcium should be used cautiously, if at all, with:

Cardiac disease

Renal disease

Respiratory conditions (e.g., sarcoidosis)

Administration. Most oral calcium supplements should be administered 1–1.5 hours after meals, unless specified otherwise on the label.

Interactions may occur with

Digitalis, resulting in potentiation (may cause arrhythmias)

Tetracycline, resulting in antagonism (inactivates the antibiotic)

PATIENT EDUCATION

Patients taking calcium should be instructed regarding:

Calcium-rich diet, especially dairy products and vitamin D-fortified milk, which can be low-fat.

Necessity for calcium supplements, usually recommended for women beginning at age 35, and especially for postmenopausal women not on estrogen therapy.

Importance of upright exercise, for example, walking at least 3–4 times per week to preserve bone mass.

Importance of outdoor activity because sunlight helps create vitamin D necessary for calcium metabolism.

Taking calcium supplements 1–1½ hours after meals, unless specified otherwise on the label.

Not taking calcium at the same time as other medicines.

IRON (FE)

Iron is the oxygen-carrying component of blood. Iron is a mineral found in meat (especially liver), egg yolk, beans, spinach, enriched cereals, dried fruits, prune juice, fish, poultry, and oysters.

Necessary for hemoglobin formation. Iron also strengthens the immune system, increasing resistance to infection.

Deficiencies (supplements recommended) with:

Hemorrhage and excessive menstrual flow
Internal bleeding, ulcers, and GI tumors
Pregnancy
Infancy
Puberty at time of growth spurt
Patients undergoing hemodialysis

Signs of deficiency may include:

Paleness of the skin and/or mucous membranes
Lethargy and weakness
Vertigo
Air hunger
Decline in mental skills
Irregular heartbeat and function
Cravings for nonfood items, for example, ice, clay, or starch (called pica)

Treatment of anemia due to iron deficiency consists of administration of iron preparations:

Oral iron products. Ferrous sulfate (Feosol, Fer-in-Sol, and others). Adults, 50–100 mg tid after meals (not with milk, coffee, or tea) infants and children, 4–6 mg/kg daily in 3 divided doses in juice or with meals (not with milk).

Injectable iron. Iron dextran (INFeD) 50–100 mg *deep* IM by the *Z-track method only.* Extreme caution is urged to prevent solution contacting the subcutaneous tissue because of its irritating effect. A fresh 2-inch needle is recommended at the time of administration. Iron dextran also can be given IV *slowly* after testing for sensitivity with a small trial dose.

Side effects of taking iron preparations can include:

Black stools
Nausea and vomiting (GI effects can be minimized by taking iron after or with meals)
Constipation or diarrhea
Anaphylactic reactions or phlebitis with IV administration of iron dextran

Contraindicated in patients with peptic ulcer, regional enteritis, or ulcerative colitis.

Parenteral iron should *not* be administered concomitantly with oral iron therapy.

Iron should *not* be administered without confirming a diagnosis of deficiency with a blood test and determining cause of deficiency.

Interactions may occur with:

Vitamin C or orange juice, taken at same time, which enhances iron absorption

Coffee or tea taken within 2 hours of iron, which reduces iron absorption by as much as 50%

Tetracycline, absorption of which is inhibited by oral iron preparations when taken within 2 hours

Antacids, which decrease iron absorption (should not be given at same time)

Symptoms of acute overdose of iron may occur within minutes or days and include:

Lethargy

Shock

Vomiting and diarrhea

Erosion of GI tract/hemochromatosis

PATIENT EDUCATION

Patients taking iron supplements should be instructed regarding:

Avoidance of self-medication without established need (blood test) and without medical supervision to determine why hemoglobin is low. Taking iron when not prescribed could mask the symptoms of internal bleeding or GI malignancy.

Black stools to be expected.

Taking iron at meals to minimize GI distress and with orange juice for better absorption.

Interactions (i.e., avoidance of coffee, tea, milk, or antacids at same time).

Caution with flavored children's tablets (overdosage can be dangerous).

Taking liquid iron preparations with drinking straw to avoid temporary stain of dental enamel.

The iron in meats is called heme iron and is better absorbed than nonheme iron in vegetables and fruits.

Nonheme iron is absorbed better if consumed with a rich source of vitamin C.

ZINC

Zinc is a component of numerous enzymes and is an essential element in metabolism. It is usually found in adequate amounts in a well-balanced diet. Rich sources include lean meat, organ meats, oysters, poultry, fish, and whole grain breads and cereals.

Necessary for:

Wound healing

Mineralization of bone

Digestion of protein

Insulin glucose regulation

Normal taste

Detoxification of alcohol in the liver

Deficiencies (supplements recommended) with:

Inadequate diet

Chronic, nonhealing wounds

Major surgery or trauma

Deficiency symptoms can include:

Poor wound healing

Reduced taste perception

Poor alcohol tolerance, glucose intolerance

Anemia, slowed growth, sterility

Dermatitis and hair loss

Toxicity (more than 2 grams/day) may cause:

Nausea, GI distress, vomiting

Interference with normal functioning of immune system

Treatment consists of 200–220 mg tablets or capsules administered with meals tid to minimize gastric distress.

Many combinations of various vitamins and minerals are available in over-the-counter products with various strengths and forms.

PATIENT EDUCATION FOR VITAMINS AND MINERALS

Patients should be instructed regarding:

Well-balanced diets and natural sources of vitamins and minerals.

Food preparation to avoid loss of vitamins.

Information regarding signs of deficiency and overdose/toxicity.

Caution taking supplements without established need or without medical supervision, especially megadoses, fat-soluble vitamins, and iron.

Proper administration to minimize side effects.

See Table 11.2 for summary of major minerals.

TABLE 11.2. SUMMARY OF MAJOR MINERALS

Name	Food Sources	Functions	Deficiency/Toxicity
Calcium (Ca)	Milk exchanges Milk, cheese Meat exchanges Sardines Salmon Vegetable exchanges Green vegetables	Development of bones and teeth Permeability of cell membranes Transmission of nerve impulses Blood clotting	Deficiency Osteoporosis Osteomalacia Rickets Toxicity none known
Potassium (K)	Fruit exchanges Oranges, bananas Dried fruits Tomatoes	Contraction of muscles Transmission of nerve impulses Carbohydrate and protein metabolism Maintaining water balance	Deficiency Hypokalemia Toxicity Hyperkalemia
Sodium (Na)	Table salt Meat exchanges Beef, eggs Milk exchanges Milk, cheese	Maintaining fluid balance in blood Transmission of nerve impulses	Deficiency Hyponatremia Toxicity Increase in blood pressure
Chlorine (Cl)	Table salt	Gastric acidity Regulation of osmotic pressure Activation of salivary amylase	Deficiency Imbalance in gastric acidity Imbalance in blood pH Toxicity Diarrhea
Magnesium (Mg)	Vegetable exchanges Green vegetables Bread exchanges Whole grains	Synthesis of ATP (adenosine triphosphate) Transmission of nerve impulses Relaxation of skeletal muscles	Deficiency (seldom) Imbalance Weakness Toxicity diarrhea
Iron (Fe)	Meat Liver Eggs Poultry Spinach Dried fruits	Hemoglobin formation Resistance to infection	Deficiency Pale Weak Lethargy Vertigo Air hunger Toxicity Vomiting Diarrhea Erosion of GI tract
Iodine (I)	Freshwater shellfish and seafood Iodized salt	Major component of thyroid hormones Regulating rate of metabolism Growth, reproduction Nerve and muscle function Protein synthesis Skin and hair growth	Deficiency Goiter Hypothyroidism Toxicity "Iodine goiter" Hyperactive, enlarged goiter

TABLE 11.2. (Continued)

Name	Food Sources	Functions	Deficiency/Toxicity

Zinc (Zn)	Meat
	Liver
	Oysters
	Poultry
	Fish
	Whole-grain bread and cereal
		Wound healing
		Mineralization of bone
		Insulin glucose regulation
		Normal taste
			Deficiency
			 Poor wound healing
			 Reduced taste
			  perception
			 Alcohol/glucose
			  intolerance
			Toxicity
			 GI distress
			 Impaired immune
			  system

Antioxidants

No discussion of nutrition would be complete without an explanation of the antioxidants, as we know them. Antioxidants are sometimes referred to as "anticancer foods," or "natural drugs," to inhibit cell destruction in damaged or aging tissues. Nucleic acids, which comprise the genetic code within the cell, usually act to regulate normal cell function and the growth and repair of damaged or aging tissues.

Free radicals attack the cells, causing damage, which prevents the transport of nutrients, oxygen, and water into the cell and the removal of waste products. This damage affects the nucleic acids in their function of growth and repair of tissue. Free radical damage is associated with several age-related diseases. For example, damage to the nucleic acids might initiate growth of abnormal cells, the first step in cancer development. Also, free radical attack to the cell membranes of the tissues lining the blood vessels can lead to cholesterol accumulation in the damaged arteries, the initial stage of atherosclerosis and heart disease. Additionally, free radicals are associated with inflammation, drug-induced organ damage, immunosuppression, and possibly other disorders as well.

The body has developed an antioxidant system response to defend itself from free radicals. An antioxidant is defined as any compound that fights against the destructive effects of free radical oxidants. This system is comprised of enzymes, vitamins, and minerals. Antioxidants function in the prevention of free radical formation by binding to, and neutralizing, destructive substances before they damage cells and tissues.

The antioxidant vitamins—vitamin C, vitamin E, and beta carotene—can function independently of enzymes. Antioxidant minerals include copper, manganese, selenium, and zinc. These minerals work with antioxidant enzymes and are essential to proper enzyme function. If the diet is inadequate in these minerals, the enzyme is not produced, or is ineffective.

Research on antioxidants is ongoing. However, statistical findings at this time indicate that "natural" antioxidants in foods are much more effective than synthetic products.

PATIENT EDUCATION

Patients asking about antioxidants should be instructed regarding:

Foods that provide antioxidant action.

Natural antioxidants in certain foods, which are more effective than synthetic products.

Worksheet 1 for Chapter 11

FAT-SOLUBLE VITAMINS

List the fat-soluble vitamins and complete all columns.

Vitamin	Sources	Cause of Deficiencies	Signs of Deficiencies	Symptoms of Overdose	Interactions and Cautions

Worksheet 2 for Chapter 11

WATER-SOLUBLE VITAMINS

List water-soluble vitamin names and complete all columns.

Vitamin and Name	Sources	Cause of Deficiencies	Signs of Deficiencies	Symptoms of Overdose	Interactions and Cautions
B_1					
B_2					
B_6					
B_{12}					
Folic acid					
Niacin					

Worksheet 3 for Chapter 11

VITAMINS AND MINERALS

List the vitamin names and mineral symbols, and complete all columns.

Vitamin with Name Mineral with Symbol	Sources	Cause of Deficiencies	Signs of Deficiencies	Symptoms of Overdose	Interactions and Cautions
C					
Potassium					
Calcium					
Iron					

A. Case Study (Vitamins and Minerals)

Miss I. M. Puny, a 30-year-old secretary, calls the physician's office asking for a prescription for iron because she feels tired and weak. The patient should be given the following information:

1. No iron medication should be taken before first taking all the following steps EXCEPT
   a. Checking hemoglobin
   b. Assessing all symptoms
   c. Trying multivitamins
   d. Determining cause of deficiency
2. Symptoms of iron deficiency may include all of the following EXCEPT
   a. Nausea and diarrhea
   b. Pale skin
   c. Air hunger
   d. Dizziness
3. Iron is found in all of the following foods EXCEPT
   a. Liver
   b. Spinach
   c. Milk
   d. Red meat
4. Oral iron products can cause all of the following EXCEPT
   a. Constipation
   b. Diarrhea
   c. Black stools
   d. Nervousness
5. Iron products should be taken with which one of the following?
   a. Coffee
   b. Tea
   c. Orange juice
   d. Milk

B. Case Study (Vitamins and Minerals)

Mr. M. I. Grate, a 40-year-old physical education instructor, comes to the health fair to get the latest advice on vitamin C supplements to prevent colds, cancer, and premature aging. He should receive the following advice:

1. Vitamin C can be found naturally in all of the following foods EXCEPT
   a. Citrus
   b. Broccoli
   c. Cabbage
   d. Cheese
2. All of the following *decrease* vitamin C levels EXCEPT
   a. Smoking
   b. Alcohol
   c. Raw vegetables
   d. Slow cooking
3. Mega doses of vitamin C can cause all of the following EXCEPT
   a. Constipation
   b. Gouty arthritis
   c. Kidney stones
   d. G I distress
4. Functions of vitamin C include all of the following EXCEPT
   a. Healing of wounds
   b. Absorption of iron
   c. Prevention of liver disease
   d. Prevention of scurvy
5. Vitamin C interacts with all of the following drugs EXCEPT
   a. Tetracycline
   b. Estrogen
   c. Aspirin
   d. Tylenol

CHAPTER 12

Skin Medications

OBJECTIVES

Upon completion of this chapter, the student should be able to:

1. Define antipruritic, emollient, demulcent, keratolytic, antiseptic, disinfectant, bactericidal, and bacteriostatic.
2. Describe application procedures for various skin preparations.
3. Identify side effects of the six major categories of skin preparations and contraindications when appropriate.
4. Compare and contrast scabicides and pediculicides.
5. Explain the factors that influence the absorption of skin medications.
6. Classify drugs according to their action: antipruritic, emollient, keratolytic, antifungal, or anti-infective.
7. Describe important patient education for all skin medications in this chapter.

The skin is the largest organ of the body. Since such a great area is involved, many conditions can affect the skin, causing annoyance and discomfort. Skin ailments can range from minor ones, such as pruritis (itching), to major ones, such as severe burns. Treatment is usually topical or local (applied to the affected area), but skin conditions are sometimes treated internally with oral medications or injections for their systemic effects.

This chapter explains *topical* medications only. Medications given parenterally or orally to relieve inflammation or itching, such as corticosteroids and antihistamines, are discussed in other chapters.

Topical skin preparations can be classified according to action in six principal categories:

1. Antipruritics relieve itching.
2. Emollients and demulcents soothe irritation.
3. Keratolytic agents loosen epithelial scales.
4. Scabicides and pediculicides treat scabies or lice.
5. Antifungals control fungus conditions.
6. Local anti-infectives prevent and treat infection.

Factors that influence the rate of absorption of medication include condition and location of the skin, heat, and moisture. If the skin is thick and callused, absorption will be slower. If the skin is moist, macerated (raw), or warm, absorption will be more rapid. Sometimes the physician will order that the skin be premoistened or plastic wrap be applied over the ointment to aid absorption; in other cases, the skin must be left exposed to the air to slow absorption and reduce systemic effects. At times, the length of time for the medication to remain on the skin is very important. Complete understanding of appropriate directions for each topical medication is vital *before administration.*

Antipruritics

Antipruritics are used short term to relieve discomfort from dermatitis (rashes) associated with allergic reactions, poison ivy, hives, and insect bites. They relieve itching by use of products singly or in combination containing:

Local anesthetics (e.g., the "-caines," such as benzocaine).

Drying agents (e.g., calamine).

Anti-inflammatory agents (e.g., corticosteroids) applied locally or given PO for systemic effect. Topical agents are preferred because of fewer adverse effects.

Antihistamines administered PO for systemic effect (antihistamines applied topically can cause hypersensitivity reactions—use only a few days).

See Chapter 26 for further information on antihistamines.

Side effects can include:

Increased chance of infection with corticosteroids

Skin irritation, rash

Stinging and a burning sensation

Allergic reactions (especially with the "-caines")

Sedation from antihistamines PO or paradoxical agitation in children

---

PATIENT EDUCATION

Patients being treated with antipruritics should be instructed to:

Use caution if they have allergies.

Avoid contact with eyes or mucous membranes.

Avoid covering with dressings unless directed by physician.

Avoid prolonged use (not longer than 1 week).

Discontinue if condition worsens or irritation develops.

Trim children's fingernails to reduce possibility of infection.

Contraindications include:

On open wounds for corticosteroids—healing delayed
For prolonged use (especially corticosteroids)
The "-caines" for allergic persons

Emollients and Demulcents

Emollients and demulcents are used topically to protect or soothe minor dermatological conditions, such as diaper rash, abrasions, and minor burns.

Keratolytics

Keratolytic agents, for example, salicylic acid, are used to control conditions of abnormal scaling of the skin, such as dandruff, seborrhea, and psoriasis, or to promote peeling of the skin in conditions such as acne, hard corns, calluses, and warts. Antifungals are also used at times for seborrheic dermatitis and dandruff. (See Table 12.2.)

Side effects can include:

Severe skin irritation, pruritis, or stinging
Irritation to eyes or mucous membranes
Photosensitivity
Systemic effects in allergic individuals (e.g., headache and GI symptoms)

Note: When podophyllum is used for genital warts, it should be removed 1–4 hours after application.

Contraindications include:

Pregnancy and lactation
Small children
For prolonged periods of time

Corticosteroid ointments and cremes are also used to treat psoriasis and seborrheic dermatitis. (See Table 12.1.)

Side effects of corticosteroid ointments and creams, especially used long term (e.g., psoriasis), can include:

Epidural thinning with frequent skin tears
Increased fragility of cutaneous blood vessels
Irritation, burning, or stinging
Ulceration, especially with occlusive dressings
Activation of latent infections

TABLE 12.1. TOPICAL MEDICATIONS FOR THE SKIN: ANTIPRURITICS, EMOLLIENTS, DEMULCENTS, AND KERATOLYTICS

Generic Name	Trade Name	Available	Comments
Antipruritics			
benzocaine	Americaine, Solarcaine	Ointment, spray	Can cause hypersensitivity reaction
calamine	Caladryl (with Benadryl)	Lotion, ointment	Drying Antihistamine
corticosteroid	Cortaid, Topicort, Cordran, Aristocort, Synalar, others	Ointment, cream, lotion, solutions	Reduced resistance to infection, impaired healing
dibucaine	Nupercainal	Ointment, cream	Potential for hypersensitivity
Emollients and Demulcents			
vitamins A and D	A & D	Ointment	
	Desitin (with zinc oxide)	Ointment	
Keratolytics			
coal tar	Zetar, Tegrin, Neutrogena	Shampoo, lotion	For dandruff, seborrheic dermatitis, or psoriasis
podophyllum	Podophyllin	Sol	For anogenital warts; systemic toxicity possible
salicylic acid	Many combinations with other keratolytics	Ointment, sol, shampoo	For dandruff, psoriasis, acne, warts, corns, calluses
sulfur	Cuticura, Clearasil	Cream, gel, lotion, shampoo, 2–5%	For acne, dandruff, scabies (stains clothing)

Note: This table lists only typical medications and does not include all of those on the market.

Contraindications with corticosteroids include:

Skin infections, bacterial or fungal, and cutaneous or systemic viral infections

Open wounds

Immunosuppressed, for example, HIV (human immunodeficiency virus) infections or receiving chemotherapy

Children

Pregnancy or lactation

Acne, rosacea, or perioral dermatitis

PATIENT EDUCATION FOR KERATOLYTICS

Patients should be instructed to:

Use only as directed, and for entire treatment period, even if improved.

Avoid contact with eyes and mucous membranes.

Avoid prolonged use.

Discontinue and seek medical aid if irritation occurs.

Avoid contact with surrounding tissues when applied as a caustic to corns or calluses.

See Table 12.1 for a summary of antipruritics, emollients, and keratolytics.

Scabicides and Pediculicides

Scabies is caused by an itch mite that burrows under the skin. It is easily transmitted from one person to another by direct contact or through contact with contaminated clothing or bed linens. Effective treatment includes laundering in hot water or dry cleaning all clothing and bedding. Sometimes concurrent treatment of close contacts is recommended.

Scabicides (benzyl benzoate or lindane) must be applied *according to directions* on the package insert, left in place the required period of time, and then rinsed thoroughly.

Pediculicides, for example, lindane (Kwell), are used in topical treatment of lice infestations. Pyrethrins (e.g. RID), is considered safer for pediculosis.

Side effects, rare when applied topically according to directions, may include:

Slight local irritation, rash, or conjunctivitis
Dermatitis with frequent application

However, with excessive or prolonged use, or with oral ingestion, or inhalation of vapors, CNS symptoms, hepatic or renal toxicity may occur. Anemia and seizures have been reported.

Contraindications include:

Acutely inflamed, raw, or weeping surfaces.
Since lindane (Kwell) can be absorbed systemically following topical application, it should be avoided during pregnancy, lactation, or with infants and small children.

However, benzyl benzoate is a safe alternative under these conditions, for scabies. Pyrethrins (e.g., RID) are a safer alternative than lindane for pediculosis.

PATIENT EDUCATION

Patients being treated with scabicides or pediculicides should be instructed to:

Follow directions carefully.
Thoroughly launder clothing and bedding.
Use caution to prevent accidental oral ingestion.
Use caution with infants who might suck thumbs.

Antifungals

Antifungals, for example, nystatin (Mycostatin), are useful in the treatment of monilial infections (candidiasis), such as thrush, diaper rash, vaginitis, athlete's foot, and jock itch.

Effective treatment includes topical administration according to directions on the package insert and good hygiene practices, including washing, drying, and exposure to air when possible.

For the treatment of candidiasis of the oral cavity, an oral suspension or oral lozenges should be administered 4 times daily for 14 days. For infants, administer after the feeding, which is followed by water to rinse mouth *before therapy.* Place one-half dose in each side of the mouth. For adults, apply *after meals* and *after rinsing* of mouth. Then the entire dose should be used to thoroughly coat inside the mouth, holding for as long as possible (e.g., several minutes), before swallowing. In both cases, the patient should be NPO for at least 1 hour after treatment.

With inadequate response to treatment, cultures should be obtained to confirm the diagnosis and assist in the selection of the most appropriate medication.

Side effects, although rare, may include:

Contact dermatitis

Itching, burning, and irritation

Contraindication or caution (under medical supervision only) applies to the use of vaginal preparations during pregnancy. Some products can cause fetal abnormalities.

PATIENT EDUCATION

Patients being treated with antifungals should be instructed to:

Carefully wash and *dry* affected areas.

Expose to air whenever possible.

Avoid tight undergarments, pantyhose, and wet bathing suits with genital fungus.

Use open sandals instead of sneakers with athlete's foot.

Follow application instructions carefully. Use for entire time, even if asymptomatic.

Remove any stains with soap and warm water.

Continue prescribed vaginal treatment even during menstruation, or if symptomatic relief occurs, until entire regime is completed.

Consult doctor before vaginal preparations are used during pregnancy.

For oral suspensions or lozenges, apply after meals and after thorough rinsing of mouth. No food or liquids for at least 1 hour after treatment.

See Table 12.2 for a summary of the antifungals.

TABLE 12.2. TOPICAL MEDICATIONS FOR THE SKIN: SCABICIDES, PEDICULICIDES, ANTIFUNGALS, ANTISEPTICS, AND BURN MEDICATIONS

Generic Name	Trade Name	Available	Comments
Scabicides and Pediculicides			
benzyl benzoate		Lotion	Apply two coats to remain 24h
lindane	Kwell	Cream, lotion, shampoo	Treat all hairy areas Toxic potential
pyrethrins	RID	Gel, shampoo, solution	For lice
Antifungals[a]			
butoconazole	Femstat	Vaginal cream	One applicator qd hs 3–6 days
clotrimazole	Myclex, Lotrimin	Lozenges, cream, lotion, sol, vaginal cream	For oral, topical, or vaginal application
ketoconazole	Nizoral	Cream, shampoo	Topical antifungal, antibacterial, antiviral (herpes simplex) also for dandruff and seborrhea
nystatin	Mycostatin	Oral suspension, lozenges, cream, lotion, ointment, vaginal tab	Apply oral suspension or lozenges PC, then NPO 1 hr
tolnaftate	Tinactin	Aerosol spray, cream, powder, sol	Avoid inhaling spray or powder
zinc undecylenate	Cruex, Desenex	Aerosol spray, powder, ointment, cream	Spray or powder: avoid inhaling
Antiviral			
acyclovir[a]	Zovirax	Ointment	Only effective first episode
Topical Anti-Infectives and Antiseptics			
hexachlorophene	Phisohex, Septisol	Sol, liquid soap	Bacteriostatic skin cleanser, surgical scrub; rinse thoroughly
povidone-iodine	Betadine, Efodine	Aq sol, tincture, liquid scrub	Bactericidal, antiseptic, surgical scrub; watch for allergies
Burn Medications			
nitrofurazone	Furacin	Cream, ointment, sol	Watch for allergies
silver sulfadiazine	Silvadene	Cream	Watch for allergies

[a]Oral preparations are discussed in Chapter 17.
Note: Other preparations are available. This is a representative list.

Antivirals

Acyclovir has an antiviral effect on herpes simplex, herpes zoster (shingles), and varicella zoster (chickenpox) viruses. Acyclovir (Zovirax) is available in oral and parenteral preparations (see Chapter 17), or in ointment applied topically. Topical therapy is substantially less effective than systemic therapy (parenteral or oral). Topical acyclovir therapy is not a cure, and does not reduce the frequency or delay the appearance of new lesions. However, topical therapy generally decreases the duration of viral shedding, the duration of pain and itching, and the time required for crusting and healing of lesions. It is effective in first episode genital herpes infection, but recurrent infections have shown little, if any, therapeutic benefit from topical therapy. The ointment should be applied as soon as possible following onset of signs and symptoms of infections. Take care not to get the ointment in the eyes. It is not effective in preventing infections.

Local Anti-Infectives

ANTISEPTICS

Antiseptics are substances that inhibit the growth of bacteria (bacteriostatic). The term is used most frequently to describe chemicals applied to body tissues, especially the skin. *Disinfectants* are included in this category, but chemicals that kill bacteria (bactericidal) are frequently too strong to be applied to body tissues and are *usually* applied to inanimate objects, such as furniture, floors, and instruments. Sometimes a chemical can be used as an antiseptic on skin and also as a disinfectant on inanimate objects by increasing the strength.

The two major antiseptics in use today are hexachlorophene and iodine, used for surgical scrubs and as bacteriostatic skin cleansers. Some iodine preparations are also bactericidal and are used in the treatment of superficial skin wounds and to disinfect the skin preoperatively. Hexachlorophene should not be used on wounds or rashes.

Side effects of hexachlorophene, which is absorbed systemically, can be serious and *rinsing thoroughly* after its use is vital to prevent:

Dermatitis and redness

Photosensitivity

Systemic effects (e.g., CNS irritability, seizures, and death)

Side effects of iodine can include:

Skin irritation or burns (Do *not* cover with a tight bandage)

Allergic reactions

Contraindications or extreme cautions for hexachlorophene include:

Not for frequent handwashing while pregnant

Not for frequent use for total body bathing

Not for routine use for infants, especially with premature or low-birth-weight infants

Not for use on burned or denuded skin or mucous membranes

Not for use with occlusive dressings

PATIENT EDUCATION

Patients being treated with local anti-infectives should be instructed to:

Rinse hexachlorophene *thoroughly.*
Avoid hexachlorophene for total body bathing, especially with small infants.
Avoid use of hexachlorophene on open skin lesions, mucous membranes, and
  genital areas.
Take care to avoid hexachlorophene or iodine in the eyes; flush thoroughly.
Avoid tight dressings over both medications.
Use caution with iodine in anyone with allergies.
Keep tincture of iodine bottles closed tightly to prevent evaporation of alcohol,
  leading to increase in strength and possible iodine burns.

Iodine cautions include:

Not for those allergic to iodine
Not covering with tight bandage

BURN MEDICATIONS

Burn treatments include topical application of medications to prevent or treat infections. The two most commonly used agents for this purpose are nitrofurazone
(Furacin) and silver sulfadiazine (Silvadene). Apply with a sterile-gloved hand.

Side effects of burn medications can include:

Pain, burning, and itching
Allergic reactions

Contraindications or extreme caution applies to newborns or to patients with:

Impaired kidney or liver function (cumulative effects)
History of allergy, especially to sulfa drugs

PATIENT EDUCATION

Patients using burn medications should be instructed to:

Use aseptic technique to prevent infection.
Watch for allergic reactions.
Keep careful intake and output record.

See Table 12.2 for a summary of scabicides, pediculicides, antifungals, antivi-
rals, antiseptics, and burn medications.

Cautions for Topical Medications

Skin medications by prescription or over-the-counter are too numerous to mention. Many patients use products without adequate instruction in administration, side effects, or precautions. The health worker has a responsibility to advise patients whenever possible to use great caution with self-medication to avoid ineffective or dangerous treatment. Both the health worker and the lay person should *read instructions completely* before administration of any medication.

PATIENT EDUCATION

Patients using topical medications should be instructed regarding:

Never taking by mouth.
Keeping out of reach of children.
Being sure labels are not obscured and are read completely.
Discontinuing at once with any side effects and seeking medical advice.
Not taking beyond time limit listed on medication container.
If allergies are known, avoiding self-medication without medical advice.

Worksheet For Chapter 12

DRUGS FOR THE SKIN

List the drugs according to category and complete all columns. Learn generic or trade names as specified by instructor.

Classifications and Drugs	Purpose	Side Effects	Contraindications or Cautions	Patient Education
Antipruritics 1. 2. 3.				
Emollients and Demulcents 1.				
Keratolytics 1. 2. 3. 4.				
Scabicides and Pediculicides 1. 2. 3.				

Classifications and Drugs	Purpose	Side Effects	Contraindications or Cautions	Patient Education
Antifungals 1. 2. 3. 4.				
Antivirals 1.				
Antiseptics 1. 2.				
Burn Medications 1. 2.				

A. Case Study for Skin Medications

Jay Skalin, a 35-year-old male, comes to the dermatologists office with a request for corticosteroid cream for an outbreak of psoriasis on his hands. He asks if he will be able to use the same medicine for his jock itch and athlete's foot and for an abrasion on his son's knee. He will need the following information.

1. Topical corticosteroids are *contraindicated* for many conditions. The *only* appropriate use listed below is for
   a. Open wounds
   b. Viral infections
   c. Fungal conditions
   d. Allergic reaction

2. Topical corticosteroids are *contraindicated* in many circumstances. Which circumstance would allow its use?
   a. With immunosuppression
   b. With children's rash
   c. With psoriasis
   d. With chemotherapy

3. Corticosteroid cream can be used for all of the following EXCEPT
   a. Jock itch
   b. Poison ivy
   c. Hives
   d. Insect bites

4. Side effects of prolonged use of corticosteroid cream can include all of the following EXCEPT
   a. Easy bruising
   b. Thick scabs
   c. Thin skin
   d. Irritation

5. Other medications to treat psoriasis include keratolytics listed below EXCEPT
   a. Zetar
   b. Tegrin
   c. Salicylic acid
   d. Lindane

B. Case Study for Skin Medications

Melody Lane goes to the physician for her 6-week postpartum check. She complains of vaginal itching and says that her baby has "white spots in his mouth." The following information would be helpful:

1. Fungal infections (candidiasis) can cause all of the following EXCEPT
   a. Thrush
   b. Acne
   c. Diaper rash
   d. Vaginitis

2. Oral candidiasis can be treated with all of the following EXCEPT
   a. Lozenges
   b. Suspension
   c. Extended-release capsules
   d. Topical application

3. Treatment for oral candidiasis includes all of the following instructions EXCEPT
   a. Treat ac
   b. Rinse first
   c. NPO after
   d. Swallow solution

4. Customary treatment of monilial vaginal infections can include all the following EXCEPT

a. Cream

b. Lotion

c. NPO after

d. IM injection

5. Treatment for vaginal monilial infections includes all of the following instructions EXCEPT

a. Avoid tight undergarments

b. Continue during menstruation

c. Discontinue when better

d. Consult M.D. if pregnant

CHAPTER 13

Autonomic Nervous System Drugs

OBJECTIVES

Upon completion of this chapter, the student should be able to:

1. Define sympathomimetic and parasympathomimetic.
2. Compare and contrast characteristics of the four categories of autonomic nervous system drugs.
3. List the most frequently used (key) drugs in each of the four categories and the purpose of administration.
4. Describe the possible side effects of each of the key drugs.

The autonomic nervous system (ANS) can be thought of as being *automatic*, self-governing, or involuntary. That is to say, we have no control over the action of the autonomic nervous system. Chemical substances called *mediators* are released at the nerve endings to transmit the nerve impulses from nerve to nerve at the synapses or from nerve to muscle at the myoneural junctions.

The autonomic nervous system is divided into the *sympathetic* and the *parasympathetic* divisions. Drugs that affect the function of the autonomic nervous system are divided into four categories:

1. Adrenergics (sympathomimetics)
2. Adrenergic blockers (beta blockers)
3. Cholinergics (parasympathomimetics)
4. Cholinergic blockers (anticholinergics)

Adrenergics

The sympathetic nervous system can be thought of as the emergency system used to mobilize the body for quick response and action. Key words to illustrate this action are *fright, fight,* and *flight.* If someone is startled in a dark place by a sudden motion, the body automatically mobilizes the sympathetic nerves to prepare the body to handle the fright by flight or a fight. The blood pressure, pulse, and respiration increase. The peripheral blood vessels constrict, sending more blood inward to the vital organs and skeletal muscles and speeding up the heart action. The bronchioles dilate to allow for a greater oxygen supply. The pupils dilate.

The chemical substances (mediators) released at the sympathetic nerve endings are called catecholamines and include epinephrine *(adrenaline),* norepinephrine, dopamine, and isoproterenol. Drugs that mimic the action of the sympathetic nervous system are called *sympathomimetic* or adrenergic.

Actions of the adrenergics include:

Cardiac stimulation
Increased blood flow to skeletal muscles
Peripheral vasoconstriction
Bronchodilation
Dilation of pupils (mydriatic action)

Uses include:

Restoring rhythm in cardiac arrest
Elevating blood pressure in shock of all kinds
Constricting capillaries (e.g., applied topically to relieve nosebleed or nasal congestion or combined with local anesthetics for minor surgery)
Dilating bronchioles in acute asthmatic attacks, bronchospasm, or anaphylactic reaction
Ophthalmic procedures (mydriatic agent)

Side effects of the adrenergics may include:

Palpitations
Nervousness or tremor
Tachycardia
Cardiac arrhythmias
Anginal pain
Hypertension
Tissue necrosis (when applied to laceration of periphery, e.g., nose, fingers, and toes)
Hyperglycemia
Headache and insomnia

Contraindications or extreme caution with adrenergics applies to:

Angina
Coronary insufficiency
Hypertension

TABLE 13.1. ADRENERGICS

Generic Name	Trade Name	Dosage	Comments
epinephrine	Adrenalin	0.1–0.5 ml 1:1,000 sol SC or IM[a] (deltoid) 0.5–1 ml 1:1,000 sol IV	For bronchospasm, asthma, cardiac arrest, anaphylaxis
ephedrine	Ephedrine	25–50 mg IM or SC 12.5–50 mg PO bid or qid, or inhalers	To raise blood pressure Nasal decongestant or bronchodilator
dopamine	Intropin	2–5 µg/kg/min IV	To raise blood pressure, cardiotonic
isoproterenol	Isuprel	10–20 mg SL q6–8h or inhalations qid 0.02–0.2 mg IV or IM	For asthma or bronchospasm; for heartblock or ventricular arrhythmias
metaraminol	Aramine	0.5–5 mg IV	To raise blood pressure in shock
norepinephrine	Levophed	2–12 µg/min IV	For severe shock

[a]Use caution with dosage. This caution applies to both dosages.

Cardiac arrhythmias
Angle-closure glaucoma
Organic brain damage
Hyperthyroidism

Caution also with administration, check dosage carefully (small amounts only). See Table 13.1. Give subcutaneous IM (deltoid), or IV.

Interactions may occur with:

CNS drugs (e.g., alcohol and antidepressants)
Propranolol (Inderal) or other beta-adrenergic blockers

See Table 13.1 for a summary of the adrenergics.

Adrenergic Blockers

Drugs that block the action of the sympathetic nervous system are called adrenergic blockers. The most commonly used drugs in this category are beta-adrenergic blockers, or beta-blockers, such as propranolol (Inderal).

Uses of the beta blockers include treatment of the following:

Hypertension
Cardiac arrhythmias
Angina pectoris
Migraine headache

Side effects of beta blockers may include:

Hypotension
Bradycardia
Fatigue or lethargy
Nausea and vomiting
Hypoglycemia
Confusion

Contraindications or extreme caution applies to use of beta-blockers with:

Congestive heart failure or atrioventricular block
Hypotension
Asthma
Diabetes

Interactions may occur with:

Digitalis
Insulin or oral antidiabetic agents
Aminophylline
Isuprel
Epinephrine
Alcohol

PATIENT EDUCATION

Patients taking beta blockers, frequently given for cardiovascular disease, should be instructed regarding:

Rising slowly from reclining position to avoid postural hypotension.
Possible slow heartbeat and reporting dizziness or excessive weakness to the physician.
Avoiding alcohol, antihistamines, muscle relaxants, tranquilizers, and sedatives because they potentiate CNS depression and sedation.
Reporting sexual dysfunction or depression to the physician for possible dosage regulation or change to different medication.

Cholinergics

The parasympathetic nerve fibers synthesize and liberate *acetylcholine* as the mediator. Drugs that mimic the action of the parasympathetic nervous system are called *parasympathomimetic* or cholinergic drugs (e.g., bethanechol, neostigmine, and pilocarpine).

TABLE 13.2. ADRENERGIC BLOCKERS

Generic Name	Trade Name	Dosage	Comments
propranolol[a]	Inderal	PO 160–480 mg qd bid or tid	Begin with smaller dose and increase gradually to optimum dose for blood pressure control
		PO 10–20 mg qid	For angina
		PO 10–30 mg qid IV 1–5 mg slowly Use **extreme** caution	For arrhythmias
		PO 80–mg initial dose, increase to 160–240 mg qd	For migraine

[a]A beta-adrenergic blocker, or beta blocker. Others available and vary with condition.

Actions of the cholinergics include:

Increased gastrointestinal peristalsis
Increased contraction of the urinary bladder
Increased secretions (sweat, saliva, and gastric juices)
Increased skeletal muscle strength
Lowered intraocular pressure
Constriction of pupils
Slowing of the heart

Uses include treatment of:

Nonobstructive urinary retention (bethanechol)
Abdominal distention (neostigmine)
Myasthenia gravis (neostigmine)
Open-angle glaucoma (pilocarpine)
As an insecticide (malathion)

Side effects may include:

Nausea, vomiting, and diarrhea
Muscle cramps and weakness
Slowing of the heart, hypotension, and bronchospasm
Sweating, excessive salivation, lacrimation and flushing
Respiratory depression
Acute toxicity or cholinergic crisis is treated with atropine sulfate IV

Contraindications or extreme caution applies to:

Benign prostatic hypertrophy (BPH)
Gastrointestinal disorders (e.g., ulcer and obstruction)
Asthma
Cardiac disorders

TABLE 13.3. CHOLINERGICS

Generic Name	Trade Name	Dosage	Comments
bethanechol	Urecholine	10–50 mg PO qid, or 2.5–5 mg subcu	For postpartum or postoperative urinary retention, **not** with benign, prostatic hypertrophy
edrophonium	Tensilon	1–2 mg IV, then 8 mg if no response	Test for myasthenia gravis
neostigmine	Prostigmin	45–150 mg PO in divided doses qd 0.5–2 mg IM or IV q 1–3h	Treatment for myasthenia gravis
pilocarpine	Isopto Carpine	Ophthalmic gtts, dose varies	To lower intraocular pressure with glaucoma

Interactions of cholinergics occur with:

Procainamide

Quinidine

See Table 13.3 for a summary of the cholinergics.

PATIENT EDUCATION

Patients taking cholinergic drugs, or exposed to insecticides containing cholinergic agents (e.g., malathion), should be instructed regarding:

Reporting immediately to physician or emergency room any symptoms of prolonged GI distress (e.g., nausea, vomiting, and diarrhea), excessive perspiration, slow heartbeat, or depressed respiration.

Avoiding combination of cholinergic medications with heart medications or antibiotics.

Cholinergic Blockers

Cholinergic blockers, or anticholinergics, are drugs that block the action of the parasympathetic nervous system. Therefore, they are also called parasympatholytic. Atropine is the classic example of a cholinergic blocker. Others are listed in Table 13.4.

Actions include:

Drying (all secretions decreased)

Decreased GI and genitourinary (GU) motility

Dilation of pupils

Uses of atropine:

Antispasmodic and antisecretory for GI or GU hypermotility

Preoperative and preanesthetic uses

Neuromuscular block and other spastic disorders

Antidote for insecticide poisoning, cholinergic crisis, or mushroom poisoning

Emergency treatment of bradycardia and atrioventricular heart block with hypotension

Dilation of pupils (mydriatic)

Prevention and treatment of bronchospasm (bronchodilator, e.g., Atrovent inhaler)

Side effects of atropine may include:

Fever or flushing

Blurred vision

Dry mouth, constipation, and urinary retention

Confusion and headache

Palpitations and tachycardia

Interactions with potentiation of sedation and drying occur with antihistamines (e.g., diphenhydramine).

Contraindications or extreme caution applies to use of atropine with:

Asthma and other chronic obstructive pulmonary disease (COPD)—atropine *inhalations* recommended rather than oral or parenteral administration, which can reduce bronchial secretions and obstruct airflow

Angle-closure glaucoma

GI or GU obstruction

Cardiac arrhythmias

Hypertension

Hypothyroidism, hepatic, or renal disease

PATIENT EDUCATION

Patients receiving cholinergic blockers should be instructed regarding:

Dried secretions (e.g., dry mouth).

Possible blurring of vision.

Reporting fast heartbeat or palpitations.

Avoiding oral anticholinergics with chronic obstructive lung disease and asthma, using inhalants only as prescribed, never OTC.

See Table 13.4 for a summary of the anticholinergics.
See Figure 13.1 for a summary of the autonomic nervous system drugs.

TABLE 13.4. CHOLINERGIC BLOCKERS

Generic Name	Trade Name	Dosage[b]	Comments
atropine	Atropine[b]	0.4–0.6 mg IM	Preoperative
		2 mg IM or IV gh	For insecticide or mushroom poisoning
		0.6–1 mg IV	For bradycardia or atrioventricular block
glycopyrrolate	Robinul	0.1 mg IM or IV	Preoperative
methantheline	Banthine	50–100 mg PO qid	For bladder spasm
scopolamine	Transderm Scop	72-hour patch	Prevent motion sickness
homatropine[a]	Isopto Homatropine	Ophthalmic gtts	Mydriatic

[a]Other anticholinergics used in ophthalmic medications are discussed in Chapter 18.
[b]Use caution to give correct dosage.

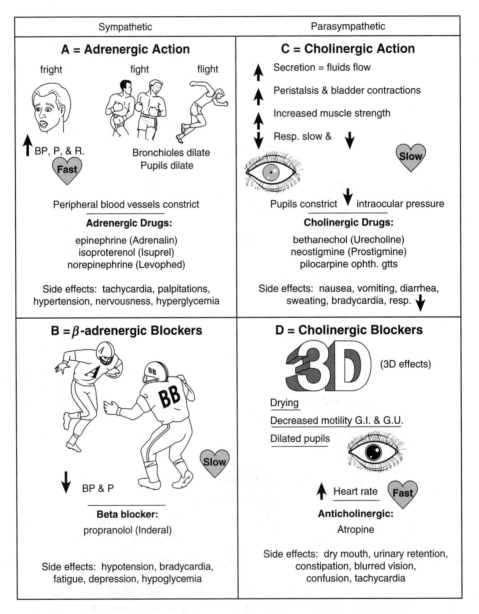

Figure 13.1 The autonomic nervous system drugs can be as simple as A, B, C, D.

Worksheet for Chapter 13

AUTONOMIC NERVOUS SYSTEM DRUGS

List the drugs according to category and complete all columns. Learn generic or trade names as specified by instructor.

Classifications and Drugs	Purpose	Side Effects	Contraindications or Cautions	Patient Education
Adrenergics 1. 2. 3. 4. 5.				
Adrenergic Blocker 1.				
Cholinergics 1. 2.				
Cholinergic Blockers 1. 2. 3. 4.				

A. Case Study for Autonomic Nervous System Drugs

Arlie Woods, a 33-year-old, receives epinephrine (Adrenalin) in the emergency room for a severe asthma attack. Health care personnel should have the following information.

1. Adrenalin has all of the following actions EXCEPT
   a. Peripheral vasodilator
   b. Dilation of pupils
   c. Bronchodilator
   d. Cardiac stimulant

2. All of the following doses of Adrenalin are appropriate EXCEPT
   a. 0.4 ml IM (deltoid)
   b. 0.3 ml subcu
   c. 5 ml SC
   d. 1 ml IV

3. Epinephrine is also used to treat all of the following conditions EXCEPT
   a. Nosebleed
   b. Hypertension
   c. Anaphylaxis
   d. Cardiac arrest

4. Side effects can include all of the following EXCEPT
   a. Tremors
   b. Hypoglycemia
   c. Tachycardia
   d. Insomnia

5. She should be told all of the following about epinephrine EXCEPT
   a. May cause sedation
   b. Avoid alcohol
   c. May cause headaches
   d. Palpitations possible

B. Case Study for Cholinergic Blockers

Milton Noteworthy was brought into the emergency room with complaints of nausea, diarrhea, and sweating. He says that he "ate mushrooms found in the woods." The following information would be helpful.

1. Mushroom poisoning mimics parasympathetic nervous system (cholinergic) action with all of the following symptoms EXCEPT
   a. Increased peristalsis
   b. Urinary retention
   c. Salivation
   d. Bradycardia

2. Treatment includes cholinergic blockers. Which of the following is *not* a cholinergic blocker?
   a. Urecholine
   b. Banthine
   c. Atropine
   d. Scopolamine

3. Which is the drug of choice to treat cholinergic toxicity (e.g., mushroom or insecticide poisoning)?
   a. Urecholine
   b. Banthine
   c. Atropine
   d. Scopolamine

4. Side effects of cholinergic blockers include all of the following EXCEPT
   a. Dry mouth
   b. Diarrhea
   c. Urinary retention
   d. Dilated pupils

5. Other side effects of cholinergic blockers can include all of the following EXCEPT
   a. Flushing
   b. Confusion
   c. Blurred vision
   d. Bradycardia

CHAPTER 14

Antineoplastic Drugs

OBJECTIVES

Upon completion of this chapter, the student should be able to:

1. Define antineoplastic, chemotherapy, palliative, proliferation, cytotoxic, and immuno-suppressive.
2. Name three characteristics associated with administration of antineoplastic drugs.
3. Name the seven major groups of antineoplastic agents.
4. List the side effects common to most of the antineoplastic agents.
5. Describe appropriate interventions in caring for patients receiving antineoplastic agents.
6. Explain precautions in caring for those receiving radioactive isotopes.
7. Describe the responsibilities of those caring for patients receiving chemotherapy.
8. Explain appropriate education for patient and family when antineoplastic agents are administered.
9. List safety factors for those who care for patients receiving cytotoxic drugs.

Antineoplastic (against new tissue formation) refers to an agent that counteracts the development, growth, or spread of malignant cells. Cancer therapy frequently includes a combination of surgery, radiation, and/or chemotherapy.

Chemotherapy is a constantly growing field in which many old and new drugs and drug combinations are used for *palliative* effects (alleviation of symptoms), or for long-term or complete *remissions* in early treatment of cancer. Antineoplastic drugs are *cytotoxic* (destructive to cells), especially to cells that are proliferating (reproducing rapidly). Unfortunately, the toxic effects of the antineoplastic drugs are not confined to malignant cells alone, but also affect other proliferating tissue, such as bone marrow, gastrointestinal epithelium, skin, hair follicles, and epithelium of the gonads, resulting in numerous adverse side effects.

Many antineoplastic agents also possess *immunosuppressive* properties, which decrease the production of antibodies and phagocytes, and reduce the inflammatory reaction. Suppression of the immune response results in increased susceptibility of the patient to infection.

Antineoplastic drugs are frequently administered in high doses on an *intermittent* schedule. Because most normal tissues have a greater capacity for repair than do most malignant tissues, normal cells may recover during the drug-free period.

Chemotherapy is *individualized* and frequently modified according to the patient's response to treatment. A *combination of several drugs* is frequently prescribed to delay the emergence of resistance, with the choice of agents based on the type of malignancy, areas involved, extent of the cancer, physical condition of the patient, and other factors. Careful planning is required to maximize the effectiveness of therapy and to minimize the side effects and discomfort for the patient. Understanding of the treatment program and possible side effects is essential for all concerned: the nurse, the patient, and the family. Preplanning includes provision for symptomatic relief, such as antiemetics, as well as reassurance and availability of support staff to answer questions, explore feelings, and allay fears. Knowledge of side effects and appropriate interventions and patient education are essential for health care workers in this area.

Antineoplastic agents can be generally classified into seven major groups: antimetabolites, alkylating agents, plant alkaloids, antitumor antibiotics, hormones, radioactive isotopes, and interferon.

Antimetabolites

Antimetabolites are used in the treatment of leukemia, osteogenic sarcoma, squamous cell carcinoma, breast cancer, and other malignancies, especially those involving the genital areas. Some antimetabolites include methotrexate, fluorouracil, cytarabine, and 6-mercaptopurine. Methotrexate has also been used for severe, resistant cases of psoriasis.

Side effects can include:

Anorexia, nausea, vomiting, and diarrhea

Ulceration and bleeding of the oral mucosa and GI (gastrointestinal) tract

Bone marrow depression, including leukopenia with infection, anemia, and thrombocytopenia with hemorrhage

Rash, itching, photosensitivity, and scaling

Alopecia (regrowth of hair may take several months)

Contraindications or extreme caution applies to:

Renal and hepatic disorders

Pregnancy

GI ulcers

Alkylating Agents

Alkylating agents are used in the treatment of a wide range of cancers, including sarcomas, lymphomas, and leukemias. Some alkylating agents include carmustine, cisplatin, and thiotepa, used for metastatic ovarian, testicular, and bladder cancer and sometimes in palliative treatment of other cancers.

Side effects can include:

Nausea, vomiting, and diarrhea

Bone marrow depression, including leukopenia, with infection, anemia, and thrombocytopenia with hemorrhage

Neurotoxicity, including headache, vertigo, and convulsions

Rash and alopecia

Loss of reproductive capacity

Contraindications or extreme caution applies to:

Debilitated patients

Pregnancy

Plant Alkaloids

Plant alkaloids are used in combination with other chemotherapeutic agents in the treatment of leukemias, Hodgkin's disease, lymphomas, sarcomas, and other malignancies. Some plant alkaloids include vinblastine and vincristine.

Side effects can include:

Neurotoxicity, including numbness, tingling, ataxia, foot drop, pain in the jaw, head, or extremities, and visual disturbances

Severe constipation or diarrhea, nausea, and vomiting

Oral or GI ulceration

Rash, phototoxicity, and alopecia

Leukopenia with vinblastine (hematologic effects rare with vincristine)

Necrosis of tissue if intravenous infiltrates into tissue

Contraindications or caution applies to pregnancy.

Antitumor Antibiotics

Antitumor antibiotics are used to treat a wide variety of malignancies, including sarcomas, Hodgkin's disease, lymphomas, and tumors of the head and testicles. Antitumor antibiotics include bleomycin, dactinomycin, mitomycin, and others.

Side effects can include:

Nausea, vomiting, and diarrhea

Bone marrow depression

Cardiotoxicity, including arrhythmias and congestive heart failure

Pneumonitis, dyspnea, and rales

Ulceration of mouth or colon

Alopecia, rash, and scaling

Contraindications or caution applies to:

Pregnancy

Liver disorders

Hormone Therapy

Corticosteroids, such as prednisone, are frequently used in combination with other chemotherapeutic agents in the treatment of leukemias and lymphomas. In addition, large doses of dexamethasone (Decadron) have been found effective in the prevention and treatment of nausea and vomiting associated with many neoplastic agents, when administered before or with chemotherapy.

Side effects with prolonged use of prednisone (see Chapter 23) include:

Fluid retention

Cushingoid features (moon face)

Fatigue and weakness

Osteoporosis

A *nonsteroidal antiestrogen,* tamoxifen, is used in the palliative treatment of advanced metastatic breast cancer or as an adjunct to surgery with negative axillary lymph nodes. Serious adverse side effects are rare and usually dose related, resembling menopausal symptoms.

Antiandrogen drugs include leuprolide acetate (Lupron Depot), a gonadotropin-releasing hormone (GnRH) analog, which is usually administered IM once monthly for prostate cancer. See Chapter 24 for more details.

Side effects can include:

Impotence and decreased libido, which are common

Hot flushes

Patients should be advised that the drug should be continued even when signs or symptoms of the disease improve.

Sex hormones, including the estrogens, progestins, and androgens, are also used as antineoplastic agents in the treatment of malignancies involving the reproductive system (e.g., cancer of the breast, uterus, or prostate). These hormones are discussed in Chapter 24.

Interferons

Interferon alfa is a complex combination of many proteins acting as a biologic response modifier. The action is complex, affecting cell proliferation and other cell functions, and immune system response. Its antiviral action is described in Chapter 17. Interferons are used in the treatment of many malignancies, for example, leukemias, lymphomas, and other cancers, especially those resistant to standard treatments. Some interferons have been designated as orphan drugs by the FDA (Food and Drug Administration) for many conditions, and research is ongoing.

Adverse side effects, sometimes severe, are experienced by almost all patients receiving interferon, varying with the dosage and condition. Most common side effects include:

Flulike syndrome—fever, fatigue, headache, muscle aches and pains

GI symptoms—anorexia, nausea, vomiting, diarrhea, and dry mouth

Nervous system effects—sleep disturbances, mental symptoms

Hematologic effects,—especially leukopenia

Dyspnea, cough, nasal congestion

Alopecia—transient

Paclitaxel

Paclitaxel (Taxol) is extracted from the bark of the Western (Pacific) yew. It is structurally different from other available antineoplastic agents. Since the tree is slow-growing and dies when the bark is removed, the supply is limited. It is used as second-line or subsequent therapy in patients with metastatic breast or ovarian carcinoma refractory to conventional chemotherapy.

Adverse side effects of Taxol are frequent and include:

Bone marrow suppression: neutropenia, leukopenia, thrombocytopenia and anemia

Hypersensitivity reactions—can be severe, with flushing, rash, dyspnea, chest pain, hypotension, bradycardia

Peripheral neuropathy

Nausea, vomiting, diarrhea

Alopecia

Since paclitaxel is so toxic, the drug is only administered IV under constant supervision of an oncologist, with frequent monitoring of vital signs, and facilities available for emergency interventions if required.

Radioactive Isotopes

Radioactive isotopes are also used in the treatment of certain types of cancer. Sometimes the radioactive material is injected into the affected site (e.g., radiogold, injected into the pleural or peritoneal cavity to treat ascites caused by cancer). Radioactive sodium iodine is administered PO or IV to treat thyroid cancer. Radioactive material is sometimes implanted in the body in the form of capsules, needles, or seeds.

Health care workers caring for patients receiving radioactive isotopes must observe special precautions to prevent unnecessary radiation exposure. Gowns and gloves should be worn when handling excreta. Other isolation procedures, such as handling of linens, will be outlined in the hospital procedure manual. This protocol should be followed with great care by all those who come in contact with patients receiving radioactive materials, for the protection of patients, as well as the health care worker.

Cautions and Responsibilities for Antineoplastic Drugs

Health care workers involved in the administration of antineoplastic agents, as well as those who care for these patients, have a number of very important responsibilities:

1. All medications should be given on time and exactly as prescribed to keep the patient as comfortable as possible. Check drug inserts on all new drugs.
2. Intravenous sites must be checked with great care because antineoplastic agents can cause extreme tissue damage and necrosis if infiltration occurs.
3. Intravenous fluids containing antineoplastic agents should not be allowed to get on the skin or into the eyes of the patient or the one administering the medication. Flush skin or eyes copiously if spills occur.
4. Antiemetics should be immediately available and administered as prescribed to minimize nausea and vomiting. Ondansetron (Zofran) and gransetron (Kytril) are newer antiemetics for this purpose.
5. Careful and frequent oral hygiene is essential to minimize the discomfort and ulceration.
6. Soft foods and cool liquids should be available to the patient as required.
7. Accurate intake and output is important for adequate assessment of hydration.
8. Careful observation and reporting of symptoms and side effects is an essential part of chemotherapy.
9. Aseptic technique is necessary to minimize the chance of infection in patients with reduced resistance to infection.
10. Careful assessment of vital signs is important to identify signs of infection, cardiac irregularities, and dyspnea.

11. The health care worker must be informed about all aspects of chemotherapy and answer the patient's questions honestly. Awareness of verbal and non-verbal communication that gives clues to the patient's needs is absolutely necessary.

12. Careful attention to detail, astute observations, appropriate interventions, and compassion are an integral part of care when the patient is receiving chemotherapy.

13. The health care worker should reassure the patient that someone will be available to help at all times. Identify these resources.

PATIENT EDUCATION

Patients being treated with antineoplastic drugs and their families should be instructed regarding:

Side effects to expect, how long they can be expected to continue, and that they are temporary.

Comfort measures for coping with unpleasant side effects, (e.g., antiemetics as prescribed).

Appropriate diet with foods that are more palatable and more likely to be tolerated (e.g., soft foods, bland foods, a variety of liquids, and especially cold foods in frequent, small quantities).

Careful aseptic technique to decrease the chance of infections and reporting any signs of infection (e.g., fever).

Careful oral hygiene with swabs to prevent further trauma to ulcerated mucosa.

Observation for bleeding in stools, urine, and gums and for bruises, and reporting this to medical personnel.

Reporting of any persistent or unusual side effects, such as dizziness, severe headache, numbness, tingling, difficulty walking, or visual disturbances.

Available community resources to assist and support the patient (e.g., Cancer Society, Hospice, or Home Health Services) as required and recommended by the physician.

How to obtain information and answers to questions regarding treatment.

The right of patients to terminate therapy if they wish.

See Table 14.1 for a summary of the antineoplastic agents.

CYTOTOXIC DRUG DANGERS TO HEALTH CARE PERSONNEL

Anyone who prepares, administers, or cares for patients receiving cytotoxic drugs should be aware of the dangers involved. The American Society of Health-Service Pharmacists (ASHP) has published a *Technical Assistance Bulletin (TAB)* that provides detailed advice on recommended policies, procedures, and equipment for safe handling of cytotoxic drugs. *(See AHFS Drug Information 96.)* It is essential

TABLE 14.1 ANTINEOPLASTIC AGENTS

Generic Name	Trade Name	Generic Name	Trade Name
Antimetabolites		**Antitumor Antibiotics**	
cytarabine	Cytosar-U	bleomycin	Blenoxane
fluorouracil	Adrucil	dactinomycin	Cosmegen
methotrexate	Rheumatrex	doxorubicin	Adriamycin
mercaptopurine	Purinethol	mitomycin	Mutamycin
Alkylating Agents		**Steroid Hormones**	
busulfan	Myleran	dexamethasone	Decadron
carmustine	BCNU	prednisone	Deltasone
chlorambucil	Leukeran	**Antiestrogen**	
cisplatin	Platinol	tamoxifen	Nolvadex
cyclophosphamide	Cytoxan	**Antiandrogen**	
thiotepa	Thiotepa	leuprolide	Lupron Depot
Plant Alkaloids		**Interferons**	Roferon A, Intron A
vinblastine	Velban	**Paclitaxel**	Taxol
vincristine	Oncovin		

Note: This listing is not complete but is representative of the most used drugs. Dosage is usually on an intermittent schedule and individualized.

that policies and procedures are followed exactly as outlined on the labels provided by the drug company. Guidelines of the individual health care agency must also be followed to the letter for the safety of all concerned.

The danger to health care personnel from handling a hazardous drug stems from a combination of its inherent toxicity and the extent to which workers are exposed in the course of carrying out their duties. This exposure may be from inadvertent ingestion of the drug on foodstuffs, inhalation of drug dust or droplets, or direct skin contact.

Recommended safe handling methods include four broad goals:

1. Protect and secure packages of hazardous drugs.
2. Inform and educate all involved personnel about hazardous drugs and train them in safe handling procedures.
3. Do not let the drugs escape from containers when they are manipulated (i.e., dissolved, transferred, administered, or discarded).
4. Eliminate the possibility of inadvertent ingestion or inhalation and direct skin or eye contact with the drugs.

Specific recommendations for cytotoxic drugs include:

1. When preparing these drugs, gloves, long-sleeved gowns, splash goggles, and disposable respirator masks are worn.
2. For administration, long-sleeved gowns and gloves are worn. Syringes and IV sets with Luer-lok fittings should be used and care taken that all fittings are secure.

3. Syringes, IV tubing and bags, gauze or any other contaminated material such as linens must be disposed of in a leakproof, puncture-resistant container that is labeled "HAZARD."

4. Gloves and gown should be worn when handling excreta from patients receiving cytoxic drugs.

5. Those who are pregnant, breast-feeding, or actively trying to conceive a child should not care for patients receiving cytotoxic drugs.

For more detailed instructions, see *ASHP Technical Assistance Bulletin on Handling Cytotoxic and Hazardous Drugs,* which is reproduced in the AHFS Drug Information book and updated based on information from OSHA (Occupational Safety and Health Administration), National Institutes of Health (NIH), National Study Commission on Cytotoxic Exposure, and the AMA (American Medical Association) Council on Scientific Affairs.

Worksheet for Chapter 14

ANTINEOPLASTIC DRUGS

Note the drugs listed according to category and complete all columns. See note on Table 14.1 regarding names of drugs.

Classifications and Drugs	Purpose	Side Effects	Contraindications or Cautions	Patient Education
Antimetabolites 1. fluorouracil 2. methotrexate 3. cytarabine 4. mercaptopurine				
Alkylating Agents 1. carmustine 2. cisplatin 3. thiotepa				
Plant Alkaloids 1. vinblastine 2. vincristine				

Classifications and Drugs	Purpose	Side Effects	Contraindications or Cautions	Patient Education
Antitumor Antibiotics 1. bleomycin 2. dactinomycin 3. mitomycin				
Steroid Hormones 1. dexamethasone 2. prednisone				
Antiestrogen				
Antiandrogen				
Interferon				

A. Case Study for Antineoplastic Drugs

Wanda Woodbirch, a 36 year old patient with leukemia, has begun chemotherapy at the oncologist's office. She will need the following information.

1. Her therapy will include all of the following EXCEPT
   - a. Individualized dosage
   - b. Intermittent schedule
   - c. Radioactive iodine
   - d. Several drugs

2. She can expect all of the following side effects EXCEPT
   - a. Nausea
   - b. Alopecia
   - c. Constipation
   - d. Photosensitivity

3. Many antineoplastic drugs cause bone marrow depression, which can result in all of the following EXCEPT
   - a. Susceptibility to infection
   - b. Increased clotting time
   - c. Anemia
   - d. Jaundice

4. The following advice is appropriate EXCEPT
   - a. Practice good oral hygiene
   - b. Exercise briskly
   - c. Eat soft foods
   - d. Watch for hematuria

5. The following should be reported to the physician EXCEPT
   - a. Fever
   - b. Dyspnea
   - c. Blood in stools
   - d. Hair loss

B. Case Study for Antineoplastic Drugs

Ila Lake, a 40-year-old patient with metastatic breast cancer, will be followed by the oncologist. The nurse or medical assistant in the office will need the following information.

1. Appropriate treatment might include any of the following drugs EXCEPT
   - a. Interferon
   - b. Lupron
   - c. Tamoxifen
   - d. Taxol

2. The patient will need a supply of all of the following EXCEPT
   - a. Analgesics
   - b. Antiemetics
   - c. Diuretics
   - d. Antidiarrhea drugs

3. Monitoring of the following is necessary EXCEPT
   - a. Vital signs
   - b. Neuro signs
   - c. Hydration
   - d. Blood sugar

4. Patient education includes all of the following EXCEPT
   - a. Careful handwashing
   - b. Adequate fluids
   - c. Brush teeth briskly
   - d. Report air hunger

5. Health care workers who handle cytotoxic drugs should observe the following precautions EXCEPT
   - a. Wear gloves
   - b. Avoid pregnancy
   - c. Wear long-sleeved gowns
   - d. Dispose of waste in dumpster

CHAPTER 15

Urinary System Drugs

OBJECTIVES

Upon completion of this chapter, the student should be able to:

1. Compare and contrast the four types of diuretics for uses, side effects, cautions, and interactions and give examples of each type.
2. Define hypokalemia, hyperkalemia, calculus, diuretic, and uricosuric.
3. Describe two interactions of other medications with Benemid.
4. Identify one medication given for chronic gout that is not uricosuric and one that is.
5. Explain the role of certain antispasmodics used to reduce contractions of the urinary bladder.
6. Identify the actions of phenazopyridine (Pyridium) and bethanechol (Urecholine).
7. Describe appropriate patient education for all medications listed in this chapter.

Diuretics

The most commonly used drugs influencing function of the urinary tract are the diuretics, which increase urine excretion. Diuretics are divided into four categories according to their action: thiazides, loop diuretics, potassium-sparing diuretics, and osmotic agents. The type of diuretic used is determined by the condition of the patient.

THIAZIDES

Thiazides are the most frequently used type of diuretic, increasing excretion of water, sodium, chloride, and potassium. An example is chlorothiazide (Diuril).

Uses of the thiazides include treatment of:

Edema from many causes (e.g., heart failure and cirrhosis)

Hypertension (blood pressure is lowered by direct arterial dilation, as well as by decreasing fluid retention)

Prophylaxis of calculus (stone) formation in those with hypercalciuria (excess calcium in the urine)

Electrolyte imbalance from renal dysfunction (metolazone is diuretic of choice)

Side effects of the thiazides may include:

Hypokalemia (potassium deficiency), may lead to cardiac arrhythmias

Hypochloremia (chloride deficiency), may lead to alkalosis

Muscle weakness or spasm

GI reactions (e.g., anorexia, nausea, vomiting, diarrhea, and cramping)

Postural hypotension, vertigo, and headache

Fatigue, weakness, and lethargy

Skin conditions (e.g., rash and photosensitivity; rare)

Hyperglycemia and increased uric acid

Contraindications or caution applies to:

Diabetes (may cause hyperglycemia and glycosuria)

History of gout (increased uric acid level)

Severe renal disease

Impaired liver function

Prolonged use (periodic serum electrolyte checks indicated, and potassium supplements recommended to prevent hypokalemia)

Elderly, especially underweight (may cause low sodium)

Interactions may occur with:

Nonsteroidal anti-inflammatory agents—risk of renal failure

Corticosteroids to increase potassium loss

Lithium, to cause lithium intoxication

Hypotensive agents, which potentiate blood pressure decrease

Digitalis with increased potential for digitalis toxicity

Probenecid (Benemid) to block uric acid retention

Alcohol, barbiturates, and opiates to increase postural hypotension

Amphetamines or quinidine, toxicity risk

PATIENT EDUCATION

Patients being treated with thiazides should be instructed regarding:

Diet including potassium-rich foods (e.g., citrus fruits and bananas) or potassium supplements (check with the physician first).
If diuretic prescribed for hypertension, a low-sodium diet (may be prescribed by the physician).
Notifying the physician of persistent or severe side effects.
Administration with food (to reduce gastric irritation) at least 6 hours before bedtime.
Rising slowly from reclining position to counteract postural hypotension.
Limitation of alcohol.
Avoiding other medications without consulting physician.

LOOP DIURETICS

These diuretics act directly on the loop of Henle in the kidney to inhibit sodium and chloride reabsorption. Potent diuretics such as furosemide (Lasix), bumetanide (Bumex) and ethacrynic acid (Edecrin) are not thiazides but act in a similar way to increase excretion of water, sodium, chloride, and potassium. Their action is more rapid and effective than that of thiazides, with a greater diuresis.

Uses of loop diuretics, such as furosemide (Lasix), bumetanide (Bumex), torsemide (Demadex), and ethacrynic acid (Edecrin), include treatment of:

Edema associated with impaired renal function or hepatic disease
Congestive heart failure
Pulmonary edema
Ascites caused by malignancy or cirrhosis
Hypertension (if thiazides ineffective, furosemide or ethacrynic acid sometimes combined with other antihypertensives)

Side effects of furosemide, bumetanide, and ethacrynic acid may include:

Fluid and electrolyte imbalance with dehydration, circulatory collapse, chest pain
Hypokalemia with weakness and vertigo (potassium supplements indicated especially for cardiac patients to prevent arrhythmias)
Hypotension (close blood pressure checks required)
GI effects, including anorexia, nausea, vomiting, diarrhea, and abdominal pain
Hyperglycemia and increased uric acid
Blood dyscrasias with prolonged use
Tinnitus, hearing impairment, and blurred vision
Rash, urticaria, pruritis, and photosensitivity

Allergic reactions to furosemide in those allergic to sulfa, since furosemide and bumetanide are *sulfonamides*

Headache, muscle cramps, mental confusion, dizziness

Contraindications or caution with bumetanide, furosemide and ethacrynic acid applies to:

Cirrhosis and other liver disease—careful monitoring required

Kidney impairment

Alkalosis and dehydration

Digitalized patients (cardiac arrhythmias possible unless potassium supplemented)

Those allergic to sulfa

Diabetes

History of gout

Pregnancy and lactation

Children under 18 years of age

Note: Torsemide (Demadex) must be given with a potassium-sparing diuretic to prevent hypokalemia and metabolic acidosis, especially in patients with cirrhosis of the liver.

Interactions are similar to those of the thiazides:

Corticosteroids—potentiate potassium loss

Lithium—toxicity risk increased

Hypotensive agents—potentiation of effects

Probenecid—may decrease diuretic effects

Alcohol, barbiturates, and opiates

Digitalis with increased potential for digitalis toxicity and arrhythmias

Additional interactions of furosemide, bumetanide, and ethacrynic acid may include:

Aminoglycosides increase chance of deafness

Indomethacin decreases diuretic effect

Salicylates with furosemide increase chance of salicylate toxicity

Anticonvulsants (e.g., phenytoin) reduce the diuretic effect of furosemide

PATIENT EDUCATION

Patients being treated with loop diuretics should be instructed regarding the same information as patients taking thiazides:

Dietary or other potassium supplements as prescribed.

Notifying the physician of side effects *immediately.*

Taking with food before 6 P.M.

Rising slowly from reclining position.

Avoiding alcohol.

Reporting sudden changes in urinary output, especially decrease.

Reporting abrupt or severe weight loss.

Limiting exposure to sunlight with furosemide, due to photosensitivity.

Not taking any other prescribed or over-the-counter drugs without consulting the physician first.

POTASSIUM-SPARING DIURETICS

Potassium-sparing diuretics such as spironolactone (Aldactone) and triamterene (Dyrenium), are sometimes administered under conditions in which potassium depletion can be dangerous. Potassium-sparing diuretics also counteract the increased glucose and uric acid levels associated with thiazide diuretic therapy.

Potassium-sparing diuretics are seldom used alone, but are usually combined with thiazide diuretics to increase the diuretic and hypotensive effects and to reduce the danger of hyperkalemia (excessive potassium retention). When combination products (e.g., Aldactazide or Dyazide) are given, supplemental potassium is usually *not* indicated, but this varies with individual circumstances and other medications taken concomitantly. Periodic serum electrolyte checks are indicated.

Side effects of potassium-saving diuretics are usually mild and respond to withdrawal of the drug, but may include:

Hyperkalemia (especially with potassium supplements), which may lead to cardiac arrhythmias

Dehydration or weakness

GI symptoms, including nausea, vomiting, and diarrhea

Fatigue, lethargy, and profound weight loss

Hypotension

Caution is indicated in patients with:

Renal insufficiency

Cirrhosis and other liver disease

Pregnancy and lactation

Interactions may occur with:

Potassium supplements to cause hyperkalemia
Beta-blockers to potentiate blocking effects
Penicillin G potassium to cause hyperkalemia

PATIENT EDUCATION

Patients being treated with potassium-sparing diuretics should be instructed regarding:

Avoidance of potassium-rich foods and salt substitutes.
Reporting signs of excessive dehydration (e.g., dry mouth, drowsiness, lethargy, and fever).
Reporting GI symptoms (e.g., nausea, vomiting, and diarrhea).
Reporting persistent headache and mental confusion.
Monitoring weight and reporting sudden, excessive weight loss.
Rising slowly from reclining position.
Taking medications after meals.

OSMOTIC AGENTS

Osmotic agents (e.g., mannitol and urea) are most frequently used to reduce intracranial or intraocular pressure. Mannitol has also been used to prevent and/or treat acute renal failure and during certain cardiovascular surgery. Mannitol is also used alone or with other diuretics to promote excretions of toxins in cases of drug poisoning.

Side effects can include:

Fluid and electrolyte imbalance
CNS symptoms, including headache, vertigo, mental confusion, nausea, and vomiting
Tachycardia, hypertension, and hypotension
Allergic reactions

Extreme caution is indicated, and kidney and cardiovascular function should be evaluated before administration of these drugs to anyone with:

Kidney failure
Cardiovascular disease
Liver disease
Pregnancy and lactation

Interactions may occur with mannitol to increase urinary excretion of other drugs. Blood levels of drugs such as lithium are lowered as a result.

TABLE 15.1. DRUGS FOR DIURESIS

Generic Name	Trade Name	Dosage (varies with condition)
Thiazide Diuretics (representative list—many others)		
chlorothiazide	Diuril	500 mg–2 g qd PO
hydrochlorothiazide	Esidrix	25–50 mg bid or tid
metolazone	Diulo, Zaroxolyn	Individualized
Loop Diuretics		
ethacrynic acid	Edecrin	50–100 mg qd or bid, varies
furosemide	Lasix	20–80 mg qd, PO, IM, or IV
bumetanide	Bumex	0.5–2 mg qd, PO, IM, or IV
torsemide	Demadex	5–20 mg qd, PO; **slow** IV IV dosage not to exceed 200 mg
Potassium-Sparing Diuretics		
spironolactone	Aldactone	50–100 mg qd
triamterene	Dyrenium	100 mg bid pc
Combination Potassium-Sparing and Thiazide Diuretics		
spironolactone and hydrochlorothiazide	Aldactazide, Spironazide	50–100 mg qd
triamterene and hydrochlorothiazide (co-triamterzide)	Dyazide, Maxzide	1 cap bid
Osmotic Agents		
mannitol	Osmitrol	Parenteral only, dose varies with condition
urea	Ureaphil	Parenteral only, dose varies with condition

PATIENT EDUCATION

Patients being treated with osmotic agents should be instructed regarding side effects to be reported to the physician immediately. The patient should be reassured that osmotic agents are always given under close medical supervision and serum electrolytes will be monitored frequently by blood tests to detect adverse reactions.

See Table 15.1 for a summary of drugs for diuresis.

Medications for Gout

Medications to treat gout include uricosuric agents and allopurinol, which lower uric acid levels.

URICOSURIC AGENTS

Uricosuric agents, such as probenecid (Benemid), act on the kidney by blocking reabsorption and promoting urinary excretion of uric acid. This type of drug is used in the treatment of *chronic* cases of gout and frequent disabling attacks of gouty arthritis. However, the uricosuric agents have no analgesic or anti-inflammatory activity and are therefore *not* effective in the treatment of acute gout. During acute attacks of gout, the probenecid dosage is supplemented with colchicine, which has anti-inflammatory action. Probenecid is a sulfonamide derivative and can cause hypersensitivity reactions in those allergic to sulfa.

Probenecid is sometimes given with penicillin to potentiate the level of the antibiotic in the blood, for example, with amoxicillin for some gonococcal infections. Probenecid is also given with cephoxitin to treat acute pelvic inflammatory disease.

Side effects of probenecid are rare but may include:

Headache

Nausea and vomiting

Kidney stones and renal colic if large volume of fluids not maintained

Hypersensitivity reactions, rash, hypotension and anaphylaxis, are rare

Contraindication applies to patients with:

History of uric acid kidney stones

History of peptic ulcer

Renal impairment

Blood dyscrasias

Interactions may occur with:

Penicillins and cephalosporins, which *potentiate* antibiotic effect

Oral hypoglycemics, which could cause hypoglycemia through potentiation

Salicylates, which antagonize uricosuric action

PATIENT EDUCATION

Patients being treated with uricosuric agents should be instructed regarding:

Drinking large amounts of fluid.

Avoiding taking any aspirin products.

Taking other medications at the same time only with physician's order.

Taking medications with food.

Reporting rash immediately.

ALLOPURINOL

Allopurinol (Zyloprim) is another medication, not a uricosuric, used to treat chronic gout. This drug acts by decreasing serum and urine levels of uric acid. It has no analgesic or anti-inflammatory activity, and therefore is *not* effective in the treatment of acute gout. **Note:** The drug of choice for acute cases of gout or gouty arthritis is *colchicine,* which is discussed in Chapter 21.

Allopurinol is also used for the prevention of renal calculi in patients with a history of frequent stone formation.

Side effects can include:

Rash

Allergic reactions, including fever, chills, nausea, vomiting, diarrhea, drowsiness, and vertigo

Severe hypersensitivity reactions rare

Contraindications or caution applies to:

Impaired renal function

History of hypersensitivity reactions

Liver disease

Pregnancy and lactation

Interactions may occur with:

Antineoplastic drugs, potentiating side effects

Alcohol and diuretics, which increase serum urate concentrations

---

PATIENT EDUCATION

Patients being treated with allopurinol should be instructed regarding:

Drinking large quantities of fluid.

Taking medication after meals.

Stopping medication and reporting rash to physician immediately.

Avoiding alcohol, which increases uric acid.

Avoiding other medications unless prescribed by physician.

Antispasmodics

Antispasmodics, which are anticholinergic in action (blocking parasympathetic nerve impulses), are used to reduce the strength and frequency of contractions of the urinary bladder. Antispasmodics, such as methantheline (Banthine), are used to increase the bladder capacity in patients with neurogenic bladder resulting in incontinence.

Other drugs, chemically similar, which exert spasmolytic effects on smooth muscle, include flavoxate (Urispas) and oxybutynin (Ditropan). They are used for the relief of symptoms such as urgency, frequency, nocturia, and incontinence. They have similar adverse side effects, especially in geriatric patients.

Side effects are anticholinergic in action and can include:

Drying of all secretions
Drowsiness and dizziness
Urinary retention
Constipation
Blurred vision
Mental confusion (especially in geriatric patients)
Tachycardia, palpitations
Nausea and vomiting
Rash, urticaria, allergic reactions

Cautions with antispasmodics for:

Geriatric patients
Hepatic or renal disease
Cardiovascular disease
Prostatic hypertrophy
Children under 5 years old—contraindicated
Pregnant or nursing women

PATIENT EDUCATION

Patients being treated with antispasmodics should be instructed regarding:

Reporting side effects that are troublesome for possible dosage adjustment.
Reporting effectiveness.
Using caution driving or operating machinery.
Avoiding alcohol or other sedatives that potentiate drowsiness.

Analgesics

Phenazopyridine (Pyridium) is an analgesic or local anesthetic for urinary tract mucosa. It is used to relieve burning, pain, discomfort, and urgency associated with cystitis; with procedures causing irritation to the lower urinary tract, such as cystoscopy and surgery; or with trauma.

Phenazopyridine is used *only for symptomatic relief* and is not a substitute for treatment of causative conditions. For treatment of urinary tract infections, anti-infective medication is required. See Chapter 17.

Side effects are rare for the most part but can include:

Headache or vertigo

Mild GI disturbances

Orange-red urine (common)—may stain fabric

Flavoxate (Urispas) also exhibits anesthetic and analgesic properties for symptomatic relief, but is not a substitute for antibiotic treatment of urinary tract infections.

Contraindications for urinary analgesics include:

Impaired kidney function

Severe hepatitis

Phenazopyridine may interfere with various urine, kidney function, or liver function tests.

PATIENT EDUCATION

Patients being treated with phenazopyridine (Pyridium) for unirary tract distress should be instructed regarding color change of urine to orange-red, which may stain fabric.

Phenazopyridine is only temporarily effective against discomfort in the lower urinary tract and is *not* effective against infection. The cause of the discomfort must be determined by examination of urine culture, and appropriate therapy, such as surgery or anti-infective medication, may be given to correct the condition.

Cholinergics

Bethanechol (Urecholine) is a cholinergic drug, stimulating parasympathetic nerves, to bring about contraction of the urinary bladder in cases of nonobstructive urinary retention, usually postoperatively or postpartum. It has been called the "pharmacological catheterization."

Side effects are cholinergic in action and usually dose related, and can include:

GI cramping, diarrhea, nausea, and vomiting

Sweating and salivation

Headache and bronchial constriction

Bradycardia

Contraindications include:

Obstruction of the GI or urinary tract

Hyperthyroidism

Peptic ulcer

Asthma

Cardiovascular disease

Pregnancy and lactation

Interactions may occur with:

Other cholinergic or anticholinesterase agents (e.g., neostigmine) administered concomitantly, which can potentiate effects, with increased possibility of toxicity

Beta-blockers, which may result in critical fall in blood pressure

Quinidine or procainamide, which antagonize cholinergic effect

Atropine, which antagonizes cholinergic effect (antidote in cases of cholinergic toxicity

Treatment of Benign Prostatic Hypertrophy (BPH)

Finasteride (Proscar) is used to reduce prostate size and associated urinary obstruction and manifestations, for example, urgency, nocturia, and urinary hesitancy in patients with BPH. Proscar 5 mg is administered daily for a minimum of 6–12 months. This therapy appears to be suppressive rather than curative, and return of the hypertrophy is likely if the drug is withdrawn.

Side effects are infrequent and mild, including impotence, decreased libido, decreased ejaculate.

Cautions: Patients should be screened first for cancer, infection or other urinary dysfunctions. Liver function abnormalities may be exacerbated. Crushed tablets should not be handled by pregnant women, (causes fetal damage).

TABLE 15.2. OTHER DRUGS AFFECTING THE URINARY TRACT

Generic Name	Trade Name	Dosage
Uricosuric Agents		
probenecid	Benemid	250–500 mg bid
sulfinpyrazone	Anturane	100–200 mg bid
Antigout Medication		
allopurinol	Zyloprim, Lopurin	200–600 mg qd
Antispasmodic		
methantheline	Banthine	50–100 mg qid PO
flavoxate	Urispas	100–200 mg tid or qid
oxybutynin	Ditropan	5 mg bid or tid Children over 5, 5 mg bid
Analgesics		
phenazopyridine	Pyridium, Azo Standard	200 mg tid pc
flavoxate	Urispas	100–200 mg tid or qid
Cholinergic[a]		
bethanechol	Urecholine	PO or SC, never IM or IV Dose according to condition Administer PO on empty stomach

[a]For bladder contraction.

Worksheet for Chapter 15

URINARY SYSTEM DRUGS

List the drugs according to category and complete all columns. Learn generic or trade names as specified by instructor.

Classifications and Drugs	Purpose	Side Effects	Contraindications or Cautions	Patient Education
Thiazides 1. 2.				
Loop Diuretics 1. 2.				
Potassium-Sparing Diuretics 1. 2.				
Combination Potassium-Sparing and Thiazide Diuretics 1. 2.				
Osmotic Agents 1.				

Classifications and Drugs	Purpose	Side Effects	Contraindications or Cautions	Patient Education
Uricosuric Agents 1.				
Antigout Medication 1.				
Antispasmodic 1. 2. 3.				
Analgesic 1.				
Cholinergic 1.				
BPH treatment				

A. Case Study for Urinary System Drugs

Peter Moore, a 60-year-old diabetic with a history of heart disease and hypertension, comes to the clinic complaining of swollen ankles, shortness of breath, weakness, and nausea. He is taking Diuril. You will need to answer his questions with the following information.

1. Diuril causes increased excretion of all of the following EXCEPT
   a. Sodium
   b. Sugar
   c. Chloride
   d. Potassium

2. Side effects of the thiazides can include all of the following EXCEPT
   a. Fatigue
   b. Nausea
   c. Muscle spasms
   d. Low blood sugar

3. He should be given all of the following advice EXCEPT
   a. Rise slowly
   b. Eat citrus
   c. Take diuretic before meals
   d. Avoid salty foods

4. Because of the edema he will probably be put on a more potent loop diuretic, such as
   a. Dyazide
   b. Osmitrol
   c. Esidrix
   d. Lasix

5. Patients like Mr. Moore taking loop diuretics should be given all of the following advice EXCEPT
   a. Avoid sunlight
   b. Avoid alcohol
   c. Take medicine at bedtime
   d. Check blood sugar

B. Case Study for Urinary System Drugs

Mrs. Reah Nell, an 85-year-old Alzheimer's patient, with cardiac arrhythmias, is brought to the physician's office by her daughter with a request for medication to decrease her mother's incontinence. She will need the following information:

1. The following medications can reduce bladder contractions EXCEPT
   a. Urecholine
   b. Urispas
   c. Ditropan
   d. Banthine

2. Side effects of the antispasmodics can include all of the following EXCEPT
   a. Constipation
   b. Drooling
   c. Blurred vision
   d. Mental confusion

3. Other side effects can include all of the following EXCEPT
   a. Nausea
   b. Dizziness
   c. Frequency
   d. Palpitations

4. Which of the following conditions would be treated with antispasmodics?
   a. Renal disease
   b. Kidney stones
   c. Prostatic hypertrophy
   d. Neurogenic bladder

5. Antispasmodics, for example, Ditropan, are contraindicated or used with caution in the following conditions EXCEPT
   a. Geriatrics
   b. Renal disease
   c. Neurogenic bladder
   d. Cardiovascular disease

CHAPTER **16**

Gastrointestinal Drugs

OBJECTIVES

Upon completion of this chapter, the student should be able to:

1. Define antiflatulent, antiemetic, laxative, and cathartic.
2. Describe side effects, contraindications, and interactions of antacids, antiulcer agents, antidiarrhea agents, antiflatulents, cathartics and laxatives, and antiemetics.
3. Compare and contrast the five types of laxatives according to use, side effects, contraindications, and interactions.
4. Identify examples of drugs from each of the seven categories of gastrointestinal drugs.
5. Explain important patient education for each category of gastrointestinal drugs.

Gastrointestinal drugs can be divided into seven categories based on the action: antacids, drugs for treatment of ulcers, management of inflammatory bowel disease, antidiarrhea agents, antiflatulents, laxatives and cathartics, and antiemetics.

Antacids

Antacids act by partially *neutralizing* gastric hydrochloric acid and are widely available in many over-the-counter preparations for the relief of indigestion, heartburn, and sour stomach. Antacids are also prescribed at times (between meals and at hour of sleep) to help relieve pain and promote the healing of gastric and duodenal ulcers. Other antiulcer agents are discussed later in this chapter. Antacids are also used at times in the management of esophageal reflux.

Antacid products may contain aluminum, calcium carbonate, or magnesium, either individually or in combination. Most antacids also contain sodium. Sodium bicarbonate alone is not recommended because of flatulence, metabolic alkalosis, and electrolyte imbalance with prolonged use. Calcium carbonate may cause acid rebound and its use is controversial.

The choice of a specific antacid preparation depends on palatability, cost, adverse effects, acid neutralizing capacity, the sodium content, and the patient's renal and cardiovascular function. Magnesium and/or aluminum antacids are the most commonly used. Magnesium can cause diarrhea and aluminum is constipating. Therefore, combinations are frequently used to control the frequency and consistency of bowel movements.

Side effects of antacids may include:

Constipation (with aluminum or calcium carbonate antacids)

Diarrhea (with magnesium antacids)

Acid rebound (with calcium carbonate)

Electrolyte imbalance

Urinary calculi and renal complications

Osteoporosis (with aluminum antacids)

Belching and flatulence (with calcium carbonate and sodium bicarbonate)

Contraindications or extreme caution applies to:

Congestive heart failure

Renal pathology or history of renal calculi

Cirrhosis of the liver or edema

Dehydration or electrolyte imbalance

Interactions with almost any other drug administered concurrently can alter the effectiveness of the other drugs. Therefore, antacids should not be taken within 2 hours of any other drug. With the following drugs, antacids may decrease effectiveness of the drug:

Antibiotics, especially tetracyclines

Digoxin, indomethacin, and iron

Salicylates and isoniazid

Antacids with the following drugs may increase action and precipitate side effects:

Dicumarol, which increases bleeding risk

Diazepam, which increases sedation

Amphetamines and quinidine, which increase cardiac irregularities

---

PATIENT EDUCATION

Patients taking antacids should be instructed regarding:

Avoiding prolonged use (no longer than 2 weeks) of OTC antacids without medical supervision because of the danger of masking symptoms of GI bleeding or GI malignancy.

Avoiding the use of antacids at the same time as any other medication because of many interactions.

Avoiding the use of antacids entirely if patient has cardiac, renal, or liver disease or fluid retention.

Patients taking medicines in the management of esophageal reflux should also be instructed regarding avoidance of constrictive clothing, treatment of obesity (if appropriate), reducing meal size, avoiding recumbency after meals, and elevating the head of the bed.

Agents for Treatment of Ulcers and Gastroesophageal Reflux Disease

Some antiulcer agents *reduce gastric acid secretion* by acting as *histamine$_2$ receptor antagonists*. Two of the drugs in this category, cimetidine (Tagamet) and ranitidine (Zantac), are used in the treatment of duodenal ulcers, gastric ulcers, GI hypersecretory conditions, short-term relief of gastroesophageal reflux (GERD), and upper GI bleeding or esophagitis. Other histamine receptor antagonists include famotidine (Pepcid) and nizatidine (Axid). Fewer adverse reactions have been reported with these two newer drugs.

Side effects, usually transient and dose related, can include:

Diarrhea, dizziness, rash, and headache
Mild gynecomastia (not with Pepcid or Axid)
Mental confusion (especially in the elderly)—not with Pepcid or Axid

Contraindications or extreme caution applies to:

Impaired renal function
Liver dysfunction
Children, pregnancy, and lactation

Interactions of Tagamet and Zantac may occur with increased blood concentrations of:

Coumarin anticoagulants
Phenytoin

Propranolol

Diazepam

Lidocaine

Theophylline

There is low potential for drug interactions with Pepcid and Axid. Interaction of Pepcid with food enhances the action slightly.

Misoprostol (Cytotec), a synthetic analog of prostaglandin E_1, inhibits gastric acid secretion and protects the mucosa from the irritant effect of certain drugs, for example, nonsteroidal anti-inflammatory drugs (NSAIDs—see Chapter 21), especially in those at risk, for example, elderly or those with a history of gastric ulcers. It is not recommended for the treatment of gastric or duodenal ulcers.

Side effects of Cytotec can include:

Diarrhea, nausea, and abdominal pain

Menstrual irregularities

Spontaneous abortion, possibly incomplete, with potentially dangerous uterine bleeding, maternal or fetal death

Contraindications include:

Women of child-bearing age

Pregnant women

Children under age 12

Interactions with food and antacids decrease the rate of absorption. Therefore, it is recommended that misoprostol be given on an empty stomach. Antacids should be given at least 2 hours away and should not be of a magnesium type.

Omeprazole (Prilosec) is a gastric antisecretory agent, unrelated to the H_2-receptor antagonists. It is used for the short-term (4–8 weeks) symptomatic relief of gastroesophageal reflux disease (GERD), for the short-term treatment of *confirmed* active duodenal ulcer, and for erosive esophagitis.

Side effects can include:

Diarrhea, constipation, nausea, vomiting, abdominal pain

Headache, dizziness

Interactions may occur with:

Diazepam

Warfarin

Phenytoin

Ampicillin

Iron

Sucralfate (Carafate), an inhibitor of pepsin, is another antiulcer agent that acts in a different way. Sucralfate is *administered on an empty stomach* and then reacts with hydrochloric acid in the stomach to form a paste that adheres to the mucosa, thus protecting the ulcer from irritation. The therapeutic effects of the drug result from local (i.e., at the ulcer site) rather than systemic activity.

Side effects of sucralfate are rare with constipation occurring occasionally.

Interactions are possible with sucralfate altering absorption and, therefore, other drugs should not be given within 2 hours of sucralfate.

Patients with recurrent or refractory peptic ulcer disease (i.e., resistance to standard antiulcer therapies: antacids, H_2-receptor antagonists, sucralfate), with failure to heal within 12 weeks, or with frequent recurrences, unrelated to NSAID, may be suffering from infection with *Helicobacter pylori*. Such infection has been treated successfully with multiple-drug regimens combining amoxicillin with omeprazole (Prilosec), or combining amoxicillin with metronidazole (antibacterial and antiprotozoal) and bismuth salicylate. This treatment and possible side effects are discussed further in Chapter 17.

PATIENT EDUCATION FOR THOSE UNDERGOING ULCER THERAPY

Patients should be instructed regarding:

Avoidance of cigarette smoking, which seems to decrease the effectiveness of medicines in the healing of duodenal ulcers.

Importance of close communication with the physician for possible dosage regulation of other medications taken at the same time.

Structuring of environment to reduce stress factors and decrease tension in order to facilitate healing of ulcers and reduce gastric motility and hypersecretion, as an adjunct to drug therapy.

Not taking antacids, if ordered, within 2 hours of taking cimetidine, ranitidine, or any other drug.

Taking medications on a regular basis and avoiding abrupt withdrawal, which could lead to rebound hypersecretion of gastric acid.

Taking sucralfate (Carafate) 1 hour before meals, on an empty stomach, and not within 2 hours of any other medicine.

Taking omeprazole (Prilosec) before meals and swallowing the capsule intact without opening, chewing, or crushing it.

Taking misoprostol (Cytotec) after meals and at bedtime, and avoiding magnesium products to lessen incidence of diarrhea.

For Inflammatory Bowel Disease

Mesalamine (Rowasa) exhibits anti-inflammatory activity in the GI tract. It is used in the management of ulcerative colitis. The exact mechanisms are unclear, but the actions include the reduction of prostaglandin concentrations in the colon, and seem to be local rather than systemic. Mesalamine is usually administered rectally as suppositories twice a day or as a retention enema at bedtime to be retained for 8 hours. The patient should be given a copy of the administration instructions provided by the manufacturer.

Side effects can include:

Abdominal pain, cramps, and/or discomfort
Headache, weakness, dizziness

Caution applies to:

Renal impairment
Allergy to sulfites (can cause anaphylaxis or asthma attack)

Antidiarrhea Agents

Antidiarrhea agents act in various ways to reduce the number of loose stools.

KAOLIN AND PECTIN

Kaolin and pectin preparations (e.g., Kaopectate) act as *adsorbents and protectants* to achieve a drying effect (i.e., decrease fluidity of stools). Sometimes paregoric (opium) is combined with these products for short-term use only.

Side effects are relatively nonexistent, other than transient constipation on occasion.

Interactions are possible, such as impaired absorption, when these agents are administered concurrently with such other medications as:

Lincomycin
Digoxin

Contraindications, without medical supervision, may occur in infants and the elderly.

PATIENT EDUCATION

Patients with diarrhea should be instructed regarding:

Avoiding self-medication for longer than 48 hours, or if fever develops, without consulting a physician.

Diet of a bland nature, excluding roughage, and including foods containing natural pectin (e.g., apple *without* peelings and without sugar added to apple).

Adequate fluid intake (especially tea *without* sugar for its astringent effect) or Gatorade to prevent dehydration.

Contacting the physician immediately if complications develop or condition worsens.

Taking other medications (e.g., antibiotics or digitalis) 2–3 hours before or after taking kaolin and pectin products.

DIPHENOXYLATE WITH ATROPINE AND LOPERAMIDE

Diphenoxylate with atropine (Lomotil), and loperamide (Imodium) act by slowing *intestinal motility*.

Side effects can include:

With Lomotil, anticholinergic effects (e.g., drying of secretions, blurred vision, urinary retention, lethargy, confusion, or flushing)

With Lomotil or Imodium, abdominal distention, nausea, or vomiting

Contraindications include:

Diarrhea caused by infection or poisoning

Young children and pregnancy

Colitis associated with broad-spectrum antibiotics

Ulcerative colitis

Cirrhosis

Caution with the elderly.

PATIENT EDUCATION

Patients taking anti-diarrhea agents should be instructed regarding:

Not exceeding the recommended dosage; short-term-only.

Adequate fluid intake and bland diet.

Reporting side effects or complications to the physician immediately, or if symptoms persist.

Not taking these medications if diarrhea caused by infection or food poisoning. In this instance kaolin and pectin preparations are preferable.

LACTOBACILLUS ACIDOPHILUS

Lactobacillus acidophilus (Lactinex) is an acid-producing bacterium in culture administered orally for simple diarrhea caused by antibiotics, infection, irritable colon, colostomy, or amebiasis. The capsules, tablets, or granules may be taken, or mixed with, cereal, food, juice, or water.

Contraindications apply to:

Anyone with a high fever
Those sensitive to milk products
Long-term use

Antiflatulents

Antiflatulents (e.g., simethicone) are used in the symptomatic treatment of gastric bloating and postoperative gas pains, by helping to break up gas bubbles in the GI tract.

No side effects have been reported.

Contraindications apply to infant colic because of limited information on safety in children.

PATIENT EDUCATION

Patients troubled with flatulence should be instructed to avoid gas-forming foods (e.g., onions, cabbage, and beans).

See Table 16.1 for a summary of Antacids, Antiulcer Agents, Antidiarrhea Agents, and Antiflatulents.

Laxatives and Cathartics

Laxatives promote evacuation of the intestine. Included in the laxative category are *cathartics*, or *purgatives*, which promote rapid evacuation of the intestine and alteration of stool consistency. Laxatives can be subdivided into six categories according to their action: bulk-forming laxatives, stool softeners, mineral oil, saline laxatives, stimulant laxatives, and hyperosmotic laxatives.

Many OTC laxatives are self-prescribed and overused by a large portion of the population. Prevention and relief of constipation is better achieved through natural methods (e.g., high-fiber diet, adequate fluid intake, good bowel habits, and exercise). Normal frequency of bowel movements varies from daily to several times weekly. When constipation occurs, the cause should be identified before laxatives are used.

TABLE 16.1. ANTACIDS, ANTIULCER AGENTS, ANTIDIARRHEA AGENTS, AND ANTIFLATULENTS

Generic Name	Trade Name	Dosage
Antacids (only a sample, many other products available)		
aluminum	Amphojel	Suspension, 320 mg /5 ml Tabs, 300–600 mg
calcium carbonate	Tums	Tabs, 500–750 mg, also liquid
aluminum-magnesium combinations	Riopan, Maalox, Gelusil, Mylanta	Suspension, tabs, dose varies with product
Agents for Ulcers and GERD		
famotidine	Pepcid	40 mg PO tabs qhs, 20 mg IV diluted
nizatidine	Axid	150 mg bid PO
ranitidine	Zantac	150 mg tabs bid
cimetidine	Tagamet	200–300 mg q6h PO or IV
sucralfate	Carafate	1 g qid 1 h ac and hs
omeprazole	Prilosec	20 mg q AM ac SR cap
misoprostol	Cytotec	200 mg tab qid pc and hs
For Inflammatory Bowel Disease		
mesalamine	Rowasa	50 mg R supp bid, retention enema 4g/60 ml q hs
Antidiarrhea Agents		
diphenoxylate with atropine	Lomotil	Sol or tabs, 2.5–5 mg qid
kaolin and pectin	Kaopectate	Suspension, 45–90 ml after each bowel movement
loperamide	Imodium	2 mg after each bowel movement solution, tabs, caps maximum 16 mg qd
lactobacillus acidophilus	Lactinex	2 caps, 4 tabs, or 1 pkg granules 3 or 4 × qd
Antiflatulent		
simethicone	Mylicon	Suspension, tabs pc and hs 150–400 mg qd in divided doses

BULK-FORMING LAXATIVES

Bulk-forming laxatives (e.g., psyllium, cellulose derivatives, karaya, malt soup extract, and bran) are the treatment of choice for simple constipation unrelieved by natural methods. These products are available in powders, flakes, granules, tablets, or liquids and *must be dissolved and/or diluted* according to manufacturers' directions (note label). The usual procedure is to dissolve the product in one *full glass* of water or juice to be taken orally and followed immediately with another glass of fluid. The proper dosage is administered 1 to 3 times per day. Laxative effect is usually, apparent within 12–24 h.

Bulk-forming laxatives are the choice for geriatric or laxative-dependent patients. Bulk-forming laxatives have been useful in maintaining regularity for patients with diverticulosis and have also been used to increase the bulk of stools in patients with chronic, watery diarrhea.

Contraindications apply to patients with acute abdominal pain, partial bowel obstruction, dysphagia, or esophageal obstruction.

PATIENT EDUCATION

Patients taking bulk-forming laxatives should be instructed regarding *dissolving all bulk-forming products completely* in one full glass of liquid and following that with another glass of fluid to prevent obstruction.

STOOL SOFTENERS

Stool softeners (e.g., docusate) are another mild form of laxative administered orally. Dosage required to soften stools varies widely depending on the condition and patient response. Stool softeners are the choice for pregnant or nursing women and children with hard, dry stools.

Side effects are rare, with occasional mild, transitory GI cramping or rash.

Contraindications include acute abdominal pain or prolonged use (more than 1 week) without medical supervision

Caution to avoid stool softeners that also contain stimulant laxatives, for example, Peri-Colace, Correctol.

PATIENT EDUCATION

Patients taking stool softeners should be instructed regarding:

Discontinuance with any signs of diarrhea or abdominal pain.
Avoiding use for longer than 1 week without medical supervision.
Interaction with mineral oil, which leads to mucosal irritation.
Taking large quantities of fluids to soften stool..

MINERAL OIL

Mineral oil may be administered orally in emulsion form for palatability (e.g., Agoral) and is usually effective in 6–8 h. Mineral oil is sometimes administered rectally as an oil-retention enema (60-150 ml).

Side effects may include:

Seepage of oil from rectum, causing anal irritation
Malabsorption of vitamins A, D, E, and K only with prolonged oral use

Contraindications for oral mineral oil include:

Children under 6 years old
Bedridden, debilitated, or geriatric patients
Patients with dysphagia, gastric retention, or hiatal hernia
Pregnancy
Prolonged use
Concomitant use of stool softeners

PATIENT EDUCATION

Patients taking mineral oil should be instructed regarding:
Avoiding frequent or prolonged use.
Caution with anyone who might have trouble swallowing or who might aspirate
the oil.

SALINE LAXATIVES

Saline laxatives (e.g., milk of magnesia) should be taken only infrequently in single doses. Saline laxatives should never be taken on a regular or repeated basis.

Side effects of saline laxatives used for prolonged periods or in overdoses can include:

Electrolyte imbalance
CNS symptoms, including weakness, sedation, and confusion
Edema
Cardiac, renal, and hepatic complications

Contraindications include:

Long-term use
Congestive heart failure or other cardiac disease
Edema, cirrhosis, or renal disorders
Those taking diuretics
Acute abdominal pain
Colostomy

PATIENT EDUCATION

Patients taking saline laxatives should be instructed regarding:

Avoiding saline cathartics with the contraindicated medical conditions
Avoiding frequent or regular use of saline cathartics

STIMULANT LAXATIVES

Stimulant laxatives (e.g., senna, cascara, phenolphthalein, aloe, and bisacodyl) are cathartic in action, producing strong peristaltic activity, and may also alter intestinal secretions in several ways. Stimulant laxatives are habit-forming, and long-term use may result in laxative dependence and loss of normal bowel function. All stimulant laxatives produce some degree of abdominal discomfort. Their use should be confined to conditions in which rapid, thorough emptying of the bowel is required (e.g., before surgical, proctoscopic, sigmoidoscopic, or radiologic examinations, or for emptying the bowel of barium following GI X-rays). Sometimes a combination of oral preparations, suppositories, and/or enemas may be ordered for these purposes.

Side effects are common, especially with frequent use, and can include:

Abdominal cramps or discomfort and nausea (frequent)
Rectal and/or colonic irritation with suppositories
Loss of normal bowel function with prolonged use
Electrolyte disturbances with prolonged use
Pink, red, or brown discoloration to urine with aloe, cascara, senna, or phenolphthalein

Contraindications include:

Acute abdominal pain or abdominal cramping—danger of ruptured appendix
Ulcerative colitis
Children, pregnancy, and lactation
Long-term use

PATIENT EDUCATION

Patients taking stimulant laxatives should be given strong warnings against frequent or prolonged use because of danger of laxative dependence and loss of normal bowel function.

HYPEROSMOTIC LAXATIVES

When administered rectally, glycerin and sorbitol exert an action that draws water from the tissues into the feces and reflexively stimulates evacuation. Glycerin rectal suppositories or enemas usually cause evacuation of the colon within 15–30 minutes. Only extremely high doses of sorbitol exert laxative action (e.g., 120 ml of a 25–30% solution rectally or 15 ml of a 70% solution orally), resulting in diarrhea. Glycerin may produce rectal irritation or cramping pain.

PATIENT EDUCATION FOR THOSE TAKING ANY LAXATIVE

Patients should be instructed regarding:

High-fiber diet to prevent constipation, including roughage, (e.g., bran whole grain cereals, and fresh fruits and vegetables).

Adequate fluid intake.

Developing good bowel habits (e.g., regular, at an unrushed time of day).

Regular exercise to develop muscle tone.

Avoiding any laxative that causes acute abdominal pain, nausea, vomiting, or fever.

Avoiding laxatives if any medical condition is present, unless prescribed by a physician. Bulk-forming laxatives are safest for long term.

Use of only the mildest laxatives (e.g., stool softeners) on a short-term, infrequent basis.

Reporting any prolonged constipation, if above measures are ineffective, to a physician for investigation.

Antiemetics

Antiemetics are used in the prevention or treatment of nausea, vomiting, or motion sickness. Many different types of products are available, varying in their actions, the condition treated, and route of administration.

The three antiemetics used most frequently to control nausea and vomiting are Emete-Con or Compazine, and Tigan, which are related to the phenothiazine or antihistamines, discussed in Chapters 20 and 26. These drugs are used for symptomatic relief, and their use must be supplemented by restoration of fluid and electrolyte balance, as well as determination of the cause of vomiting.

Prochlorperazine (Compazine) is a phenothiazine that shows a high incidence of extrapyramidal reactions, especially in psychiatric patients receiving phenothiazines long term or in children. It is not recommended for children under 12. Caution with the elderly.

For preoperative preventive antiemetic effect or postoperative treatment for nausea and vomiting, a phenothiazine (e.g., Phenergan) is usually the drug of choice. Ondansetron (Zofran) and gransetron (Kytril) are also used preoperatively and for nausea with chemotherapy.

For treatment of motion sickness, preventive drugs such as dimenhydrinate (Dramamine) or scopolamine are used. For greatest effectiveness, the Transderm-Scop patch is applied behind the ear 4 h before anticipated exposure to motion and is effective up to 72 h. Dramamine is administered orally 30 min before exposure to motion. Both of these drugs are also available for intramuscular injection in patients who have already developed motion sickness.

Meclizine (Antivert) is an antihistamine used in the prevention and treatment of nausea, vomiting, and/or vertigo associated with motion sickness, and in the symptomatic treatment of vertigo associated with the vestibular system (e.g., Meniere's disease). The onset of action is about 1 hour and effects persist 8–24 hours after a single oral dose. Although meclizine produces fewer adverse anticholinergic effects than scopolamine, it can cause drowsiness, but to a lesser degree than dimenhydrinate (Dramamine). It is not recommended for children under 12.

Side effects of the antiemetics vary with the drug and dosage, but the most common include:

Confusion, anxiety, restlessness

Sedation, drowsiness, vertigo, weakness, depression

Dry mouth and blurred vision

Extrapyramidal reactions (involuntary movements), especially in children and the elderly with Compazine

Cardiac arrhythmias and hypertension with IV administration

Contraindications or extreme caution with antiemetics apply to:

Children and adolescents (increased risk of Reye's syndrome)—especially Compazine

Pregnancy and lactation

Debilitated, emaciated, or geriatric patients

Angle-closure glaucoma

Prostatic hypertrophy

Cardiac arrhythmias or hypertension

Seizure disorders

Interactions resulting in potentiation of a sedative effect occur with:

CNS depressants, including tranquilizers, hypnotics, analgesics, antipsychotics

Alcohol

Muscle relaxants

Metoclopramide (Reglan), a dopamine-receptor antagonist, is an antiemetic and a stimulant of upper GI motility. It accelerates gastric emptying and intestinal transit. It is used in a variety of GI motility disorders, especially gastric stasis, *short-term (up to 12 weeks)* treatment of gastroesophageal reflux disease (GERD), and for the prevention of cancer chemotherapy-induced emesis.

Side effects of metoclopramide can include:

Restlessness, drowsiness, fatigue, lassitude

Depression—can be severe

Extrapyramidal reactions, especially in children and young adults, or *irreversible* tardive dyskinesia, especially in geriatric women with long-term therapy

Caution or contraindications include:

Children or young adults

Geriatric patients, especially long term

Cisapride (Propulsid), a dopamine-receptor antagonist less potent than metoclopramide (Reglan), also stimulates upper GI motility. It is used in the symptomatic treatment of gastroesophageal reflux disease (GERD).

Side effects of cisapride can include:

Diarrhea, abdominal pain, constipation, flatulence, and rhinitis with 20 mg dosage

Rare cases of serious cardiac arrhythmias

Interactions

Antagonistic to cisapride:

Erythromycin, clarithromycin, and fluconazole

Anticholinergics

Cisapride can potentiate the effects of:

Benzodiazepines and alcohol-increased sedation

Anticoagulants—increased coagulation time

Contraindications:

Cardiac disease or arrhythmias

GI hemorrhage or obstruction

Concomitant administration with ketoconazole or miconazole—increases risk of cardiac arrhythmias

See Table 16.2 for a summary of laxatives and antiemetics.

PATIENT EDUCATION

Patients being treated with antiemetics should be instructed regarding:

Taking these medications under medical supervision.

Determining the cause of nausea and vomiting.

Reporting effectiveness or complications.

Administering only as directed.

Not combining with any other CNS depressants, alcohol, or muscle relaxants unless prescribed by a physician (e.g., with cancer patients).

TABLE 16.2. LAXATIVES AND ANTIEMETICS

Generic Name	Trade Name	Dosage
Laxatives (only a sample, many other products available)		
Bulk-forming psyllium	Metamucil, Konsyl-D, Fiberall, others	Powder, 1 tsp, dissolve in full glass of fluid 1–3 × day
Stool softener docusate	Surfak, Doxidan, Dialose, Colace, others	Oral caps, liquid 50–360 mg qd
Mineral oil	Agoral, Kondremul	15–45 ml PO
Saline laxatives	Milk of Magnesia	300–600 mg tabs 30–60 ml suspension
Stimulant laxatives cascara sagrada fluid extract		0.5–1.5 ml single dose
senna	X-prep, Senokot	7.5 mg or 5 ml single dose, 8.6 mg tab, or 7.5 mg sol
bisacodyl	Dulcolax	5–15 mg tabs 10 mg supp
phenolphthalein	Ex-Lax	30–270 mg tabs, only PRN
combinations	Correctol, Feen-A-Mint	Only single dose, not on reg. basis
Hyperosmotic Laxatives		
glycerin	glycerin supp. or enema	2–3 supp PRN 5–15 ml PRN
sorbitol	D-Glucitol	15 ml of 70% sol PO 120 ml of 25–30% sol R
Antiemetics		
benzquinamide	Emete-Con	50 mg IM q3–4h PRN
prochlorperazine	Compazine	PO, IM, IV, or supp, 25 mg 5–10 mg PO or IM qid
trimethobenzamide	Tigan	PO, IM, or supp 250 mg tid or qid
promethazine	Phenergan	Tabs, syrup, IM, or supp 25 mg
dimenhydrinate	Dramamine	PO or IM 50–100 mg q4h PRN for motion sickness
scopolamine	Transderm-Scop	0.5 mg patch q72h for motion sickness
meclizine	Antivert	25–50 mg qd, 1 h before motion 25–100 mg div. doses/Meniere's
metoclopramide	Reglan	PO, IM, IV, stimulates upper GI motility, dose varies with condition, see cautions
cisapride	Propulsid	10–20 mg qid ac and hs, stimulates upper GI motility

Worksheet for Chapter 16

GASTROINTESTINAL DRUGS

List the drugs according to category and complete all columns. Learn generic or trade names as specified by instructor.

Classifications and Drugs	Purpose	Side Effects	Contraindications or Cautions	Patient Education
Antacids 1. aluminum 2. calcium carbonate 3. aluminum/magnesium				
Antiulcer Agents 1. Tagamet and Zantac 2. Pepcid and Axid 3. Carafate 4. Cytotec 5. Prilosec				
For Inflammatory Bowel Disease Rowasa				
Antidiarrhea Agents 1. Kaopectate 2. Lomotil 3. Imodium 4. Lactinex				
Antiflatulent 1. Simethicone				

Classifications and Drugs	Purpose	Side Effects	Contraindications or Cautions	Patient Education
Bulk-forming Laxative 1.				
Stool softeners 1. 2.				
Saline Laxative 1.				
Stimulant Laxatives 1. 2. 3. 4.				
Antiemetics 1. 2. 3. 4. 5. 6.				
For Vertigo/Meniere's 1.				
Stimulate Upper GI Motility 1. 2.				

A. Case Study for Gastrointestinal Drugs

Homer Hill, a 55-year-old salesman, has been taking antacids for years for recurrent gastric distress. X-ray has confirmed a gastric ulcer. The following information will be helpful.

1. All of the following can result from antacids EXCEPT
   a. Gastric acid decrease
   b. Urinary calculi
   c. Constipation
   d. Diarrhea
2. All of the following are antiulcer drugs EXCEPT
   a. Axid
   b. Pepcid
   c. Rowasa
   d. Cytotec
3. All of the following are true of sucralfate (Carafate) EXCEPT
   a. Taken before meals
   b. Decreases gastric acid
   c. Coats the stomach
   d. Action is local
4. The following are true of Tagamet and Zantac EXCEPT
   a. Reduces gastric acid
   b. Used long-term for GERD
   c. Can cause confusion in elderly
   d. Can cause dizziness
5. Patients with recurrent, resistent peptic ulcers might be treated with a combination of all of the following EXCEPT
   a. Prilosec
   b. Amoxicillin
   c. Metronidazole
   d. Gentamycin

B. Case Study for Gastrointestinal Drugs

Ila Park, a 70-year-old woman, has been taking cathartics for years and they are now ineffective. She requests a new one she can take daily. She needs the following information.

1. The only laxative that should be taken daily is
   a. Dulcolax
   b. Senokot
   c. Metamucil
   d. Milk of Magnesia
2. Stimulant laxatives can cause all of the following EXCEPT
   a. Electrolyte imbalance
   b. Reduced peristalsis
   c. Dependence
   d. Cramping
3. The following is true of bulk-forming laxatives EXCEPT
   a. Given with liquids
   b. Useful for diverticulosis
   c. Used for chronic diarrhea
   d. Give only pc
4. The following is true of mineral oil (e.g., Kondremul) EXCEPT
   a. Can cause anal irritation
   b. Used with stool softener
   c. Can cause vitamin deficiency
   d. Contraindicated with dysphagia

5. Patient education includes all of the following EXCEPT
   a. Increase fluids
   b. High fiber diet
   c. Stool softeners used short term
   d. Milk of magnesia used long term

CHAPTER **17**

Anti-Infective Drugs

OBJECTIVES

Upon completion of this chapter, the student should be able to:

1. Define C & S, broad-spectrum, resistance, hypersensitivity, anaphylaxis, direct and indirect toxicity, and superinfection.
2. Identify side effects, contraindications, and interactions common to each category of anti-infectives.
3. Explain the unique features of patient education appropriate for each category of anti-infectives.
4. Describe general instructions that should be given to every patient undergoing anti-infective therapy.

Treatment of infection with medication is complicated by the great variety of these medications available and differing modes of action of the various drugs (e.g., bacteriostatic versus bactericidal). The first step in treatment is identification of the causative organism and the specific medication to which it is sensitive. *Culture and sensitivity tests (C & S)* will be ordered, based on symptoms (e.g., wound, throat, urine, or blood). It is imperative to obtain the appropriate specimen before administering medication. Results of C & S will not be available for 24–48 h. In the meantime, the physician will sometimes order a *broad-spectrum* antibiotic, one that is effective against a large variety of organisms.

Sometimes organisms build up *resistance* to drugs that have been used too frequently, and then the drugs are no longer effective. This explains why antibiotics are seldom used for the common cold, which is usually caused by a virus rather than bacteria anyway. Organisms can also become resistant if infections have been treated incompletely, as when the medication is discontinued before the required number of days to be fully effective.

As more anti-infective drugs become available and increased public awareness demands antibiotic treatment, many organisms are becoming resistant to more antibiotics, as shown by surveillance data from the U.S. Centers for Disease Control and Prevention (CDC). An example of an organism resistant to most antibiotics is methicillin-resistant *Staphylococcus aureus* (MRSA). Vancomycin IV is one of the very few drugs effective against MRSA, but can cause serious

269

adverse side effects, including ototoxicity and nephrotoxicity. The CDC also reports outbreaks of tuberculosis resistant to standard drug therapy. (See Antituberculosis Agents.) Some strains of organisms causing pneumonia, gonorrhea, and influenza are also becoming resistant to many antibiotics, for example, penicillins, tetracyclines, and others.

Therefore, it is the responsibility of the health care worker to explain *resistance* to the patient and discourage insistence on antibiotics when inappropriate, for example, for minor infections in otherwise healthy individuals.

Selection of anti-infective drugs is based on several factors:

1. *Status of hepatic and/or renal function.* Lower doses or alternate drugs might be indicated with impairment.
2. *Age of the patient.* Some anti-infectives are more toxic in children or the elderly. Lower doses or alternate drugs might be indicated.
3. *Pregnancy or lactation.* Some anti-infectives can cross the placenta and cause damage to the developing fetus, e.g. tetracycline or streptomycin. Others can be carried in breast milk and can cause toxicity to the infant.
4. *Likelihood of organisms developing resistance.* Sometimes a combination of drugs is used to decrease the chance of developing resistance to a single drug. Examples of combination therapy include sulfamethoxazole and trimethoprin combined to treat urinary tract infections. Another example is the combination of three or more drugs to treat tuberculosis.

Adverse reactions to anti-infectives are divided into three categories:

1. *Allergic hypersensitivity.* Overresponse of the body to a specific substance. A *mild* reaction with only rash, urticaria (hives), or mild fever is usually treated with corticosteroids or antihistamines, and the medication is *discontinued.* Sometimes severe reactions occur with the first administration of a specific medication (e.g., penicillin), or they may follow a mild reaction. *Severe* reactions may be manifested as *anaphylaxis,* a sudden onset of dyspnea, chest constriction, shock, and collapse. Unless treated promptly with epinephrine, corticosteroids, and CPR (cardiopulmonary resuscitation) death may result.
2. *Direct toxicity.* Results in tissue damage, such as ototoxicity (hearing difficulties or dizziness), nephrotoxicity (kidney problems), hepatotoxity (liver damage), or blood dyscrasias (abnormalities in blood components). Sometimes the damage is permanent, or it may be reversible when the medication is discontinued. The health worker's responsibility involves assessment of physical condition and laboratory reports, and *discontinuance* of medication at the first sign of toxicity.
3. *Indirect toxicity, or superinfection.* Manifested as a new infection with different resistant bacteria or fungi as a result of killing the normal flora in the intestines or mucous membranes especially with broad-spectrum antibiotics. Symptoms of superinfections can include diarrhea, vaginitis, stomatitis, or glossitis. Treatment consists of antifungal medications. Including buttermilk or yogurt in the diet, or administering Lactinex (see Chapter 16), helps to restore normal intestinal flora. With the other two types of adverse reactions, the medication is discontinued. With superinfections, the medication is *usu-*

ally continued, the symptoms are treated, and sometimes the dosage is adjusted. With severe colitis, the medication is discontinued and aggressive treatment is required.

It would be impractical to list all the anti-infective agents on the market. Therefore, only a few examples of the most frequently used drugs are listed in each category. The antibiotics are divided into categories including aminoglycosides, cephalosporins, chloramphenicol, erythromycins, penicillins, quinalones and tetracyclines. In addition, antifungals, antituberculosis agents, sulfonamides, and urinary anti-infectives are also listed. Miscellaneous anti-infective agents, including some drugs used to treat opportunistic infections associated with AIDS (autoimmune deficiency syndrome) are included. Antiviral drugs, used to treat HIV (human immunodeficiency virus) and other viral infections, are also described. We have omitted the amebicides, anthelmintics, and antimalarial drugs, but urge those in the public health or pediatric fields to investigate these drugs as appropriate to their practice.

Aminoglycosides

Aminoglycosides are used to treat many infections caused by gram-negative bacteria (e.g., *Escherichia Coli, Pseudomonas* and *Salmonella*) as well as many gram-positive bacteria (e.g., *Staphylococcus aureus*). Aminoglycosides are used in the *short-term* treatment of many serious infections (e.g., septicemia) *only* when other less toxic anti-infectives are ineffective or contraindicated. Examples of aminoglycosides include amikacin, gentamicin, and tobramycin. Because of poor absorption from the GI tract, aminoglycosides are usually administered parenterally, (i.e., IM or IV).

Organisms *resistant* to aminoglycosides, especially gentamicin, are increasing in number.

Serious side effects, especially in the elderly, dehydrated patients, or those with renal or hearing impairment, can include:

Nephrotoxicity, including pathologic kidney condition
Ototoxicity, both auditory (hearing loss) and vestibular (vertigo)
Neuromuscular blocking, including respiratory paralysis
CNS symptoms including headache, tremor, lethargy, numbness, seizures
Blurred vision, rash, or urticaria

Contraindications or extreme caution applies to patients with:

Tinnitus, vertigo, and high-frequency hearing loss
Reduced renal function
Dehydration
Pregnant or nursing women
Infants

Interactions may occur with:

Other ototoxic drugs (e.g., amphotericin B, cephalosporins, polymixin B, bacitracin, and vancomycin)

General anesthetics or neuromuscular blocking agents (e.g., succinylcholine or curare), which can cause respiratory paralysis

Antiemetics—may mask symptoms of vestibular ototoxicity

PATIENT EDUCATION

Patients being treated with aminoglycosides should be instructed regarding:

Extreme importance of close medical supervision during therapy.
Careful observation of intake and urinary output.
Prompt reporting of any side effects, especially kidney or hearing problems.

Cephalosporins

Cephalosporins are semisynthetic antibiotic derivatives produced by a fungus. They are related to the penicillins and *some* patients allergic to penicillin are also allergic to cephalosporins. In general, cephalosporins are broad-spectrum, active against many gram-positive and gram-negative bacteria. However, there are many different cephalosporins and they vary widely in their activity against specific bacteria. Cephalosporins are classified as first, second, or third generation, according to the organisms susceptible to their activity. First-generation drugs, for example, cephalexin, are usually effective against gram-positive organisms, such as those causing some pneumonias or some urinary tract infections. Second-generation drugs, for example, cefaclor, are usually effective against many gram-positive and gram-negative organisms, such as many strains causing influenza. Third-generation drugs, for example, ceftriaxone, are usually effective against more gram-negative bacteria than the others and are sometimes used for sexually transmitted diseases such as chancroid or gonorrhea.

A culture and sensitivity is essential to determine which cephalosporin is appropriate. Different drugs are used to treat different infections of the respiratory tract, skin, urinary tract, bones and joints, septicemias, some sexually transmitted diseases, and endocarditis. They are also used prophylactically, especially in high-risk patients, for many types of surgery.

Side effects can include:

Hypersensitivity, including rash, edema, or anaphylaxis (especially in those allergic to penicillin)
Blood dyscrasias (e.g., increased bleeding time or transient leukopenia)
Renal toxicity, especially in older patients
Mild hepatic dysfunction
Nausea, vomiting, and diarrhea

Phlebitis with IV administration and pain at site of IM injection
Respiratory distress

Contraindications or extreme caution applies to:

Renal impairment
Known allergies, especially to penicillin (3–6% cross-sensitivity)
Prolonged use possibly leading to superinfections or severe colitis
Pregnant or nursing women
Children—mild hearing loss reported

Interactions can include:

Increased effectiveness with probenecid
Disulfiram-like reactions (flushing, tachycardia, shock) with alcohol ingestion

---

PATIENT EDUCATION

Patients being treated with cephalosporins should be instructed regarding:

Possible allergic reactions.
Avoidance of alcohol.
Reporting any side effects to physician.
Including buttermilk or yogurt in diet to restore normal intestinal flora.
Taking without regard to meals but with food if stomach upset occurs.
Attention to signs of abnormal bleeding (checking stools and urine for blood).

Chloramphenicol

Chloramphenicol (Chloromycetin) is potentially very toxic and therefore is used only to treat serious infections caused by susceptible organisms when less toxic drugs are ineffective. It is used for typhoid fever, meningitis *(Hemophilus influenzae),* rickettsial infections (e.g., Rocky Mountain spotted fever), or bacteremia when other antibiotics have proven ineffective. Patients should be hospitalized during chloramphenicol therapy for appropriate lab tests and observation.

Serious side effects can include:

Bone marrow depression, leading to bleeding and infections
Aplastic anemia, which can be fatal
Circulatory collapse, which can lead to death
Visual disturbances
Neuritis, headache, and confusion
Hypersensitivity reactions

Contraindications include:

Infants

Pregnant or nursing women

Impaired renal or hepatic function

Interactions can occur with:

Potentiation of dicumarol, phenytoin, and tolbutamide

Antagonistic response to vitamin B_{12}, folic acid, or iron preparations

---

PATIENT EDUCATION

Patients being treated with chloramphenicol should be instructed regarding the very serious potential side effects and given explanations regarding its use when absolutely necessary under close medical supervision.

Erythromycins

Erythromycins are used in many infections of the respiratory tract and for skin conditions such as acne or for some sexually transmitted infections when the patient is allergic to penicillin. Erythromycins are considered among the least toxic antibiotics and are therefore preferred for treating susceptible organisms under conditions in which more toxic antibiotics might be dangerous (e.g., in patients with renal disease, pregnant patients, or small infants).

Organisms resistant to erythromycins, for example, some strains of streptococcus A, are increasing in number.

Side effects of a serious nature are rare, and mild side effects, usually dose related, can include:

Anorexia, nausea, vomiting, diarrhea, and cramps

Urticaria and rash

Superinfections

Contraindications or caution applies to patients with:

Liver dysfunction

Alcoholism

Interactions may occur with potentiation of the following drugs and possible toxicity:

Carbamazepine (Tegretol)—ataxia, dizziness, drowsiness

Cyclosporine (immunosuppressant with kidney/liver transplants)

Theophylline

Terfenadine (Seldane) or astemizole (Hismanal)—may cause *serious* cardiac effects

Triazolam (Halcion)—potentiation of sedative effect of other benzodiazepines theoretically possible also

Warfarin—may prolong prothrombin time and bleeding

Digoxin

PATIENT EDUCATION

Patients being treated with erythromycins should be instructed regarding:

Common GI side effects to be expected.

Importance of reporting side effects for possible dosage adjustment or prescription of medication for symptomatic relief.

Taking medication with full glass of water 1 hour before or 2 hours after meals, unless stomach upset (some forms can be taken without regard to meals).

Including yogurt or buttermilk in diet to help regulate intestinal flora and reduce incidence of diarrhea.

Not taking with other medications (see Interactions).

Penicillins

Penicillins are antibiotics produced from certain species of a fungus. They are used to treat many streptococcal and some staphylococcal and meningococcal infections, including respiratory and intestinal infections. Penicillin is the drug of choice for treatment of gonorrhea and syphilis, and is also used prophylactically to prevent recurrences of rheumatic fever or endocarditis.

Amoxicillin has also been used to treat *Helicobacter pylori* infection associated with peptic ulcer disease, sometimes combined only with omeprazole (Prilosec), a gastric antisecretory agent. Other clinicians recommend that amoxicillin be combined with bismuth salicylate and metronidazole to treat *H. pylori* infection.

Some semisynthetic penicillins have a wider spectrum of activity and are called extended-spectrum penicillins, for example, carbenicillin and ticarcillin.

Some organisms, including both gram-positive and gram-negative bacteria, for example, that cause gonorrhea, have become *resistant* to many forms of penicillin. Culture and sensitivity tests are essential to determine appropriate forms of medication.

Serious side effects of penicillins can include:

Hypersensitivity reactions ranging from rash to fatal anaphylaxis

Superinfections (especially with oral ampicillin)

Nausea, vomiting, and diarrhea

Blood dyscrasias, which are reversible with discontinuance of drug

Renal and hepatic disorders

CNS effects, for example, confusion, anxiety, seizures (especially with penicillin G)

Contraindications or extreme caution applies to patients with:

History of allergy, especially to any drugs (anaphylaxis has been reported with parenteral, oral, or intradermal skin testing)

Impaired renal function

Treatment for severe reactions includes discontinuance of the drug, immediate administration of appropriate medications (e.g., epinephrine and corticosteroids), and maintenance of a patent airway. Administration of antihistamines with penicillin will <u>not</u> prevent hypersensitivity reaction.

Interactions include:

Potentiation of penicillin with probenecid (Benemid) and with anti-inflammatory drugs such as phenylbutazone, indomethacin, and the salicylates given concomitantly (at the same time)

Antagonistic effect (delayed absorption) of oral penicillins when given with antacids or with food

Antagonistic effect of some other anti-infectives on penicillin

Penicillin V or ampicillin may inhibit the action of estrogen-containing oral contraceptives

---

PATIENT EDUCATION

Patients being treated with penicillin should be instructed regarding:

Discontinuance of medication and *immediate* reporting of any hypersensitivity reactions (e.g., rash, swelling, or difficulty breathing).

Taking medication on time as prescribed on empty stomach, 1 hour before or 2 hours after meals, with full glass of water.

Avoidance of antacids and alcohol.

Effectiveness of estrogen contraceptives may be affected.

Quinolones

A newer type of anti-infective agent, quinolones, such as ciprofloxacin (Cipro), is used in adults for the treatment of some infections of the urinary tract, lower respiratory tract, GI tract, skin, bones, and joints.

Strains of organisms *resistant* to the quinolones, for example, ciprofloxacin, have been reported with increasing frequency. Therefore, culture and sensitivity tests should be administered to identify the causative organism and sensitivity before the drug is administered.

***Side effects of ciprofloxacin* can include:**

Nausea, vomiting, diarrhea, abdominal pain, colitis (especially geriatric patients)
CNS effects: headache, dizziness, confusion, irritability, seizures, anxiety
Crystalluria—drink liberal quantities of fluids
Superinfection—treat infection appropriately, may need to stop drug
Hypersensitivity reactions or rash—rare
Phototoxicity—severe sunburn

***Contraindications* or caution applies to:**

Elderly, especially with GI disease or arteriosclerosis
Children or adolescents
Pregnancy and lactation
Severe renal impairment
Seizure disorders

***Interactions* may occur with:**

Theophylline—can potentiate serious or fatal CNS effects, cardiac arrest, or respiratory failure
Probenicid—increased blood levels of Cipro
Antacids—decreased absorption
Coumarin—increased risk of bleeding

PATIENT EDUCATION

Patients taking Cipro should be instructed regarding:

Not taking other medication without physician's approval.
Drinking liberal quantities of fluids.
Restricting caffeine intake—see CNS effects.
Avoiding excessive exposure to the sun.
Reporting all side effects, especially rash or hypersensitivity signs.
Geriatric patients should follow above instructions, especially reporting GI effects or CNS effects (see Side Effects above).

See Table 17.1 for a summary of the aminoglycosides, cephalosporins, chloramphenicols, erythromycins, penicillins, and quinalones.

TABLE 17.1. ANTI-INFECTIVE AGENTS: AMINOGLYCOSIDES, CEPHALOSPORINS, CHLORAMPHENICOL, ERYTHROMYCINS, PENICILLINS, AND QUINOLONES

Generic Name	Trade Name	Average Dosage
Aminoglycosides		
gentamicin	Garamycin	IM, IV 1 mg/kg body weight q8h
neomycin	Mycifradin	Oral sol, tab, IV 40–88 mg qd in divided doses
tobramycin	Nebcin	IM, IV 1 mg/kg body weight q8h
Cephalosporins		
cephalexin	Keflex	Cap, liquid, tab 250 mg q6h
cefaclor	Ceclor	250 mg q8h
ceftriaxone	Rocephin	IV, deep IM 1–2 g qd
cefazolin	Kefzol, Ancef	IM, IV, 250 mg q8h to 1.5 g q6h
Chloramphenicol		
chloramphenicol	Chloromycetin	Oral 50 mg/kg body weight qd IV 50 mg/kg body weight qd in divided doses q6h
Erythromycins		
erythromycin	E-Mycin, Ilosone	Tab, cap 250–500 mg q6h
	EES, ERYC	Tab, suspension 400 mg q6h
clarithromycin	Biaxin	250–500 mg q 12h
Penicillins		
amino-penicillins	Amoxicillin, Ampicillin, Augmentin	Cap, tab, suspension 250–500 mg q6–8h
carbenicillin	Geopen	IV 400–500 mg/kg body weight qd, div. doses
	Geocillin	382-764 mg PO qid
ticarcillin	Ticar	IV div. doses 200–300 mg/kg body weight qd
penicillin G procaine	Bicillin, Crystacillin, Wycillin	Deep IM 600,000–2.4 million U
penicillin V	V-Cillin K, Pen-Vee K	Tab 250–500 mg q6h
Quinolones		
ciprofloxacin	Cipro	250–500 mg tab q12h

Note: Average doses only are listed. In severe infections, higher doses may be indicated. Many other anti-infectives are available. Only a few are represented here. Pediatric doses are computed according to weight of the child and condition.

Tetracyclines

Tetracyclines are broad-spectrum antibiotics used in the treatment of infections caused by rickettsia, chlamydia, or some *uncommon* bacteria. Diseases such as Rocky Mountain spotted fever, atypical pneumonia, some sexually transmitted diseases, and some severe cases of inflammatory acne are treated with tetracycline. However, some organisms are showing increasing resistance to the tetracyclines, and therefore they should be used only when other antibiotics are ineffective or contraindicated.

Side effects can include:

Nausea, vomiting, and diarrhea (frequently dose related)
Superinfections such as vaginitis and stomatitis
Photosensitivity, with exaggerated sunburn
Discolored teeth in fetus or young children
Retarded bone growth in fetus or young children
Hepatic or renal toxicity (rare)
CNS symptoms (rare) such as vertigo and cerebral edema
Thrombophlebitis possible with IV therapy
Allergic reactions rare

Contraindications include:

Pregnancy, lactation, and children under age 8
Patients exposed to direct sunlight
Caution in patients with liver or kidney disease
Patients with esophageal obstruction or dysfunction

Interactions may occur with the following antagonists (which decrease absorption):

Antacids, calcium supplements, or magnesium laxatives
Iron preparations
Antidiarrhea agents containing kaolin, pectin, or bismuth
Dairy products

PATIENT EDUCATION

Patients being treated with tetracyclines should be instructed regarding:

Avoiding exposure to sunlight.
Avoiding this medication if pregnant or nursing or a child under 8 years of age.
Administration preferable on an empty stomach with full glass of water, 1 hour before or 2 hours after meals, unless there is gastric distress.
Avoiding iron, calcium, magnesium, and antidiarrhea agents or dairy foods within 3 h of taking tetracyclines.
Not taking at bedtime to prevent irritation from esophageal reflux.
Discarding any expired drug—nephrotoxicity can result from taking outdated drug.

Antifungals

Antifungal agents are used to treat specific susceptible fungi. The medications are quite different in action and purpose, and are treated separately.

AMPHOTERICIN B

Amphotericin B is administered IV for the treatment of severe systemic, potentially fatal infections caused by susceptible fungi. It is sometimes considered the drug of choice to treat severe fungal infections resulting from immunosuppressive therapy (e.g., antineoplastic agents) or in patients with acquired immunodeficiency syndrome (AIDS), or those with severe illness (e.g., meningitis). *Severe side effects* are expected, and therefore close medical supervision (hospitalization) is usually required so that measures are available to provide symptomatic relief (e.g., antipyretics, antihistamines, and antiemetics).

Side effects commonly include several of the following:

Headache, chills, fever, hypotension, tachypnea

Malaise, muscle and joint pain, and weakness

Anorexia, nausea, vomiting, and cramps

Nephrotoxicity occurs to some degree in most patients

Anemia

Hypokalemia—can lead to congestive heart failure

FLUCONAZOLE

Fluconazole is usually limited to severe candidial infections unresponsive to conventional antifungal therapy. Because of good patient tolerance, and oral dosage, the drug is appropriate for patients requiring prolonged antifungal therapy. It is used in the treatment of oropharyngeal and esophageal candidiasis and serious systemic candidial infections (e.g., urinary tract infections and pneumonia). Patients with recurrent candidiasis, especially those who are immunodeficient, may require maintenance therapy to prevent relapse.

Side effects can include:

Moderate nausea, vomiting, abdominal pain, diarrhea

Rash

Hepatic abnormalities

Dizziness and headache

Contraindications or extreme caution applies to:

Children under 13

Pregnant or nursing women

Seizure disorders receiving phenytoin

Interactions may occur with:

Coumarin anticoagulants—increased prothrombin time could cause hemorrhage
Astemizole and Terfenadine antihistamines—serious cardiac effects possible
Oral antidiabetic agents—hypoglycemia can result

GRISEOFULVIN

Griseofulvin is administered PO in the treatment of *specific* fungi causing *tinea* infections (e.g., ringworm or athlete's foot) that do not respond to topical agents.

Side effects can include:

Headache—frequent initially
Thirst, nausea, vomiting, and diarrhea
Hypersensitivity reactions—rash, urticaria
Photosensitivity
Hepatic toxicity or renal abnormalities

Contraindications include:

Children under 2
Pregnancy—or women who may become pregnant while taking the drug
Liver dysfunction
Porphyria

Interactions may occur with:

Alcohol, causing flushing and tachycardia
Phenobarbital, which is antagonistic to griseofulvin action
Coumarin anticoagulants—decreased prothrombin time
Oral contraceptives—may decrease contraceptive efficacy

NYSTATIN

Nystatin (Mycostatin) is used orally in the treatment of intestinal candidiasis. It is also used as a fungicide in the topical treatment of skin and mucous membranes, for example, diaper area, mouth, or vagina (see Skin Medications).

Side effects are rare but may include nausea, vomiting, and diarrhea with high oral doses occasionally.

Caution with pregnant or nursing women.

PATIENT EDUCATION

Patients on antifungal therapy should be instructed regarding:

Taking the medication for prolonged periods as prescribed, even after symptoms
  have subsided.
Reporting relapses promptly to physician.
Reporting side effects immediately to the physician for possible dosage adjustment or symptomatic treatment.
Not taking any other medications at the same time without physician approval
  (see Interactions).

Antituberculosis Agents

Antituberculosis agents are administered for two purposes: (1) to treat asymptomatic infection (no evidence of clinical disease), for instance, after exposure to
active tuberculosis and/or significantly positive PPD (purified protein derivative)
skin test; (2) for treatment of active clinical tuberculosis and to prevent relapse.

For asymptomatic tuberculosis, the *treatment* consists of daily administration of
isoniazid (INH) alone for 6–12 months to prevent development of the disease.

However, treatment of clinical tuberculosis has changed for two reasons:

1. Because of the increasing incidence of tuberculosis, particularly among certain high-risk populations (e.g., HIV-infected individuals, socioeconomically
   disadvantaged racial/ethnic minorities, homeless individuals).
2. Because organisms have become resistant to many antituberculosis drugs due
   to patient noncompliance or failure to complete the former 18–24-month conventional treatment.

Therefore, the CDC recommends the following treatment regimen:

1. A four-drug initial regimen of isoniazid, rifampin, pyrazinamide and ethambutol or streptomycin given daily for 2 months. This is followed by daily,
   twice-weekly or 3-times weekly therapy with isoniazid and rifampin for a
   total of 6–9 months minimum treatment, if results of susceptibility tests
   demonstrate that the organisms are sensitive to these drugs. If resistance to
   any of the drugs is found, treatment is changed accordingly.
2. In areas with a high incidence of multidrug-resistant tuberculosis, especially
   in health care and correctional facilities, and with immunocompromised
   patients, initial therapy with five or six drugs may be indicated. The use of
   multiple agents rapidly decreases infectiousness and may delay or prevent
   emergence of resistant organisms. Patients with HIV infection should be
   treated a minimum of 9 months and for 6 months after negative cultures.
3. In addition, the CDC recommends that directly observed (supervised) treatment be used whenever possible to ensure compliance.

4. Safe use of all these drugs during pregnancy has not been established. The CDC recommends that tuberculosis during pregnancy be treated initially with isoniazid, rifampin, and ethambutol. Streptomycin is not included because it may cause congenital ototoxicity.

Side effects of *INH and rifampin* are usually more pronounced in the first few weeks of therapy and can be treated symptomatically. Dosage regulations are sometimes required in cases of acute toxicity, but the medication must *not* be discontinued. Side effects can include:

Nausea, vomiting, and diarrhea

Dizziness, blurred vision, headache, and fatigue

Numbness, weakness of extremities

Hepatic toxicity—especially those over 35 and children (see Cautions)

Excretions colored red-orange with rifampin

Hypersensitivity reaction, with flulike symptoms (sometimes with rifampin)

Contraindications or caution applies to:

Chronic liver disease or alcoholics, periodic laboratory tests required

Impaired renal function

Children's doses of INH and rifampin should be limited to 10 and 15 mg/kg respectively to decrease likelihood of hepatic toxicity

Interactions of INH and rifampin include:

Antagonism by oral hypoglycemics, corticosteroids, digitalis, anticoagulants, and estrogen (serum levels of these drugs are reduced when taking rifampin)

Potentiation by phenytoin (Dilantin); increased action (possible toxicity) when taken with isoniazid

Alcohol, which increases possibility of liver toxicity

Side effects of ethambutol can include:

Optic neuritis—with visual problems

Dermatitis, pruritis, headache, malaise, fever, confusion, joint pain

GI symptoms, peripheral neuritis rarely

Cautions and contraindications:

Visual testing should be performed prior to and during therapy

Impaired renal function—reduced doses indicated

Diabetes, especially diabetic retinopathy

Ocular defects

Children under 13—and only in children whose visual acuity can accurately be determined and monitored

Pregnancy—caution

Side effects of pyrazinamide can include:

Hepatic toxicity

Gout—increased uric acid

Hypersensitivity

GI disturbances

Cautions and contraindications include:

Renal failure or history of gout

Diabetes

Severe hepatic disease

Children—potential toxicity

Pregnant or nursing women

Side effects of streptomycin, common to all aminoglycosides, include:

Ototoxicity

Nephrotoxicity

Streptomycin is administered by deep IM injection, alternating sites. Although not authorized by the manufacturer, it has been administered IV without adverse side effects.

PATIENT EDUCATION

Patients taking antituberculosis agents should be instructed regarding:

Taking rifampin on empty stomach for maximum absorption, or with food if nauseated.

Taking prescribed medication for *lengthy required period of time* even though asymptomatic.

Reporting side effects for possible dosage adjustment or prescription of other palliative medications to relieve discomfort.

Importance of frequent medical and laboratory checks.

Red-orange color of urine, feces, sputum, sweat, and tears with use of rifampin.

Interactions with other drugs, (e.g., *birth control pills may be ineffective*).

Avoidance of alcohol.

Importance of visual testing periodically with ethambutol.

See Table 17.2 for a summary of tetracyclines, antifungal, and antituberculosis agents.

TABLE 17.2. ANTI-INFECTIVE AGENTS: TETRACYCLINES, ANTIFUNGALS, AND ANTITUBERCULOSIS AGENTS

Generic Name	Trade Name	Average Dosage	Comments
Tetracyclines			
tetracyclines HCL	Achromycin V	Cap, tab, 500 mg–lg div. doses 1–2 weeks	Phototoxicity, discolored teeth in infants and children
oxytetracycline	Terramycin	Cap, tab, suspension, IM, IV 1–2 g qd div. doses	Phototoxicity, discolored teeth in infants and children
Antifungals			
amphotericin B	Fungizone	IV dose varies with condition	Special IV cautions, protect from light
fluconazole	Diflucan	100–400 mg PO or IV qd	Prolonged or maintenance doses usually
griseofulvin	Grisactin, Fulvicin	Cap, tab, suspension 250 mg–1 g qd	
nystatin	Mycostatin	Tab, suspension 500,000–1 million U tid	
Antituberculosis Agents			
isoniazid	INH	Tab 1 dose qd 5–10 mg/kg	Preventive alone, or as treatment with other medications
ethambutol	Myambutol	Tab 1 dose qd 15–25 mg/kg	Always with other medications
rifampin	Rifadin	600 mg cap qd	Always with other medications
pyrazinamide	Pyrazinamide	20–35 mg/kg div. doses	Initial phase with other drugs
streptomycin	Streptomycin	25–30 mg/kg (up to 1.5 g) IM 2–3 times wk	With other medications Initial phase

Note: Other anti-infectives are available. Only a few are represented here. Pediatric doses are computed according to weight and condition of child.

Miscellaneous Anti-Infectives

Clindamycin has a wider spectrum of activity than lincomycin, from which it is derived. It is used in the treatment of serious respiratory tract infections, septicemia, osteomyelitis, serious infections of the female pelvis caused by susceptible bacteria, and for *Pneumocystis carinii* pneumonia associated with AIDS (see AIDS section in this chapter).

Side effects that frequently occur can include:

Nausea, vomiting, diarrhea, colitis

Rash, pruritis, fever, and occasionally anaphylaxis

Local effects—minimize by deep IM or frequent IV catheter change

Cautions include:

History of GI disease
Elderly
Children
Pregnancy and lactation—contraindicated

Vancomycin is structurally unrelated to other available antibiotics. IV vancomycin is used in the treatment of potentially life-threatening infections caused by susceptible organisms that cannot be treated with other less toxic anti-infective agents. It is the drug of choice for methicillin-resistant *Staphylococcus aureus* (MRSA), some severe cases of colitis, or some endocarditis. However, the CDC reports a 20-fold increase in the percentage of vancomycin-resistant enterococci. Therefore, use of vancomycin should be restricted to cases where it is absolutely necessary and it should not be used prophylactically.

Side effects can include:

Ototoxicity or nephrotoxicity with IV use—discontinue with tinnitus, may precede deafness
Local effects—give only IV with care, can cause necrosis or thrombophlebitis
Rash, anaphylaxis, vascular collapse (hypersensitivity reactions reported in 5–10% of patients)
Pseudomembranous colitis—mild to life-threatening

Caution with:

Elderly
Hearing impaired
Renal impairment
Contraindicated with pregnancy and lactation

Antivirals

The antiviral *(acyclovir)* is used predominantly in the treatment of herpes simplex, herpes zoster (shingles) and varicella zoster (chickenpox) infections. Acyclovir does not cure or prevent further occurrence of blisterlike lesions. Topical application appears effective only with initial infections in relieving discomfort and shortening healing time of lesions (see Skin Medications.) Oral treatment is most effective in initial treatment of herpes to relieve pain and to speed healing of lesions, and is also used to treat recurrent infections in some patients. In immunocompromised patients and children, parenteral treatment is recommended.

Side effects are not common, but can include:

Impaired renal function, especially with rapid IV infusion
Lethargy, tremors, confusion, and headache, especially with older adults

Rash, urticaria, and inflammation at injection site
Nausea, vomiting, abdominal pain, and diarrhea

Contraindications or caution with:

Children, pregnant or nursing women
Renal or hepatic disease
Dehydration
Neurologic abnormalities

PATIENT EDUCATION

Patients being treated with acyclovir should be instructed regarding:

The fact that acyclovir is usually effective only with *initial* infection in relieving pain and shortening healing of lesions, but is *not* a cure and there will be recurrences of lesions.
Reporting side effects.
Taking medicine only as prescribed.
Storing capsules and tablets in tight, light-resistant container at 15–25°C..

Another antiviral, *amantadine,* is used for the prophylaxis and symptomatic treatment of respiratory infections caused by influenza A virus strains, especially with high-risk patients. It has no effect on influenza B or other viruses. Amantadine is also used in the treatment of parkinsonian syndrome (see Chapter 22). Prophylactic use should not be considered a substitute for vaccination.

Side effects of amantadine can include:

CNS symptoms—dizziness, nervousness, confusion, anxiety, headache, weakness, tremor, insomnia
Bluish mottling of skin on legs, eczema
Anorexia, nausea, constipation, and dry mouth
Hypotension, edema, urinary retention, dyspnea
Visual disturbances

Contraindications or caution applies to:

Those with mental disorders
Seizure disorders
Cardiovascular disorders, hypotension
Renal impairment or liver disease
Elderly—need reduced dosage
Pregnant or nursing women

Interactions with anticholinergics may increase potential for adverse side effects.

A drug with the broadest spectrum of antiviral activity, *ribavirin*, is used via nasal and oral inhalation for the treatment of children with severe lower respiratory tract infections. It has also been used orally or parenterally in the treatment of other severe viral infections in adults, for example, Lassa fever and Hantavirus. Research in other conditions is ongoing.

Side effects can include:

Respiratory complications
Hypotension, cardiac arrest
Anemia
Rash, conjunctivitis

Contraindicated during pregnancy or lactation. Health care workers and visitors who are pregnant or lactating should be warned about the serious risk of close contact with patients receiving ribavirin inhalation therapy.

Interactions include:

Digitalis or diuretics—potential for toxicity increased
Zidovudine—antiviral action against HIV antagonized

Treatment of Human Immunodeficiency Virus/AIDS Infections

Several drugs are currently used in the management of HIV and AIDS infections. Research in the long-term efficiency and safety of these drugs is ongoing. Some drugs are used specifically for their antiretroviral activity, for example, *zidovudine* (Retrovir). Other drugs are used in the management of opportunistic infections associated with AIDS infection. There is no cure for HIV infections and HIV cannot be eliminated from infected patients at this time.

Zidovudine currently is considered the antiretroviral drug of choice for the initial management of HIV infections. Research has shown that zidovudine therapy can reduce the rate of progression to *acquired immunodeficiency syndrome* (AIDS) and decrease the incidence and severity of opportunistic infections. Patients with asymptomatic HIV infections are monitored closely. The CDC recommends that zidovudine therapy be initiated in asymptomatic patients with CD4+ T-cell counts less than 200. However, many clinicians recommend zidovudine therapy for patients with CD4+ T-cell counts lower than 500. No zidovudine therapy is currently recommended for those with CD4+ T-cell counts over 500. Health care workers reportedly have a 1 in 250 (0.4%) chance of becoming seropositive for HIV after a single needlestick injury. However, the use of prophylactic therapy in such cases is controversial because of the lack of proof of efficacy and possibility of severe adverse effects of zidovudine including carcinogenic potential.

Side effects of zidovudine (AZT) are common and can include:

Anemia and/or granulocytopenia—can be severe
Headache, insomnia, lethargy, fatigue
Nausea, vomiting, abdominal pain, diarrhea
Hepatic dysfunction
Muscle pain or muscle weakness
Adverse side effects in *asymptomatic* patients have been greatly reduced by decreasing the dosage to 500 mg per day
Other adverse side effects have been reported, but could be the result of the disease itself rather than drug related

Caution applies to all patients and close clinical supervision is required.

Those with impaired renal or hepatic function are at increased risk of toxicity. Long-term safety and efficacy have not been fully established.

Interactions that may potentiate adverse side effects include:

Probenecid—flulike symptoms
Acetaminophen—increased risk of granulocytopenia

PATIENT EDUCATION

Patients taking zidovudine should be instructed regarding:

No cure for HIV and opportunistic infections may develop.
Taking the drug in an upright position with full glass of water.
Taking the drug exactly as prescribed. If ordered q4h, must be taken around the clock.
Reporting any change in health status.
Not exceeding the prescribed dosage.
Not sharing the drug with others.
Not taking any other drugs unless prescribed, for example, acetaminophen contraindicated.
Zidovudine does not reduce the risk of transmission of HIV to others through sexual contact or blood contamination.

Zalcitabine (HIVID) is another antiviral oral drug combined with zidovudine for the management of advanced AIDS (T-cell counts of 300 or less) with significant clinical deterioration. The FDA recommends that zalcitabine be given only with zidovudine and not administered alone.

Side effects of zalcitabine are common and include:

Peripheral neuropathy (severe pain and/or numbness in the feet)
Rash or oral ulcers—could be dose related
Other reported effects could be caused by the disease rather than the drug

Cautions apply to:

Patients with pancreatic, renal, or hepatic disorders
All patients receiving zalcitabine should be monitored with frequent blood tests

---

PATIENT EDUCATION

Instructions for those taking zalcitabine are the same as zidovudine (see above) plus the following:

Report pain or numbness in feet immediately.
Take medication on an empty stomach.

TREATMENT OF THE OPPORTUNISTIC INFECTIONS OF AIDS

- *Interferons* are antiviral drugs sometimes used in the palliative treatment of AIDS-related *Kaposi's sarcoma* in selected adults who meet certain criteria, that is, are otherwise asymptomatic and not severely immunocompromised. Investigation continues into the efficacy for this purpose. However, interferon has also been used in the treatment of chronic hepatitis B and in some leukemias and other malignancies. Adverse side effects are common and varied, depending on dosage and condition treated (see Antineoplastic Drugs).
- *Pneumocystis carinii* pneumonia treatment:
  Co-trimoxazole (oral or IV), For prevention in all HIV-infected children, and in asymptomatic adults with CD4+ T-cell counts less than 200. For *treatment* of adults and children. See Side Effects, Contraindications, and Interactions under Sulfonamides in this chapter.
  Pentamidine aerosolized oral inhalation (antiprotozoal agent), for *prevention* in HIV-infected children, and in adults with CD4+ T-cell counts less than 200. For *treatment* of adults and children in patients whose infection does not respond to co-trimoxazole or who cannot tolerate co-trimoxazole because of allergies or adverse side effects.

Side effects of pentamidine can include:

Nephrotoxcity
Cough and bronchospasm

Cautions: Health care personnel who administer pentamidine inhalation therapy to HIV-infected patients should be aware of the possibility of exposure to tuberculosis in cough-inducing procedures. Antituberculosis therapy should be initiated prior to pentamidine treatment in potentially infectious tuberculosis patients. Use of high-efficiency particulate air filter respirators by health care personnel in such settings is imperative, as well as appropriate isolation procedures.

Contraindicated (pentamidine) in pregnancy and lactation.

Clindamycin combined with primaquine (alternate treatment). See Side Effects and Cautions of clindamycin under Miscellaneous Anti-infectives in this chapter.

Trimetrexate (Neutrexin)—alternate treatment for patients who have exhibited intolerance to co-trimoxazole. Trimetrexate is a folate antagonist and must be administered with leucovorin to counteract myelosuppression (inhibiting bone marrow function).

Side effects of Neutrexin, with severe toxicity, can include:

Myelosuppression, especially drop in WBC (white blood cell) counts, if not given concurrently with leucovorin

Liver enzyme elevation, fever, rash

Renal or GI effects

Contraindications include:

Pregnant or nursing women

Children under 18

Interactions include:

Zidovudine—discontinue during trimetrexate and leucovorin therapy, may resume afterwards

Erythromycin, rifampin, fluconazole, cimetidine, and acetaminophen are antagonistic to Neutrexin

- *Toxoplasmosis treatments:*

  Co-trimoxazole (Bactrim, Septra) or *pyrimethamine with sulfadoxine* (Fansidor). See Sulfonamides section for side effects of both of these combination drugs.

  Clindamycin. See Side Effects and Cautions of clindamycin under Miscellaneous Anti-Infectives in this chapter.

- Cytomegalovirus retinitis treatment:

  Two antiviral agents used to treat this condition are *foscarnet* and *ganciclovir.*

Side effects of foscarnet are common and can be severe, including:

Nephrotoxicity

Nausea, vomiting, and diarrhea

Electrolyte imbalance and cardiac abnormalities

Coughing and dyspnea

Side effects of ganciclovir are frequent, but usually reversible, including:

Blood dyscrasias—neutropenia and thrombocytopenia
Headache, confusion, seizure
Hepatic or renal effects

Sulfonamides

Sulfonamides are among the oldest anti-infectives. The increasing resistance of many bacteria has decreased the clinical usefulness of the drugs. However, they are used most effectively in combinations with other drugs, for example, with trimethoprim (co-trimoxazole) or with pyrimethamine (Fansidor). In combinations such as these, resistance develops more slowly. Co-trimoxazole (Bactrim, Septra) is used for urinary tract infections, especially acute, complicated UTIs, enteritis (e.g., travelers' diarrhea), otitis media, and in the treatment of *Pneumocystis carinii* pneumonia in AIDS patients or prevention of that disease in HIV-infected children (see treatment of HIV/AIDS in this chapter. Both of the above-mentioned sulfonamide combination drugs are also used in the treatment of toxoplasmosis in AIDS patients.

Side effects with sulfonamides are numerous and sometimes serious, and can include:

Rash, pruritis, dermatitis, and photosensitivity
Nausea, vomiting, and diarrhea
High fever, headache, stomatitis, and conjunctivitis
Blood dyscrasias
Hepatic toxicity with jaundice
Renal damage with crystalluria and hematuria
Hypersensitivity reactions, which can be fatal

Contraindications include:

Impaired hepatic function
Impaired renal function or urinary obstruction
Blood dyscrasias
Severe allergies or asthma
Pregnancy or lactation

Interactions include:

Potentiation of anticoagulants and oral antidiabetics
Antagonism of local anesthetics (e.g., procaine may inhibit antibacterial action of sulfa), and digitalis and phenytoin (Dilantin; sulfonamides may inhibit action)

PATIENT EDUCATION

Patients taking sulfonamides should be instructed regarding:

Importance of drinking large amounts of fluid to prevent crystalluria.
Discontinuance of sulfa at first sign of rash.
Reporting any side effects to physician *immediately.*
Avoiding exposure to sunlight.
Ingestion of sulfa with food, which delays, but does not reduce, absorption of the
    drug.
Orange urine with Azulfidine and Azo Gantanol (contain pyridium).

Urinary Anti-Infectives

Urinary anti-infectives are usually bacteriostatic instead of bactericidal in action. Nitrofurantoin (Furadantin and Macrodantin) are the most commonly used for initial or recurrent urinary tract infections caused by susceptible organisms. Treatment must continue for an adequate period of time to be effective and minimize recurrence of infection.

Side effects can include:

Nausea and vomiting, which are less frequent if taken with milk or food
Numbness and weakness of lower extremities
Headache, dizziness, and weakness of muscles
Respiratory distress with prolonged use
Brown urine
Anemia

Contraindications or caution applies to:

Renal impairment
Anemia
Diabetes
Electrolyte abnormalities
Asthma
Pregnancy and lactation
Children under 12

Interactions (antagonistic) with:

Benemid and magnesium
Antacids, decreasing the effectiveness of these drugs

PATIENT EDUCATION

Patients taking urinary anti-infectives should be instructed regarding:

Importance of taking medication for required number of days and follow-up urine culture.
Reporting side effects.
Taking medication with milk or food to reduce incidence of nausea and vomiting.
Avoiding antacids.

See Table 17.3 for a summary of the miscellaneous anti-infectives, drugs for HIV/AIDS, sulfonamides, and urinary anti-infectives.

Other anti-infective agents in these categories are available. This is a representative sample of drugs most commonly in use. Research is ongoing with these and other new drugs and the FDA has developed procedures to expedite the review and approval of certain new drugs. When these drugs are being investigated for the treatment of life-threatening or other serious conditions, for example, HIV infections, including AIDS, the drugs are classified as investigational new drugs (INDs). Revised government regulations require that INDs receive the highest priority for review in order to make promising new drugs available as soon as possible. Since the status of these drugs changes so rapidly, current information may not be available in the *PDR* or the *American Hospital Formulary Service Drug Information* reference books. However, it is your responsibility to review all the information obtained from the pharmacist or drug insert before administering any new drugs. The risks are especially great with drugs that have been on the market only a short time, and side effects can be severe, even life-threatening.

PATIENT EDUCATION

Patients taking antibiotics should be instructed regarding:

Unless directed otherwise, taking all antibiotics with a full glass of water on empty stomach, at least 1 h before meals and 2 h after meals.
Not taking with fruit juice.
Not taking with antacids.
Not taking with alcohol.
If side effects occur, discontinuing medication and consulting the physician or pharmacist.
Reporting rash, swelling, or breathing difficulty to the physician *immediately*.
Taking antibiotics at prescribed times to maintain blood levels.
Taking entire prescription *completely; not* discontinuing when symptoms of infection disappear.
Not taking any other medications, prescriptions, or over-the-counter drugs at the same time as antibiotics without checking first with the physician or pharmacist regarding interactions.

TABLE 17.3. MISCELLANEOUS ANTI-INFECTIVE AGENTS, ANTIVIRALS, DRUGS FOR HIV/AIDS, SULFONAMIDES, AND URINARY ANTI-INFECTIVES

Generic Name	Trade Name	Dosage
Miscellaneous Anti-infectives		
clindamycin	Cleocin	PO 150–450 mg q6h Ped 8–25 mg/kg qd, div. doses IM/IV 600 mg–2.7 g qd, div. doses
vancomycin	Vancocin	IV 500 mg q6h, Slow careful IV Ped 10–15 mg/kg q8–12h, not to exceed 2 g qd PO 0.5–2g qd div. doses, adults
Antiviral		
acyclovir	Zovirax	Caps or tabs 200-800 mg 5 × qd, q4h IV 5 mg/kg q8h
amantadine	Symadine, Symmetrel	100–200 mg qd
ribavirin	Virasole	Pwdr/sol-inhalation Oral, IV—dose varies
Drugs for HIV (Antivirals–Slow HIV Progression)		
zalcitabine (ddc)	HIVid	PO 0.75 q8h ac
zidovudine (AZT)	Retrovir	100–200 mg caps q4h 500–600 mg IV qd
Drugs for Opportunistic Diseases of AIDS		
co-trimoxazole	Bactrim, Septra	Adults or peds 15–20 mg/kg/day PO or IV div. doses
clindamycin	Cleocin	1.2–3.6g qd PO or IV, div. doses
foscarnet	Foscavir	Slow IV, dose varies
ganciclovir	Cytovene	Slow IV, dose varies
pentamidine	NebuPent	Aerosol inhalation, dose varies
trimetrexate	NeuTrexin	IV dose varies
interferon	Roferon A, Intron A	Dose varies ■ Always check **current** literature for dosage and side effects. ■ Other drugs and combinations are being used investigationally in the treatment of HIV- and AIDS-related diseases.
Sulfonamides		
sulfasalazine	Azulfidine	Tab, suspension 1–2 g qd in div. doses
sulfasoxazole	Gantrisin	Tab, creams, IV, IM 2–4 g daily in div. doses
co-trimoxazole	Septra, Bactrim	Tab, suspension, IV 160 mg q12h or 15–20 mg/kg qd in div. doses
Urinary Anti-Infective		
nitrofurantoin	Macrodantin, Furadantin	Cap, tab, suspension, IV 50–100 mg qid
trimethoprim	Proloprim	100 mg tab q12h

Worksheet for Chapter 17

ANTI-INFECTIVE DRUGS

List the drugs according to category and complete all columns. Learn generic or trade names as specified by instructor.

Classifications and Drugs	Purpose	Side Effects	Contraindications or Cautions	Interactions/ Patient Education
Aminoglycosides 1. 2. 3.				
Cephalosporins 1. 2. 3.				
Chloramphenicol 1.				
Erythromycins 1.				
Penicillins 1. 2. 3.				
Quinalones 1.				

Classifications and Drugs	Purpose	Side Effects	Contraindications or Cautions	Interactions/ Patient Education
Tetracyclines 1. 2.				
Antifungals 1. 2. 3.				
Sulfonamides 1. 2.				
Urinary Anti-infectives 1. 2.				
Miscellaneous 1. Vancomycin				
Anti-TB 1. 2. 3. 4. 5.				
Antiviral 1. 2. 3.				
Drugs for HIV/AIDS				

A. Case Study for Anti-Infective Drugs

Mrs. Madre, a 19-year-old pregnant woman, allergic to penicillin, calls her physician and requests some tetracycline for her acne and some Keflex for a "sore throat." The following information would be useful to her.

1. Tetracycline is contraindicated under all of the following circumstances EXCEPT
   a. Pregnancy
   b. Children under 8
   c. Working indoors
   d. Nursing a baby

2. Sometimes organisms build up resistance to drugs. The following practices could lead to resistance EXCEPT
   a. Too frequent antibiotic use
   b. Combination antibiotics
   c. Antibiotic for minor URI
   d. Stopping drug after 2 days

3. If she has fever, productive cough, or trouble swallowing, the physician might order a throat culture to determine all of the following EXCEPT
   a. Causative organisms
   b. Possible allergies
   c. Resistance to drugs
   d. Drug sensitivity

4. Those allergic to penicillin might also be sensitive to cephalosporins. The following are signs of allergic reaction EXCEPT
   a. Rash
   b. Hives
   c. Trouble breathing
   d. Vomiting

5. Cephalosporins can cause superinfections manifested by all of the following EXCEPT
   a. Diarrhea
   b. Vomiting
   c. Sore mouth
   d. Vaginitis

B. Case Study for Anti-Infective Drugs

Tom Brown, a 35-year-old prison guard, has a positive skin test for tuberculosis. Infection is confirmed by sputum test. The following information will be important to him.

1. He will need to take medicines for a minimum of
   a. 1 month
   b. 3 months
   c. 9 months
   d. 2 years

2. Family members with negative tests will be treated prophylactically with which one of the following medications?
   a. Rifampin
   b. Isoniazid
   c. Ethambutol
   d. Streptomycin

3. While taking the antituberculosis drugs, which of the following should be avoided?
   a. Milk
   b. Orange juice
   c. Alcohol
   d. Sunlight

4. He will take at least four drugs initially, including all of the following EXCEPT
   a. Isoniazid
   b. Rifampin
   c. Pyrazinamide
   d. Zidovudine

5. Side effects of INH and rifampin are more pronounced at first and can include all of the following EXCEPT
   a. Diarrhea
   b. Dizziness
   c. Hearing problems
   d. Nausea and vomiting

CHAPTER 18

Eye Medications

OBJECTIVES

Upon completion of this chapter, the student should be able to:

1. Define mydriatic, miotic, and cycloplegic.
2. Demonstrate the administration technique for instillation of ophthalmic medication to reduce systemic absorption.
3. List the five categories of ophthalmic medication.
4. Identify side effects, contraindications, and interactions for each category of ophthalmic medication.
5. Explain appropriate patient education necessary for each category of eye medication.

Medications for the eye can be classified into five categories: anti-infectives, anti-inflammatory agents, antiglaucoma agents, mydriatics, and local anesthetics.

Anti-Infectives

Many anti-infective ophthalmic topical ointments and solutions are available for treatment of superficial infections of the eye caused by susceptible organisms. It is important to determine the causative organism so that the appropriate medication is used. Ophthalmic antibiotic preparations include erythromycin, gentamycin, neomycin, polymixin B and others. Resistance and cross-resistance have been demonstrated with many antibiotics. Always check the latest literature regarding resistant organisms and check the patient's history regarding allergies. See chapter 17 for further details on resistance and allergies.

Side effects can include hypersensitivity reactions such as conjunctivitis, burning, rash, and urticaria in allergic persons.

Contraindications apply to anyone allergic to the drug.

Interactions may occur with corticosteroids, which can accelerate the spread of infection.

Antiviral ophthalmic preparations, used topically in the treatment of herpes simplex, keratitis, or conjunctivitis include vidabrine (Vira-A) ophthalmic ointment. This ointment should be applied inside the lower conjunctival sac of the infected eye 5 times daily at 3-hour intervals.

PATIENT EDUCATION

Patients being treated with anti-infective opthalmic preparations should be instructed regarding:

Using only as directed. Check dosage for frequency.

Careful instillation into the lower conjunctival sac to avoid contamination of the tip of the dropper or ointment tube (see Figure 18.1).

Possible hypersensitivity reactions in patients with allergies of any kind.

Discontinuance of the medication and reporting immediately to a physician any signs of sensitivity (e.g., burning and itching).

Careful handwashing to prevent spread of infection to other eye or other persons.

Anti-Inflammatory Agents

Anti-inflammatory ophthalmic agents are used to relieve inflammation of the eye or conjunctiva in allergic reactions, burns, or irritation from foreign substances. Various topical forms of the corticosteroids are also useful in the acute stages of eye injury to prevent scarring, but are not used for extended periods because of the danger of masking the symptoms of infection or slowing the healing process. Application of ophthalmic corticosteroids topically does not generally cause systemic effects. However, systemic absorption can be minimized by gentle pressure on the inner canthus of the eye following instillation of corticosteroid ophthalmic drops or ointment.

Side effects of corticosteroids can include:

Increased intraocular pressure (depends on dose, frequency, and length of treatment)

Reduced resistance to bacteria, virus, or fungus

Delayed healing of wounds

Stinging or burning

Contraindications or extreme caution applies to:

Acute bacterial, viral, or fungal infections

Primary open-angle glaucoma

Diabetes

Pregnancy

Prolonged use

TABLE 18.1.   ANTI-INFLAMMATORY CORTICOSTEROID OPHTHALMIC DRUGS

Generic Name	Trade Name	Dosage
prednisolone	Many combinations with antibiotics	Oint, sol, susp varies with condition
dexamethasone	Many combinations with antibiotics	Oint, sol, susp varies with condition

Note percent and dose ordered **carefully!**

PATIENT EDUCATION

Patients being treated with corticosteroid ophthalmic drugs should be instructed regarding:

Following directions carefully regarding time and amount.

Lowered resistance to infection—do not use long term.

Administration (i.e., pressure on tear duct at inner corner to reduce systemic absorption, (see Figure 18.2).

See Table 18.1 for a summary of anti-inflammatory ophthalmic drugs.

Antiglaucoma Agents

Glaucoma is an abnormal condition of the eye in which there is increased intraocular pressure (IOP) due to obstruction of the outflow of aqueous humor. There are two main types of glaucoma:

1. *Acute (angle-closure) glaucoma.* Characterized by a sudden onset of pain, blurred vision, and a dilated pupil. If untreated, blindness can result in a few days. Treatment consists of miotics (e.g., pilocarpine), osmotic agents (e.g., mannitol), (see Diuretics Chapter 15) carbonic inhibitors (e.g. Diamox) and surgery to open a pathway for release of aqueous humor.

2. *Chronic (open-angle) glaucoma.* Much more common, often bilateral, and develops slowly over a period of years with few symptoms except a gradual loss of peripheral vision and possibly blurred vision. Halos around lights and central blindness are late manifestations. *Treatment* consists of miotics, carbonic anhydrase inhibitors, and a local beta-adrenergic blocker, such as timolol (Timoptic) eye drops; sometimes epinephrine eye drops are given *with the miotics.* (**Note:** Epinephrine ophthalmic drops are *contraindicated in angle-closure glaucoma.*)

Antiglaucoma drugs, given to lower intraocular pressure, can be divided into four main categories based on their mode of action:

1. *Carbonic anhydrase inhibitors.* Act by decreasing the formation of aqueous humor.
2. *Miotics.* Act by increasing the aqueous outflow.
3. *Beta-adrenergic blockers,* for example, timolol.
4. *Sympathomimetics,* for example, dipivefrin, a prodrug of epinephrine, usually combined with other antiglaucoma drugs .

Drugs in different categories are sometimes given concomitantly.

CARBONIC ANHYDRASE INHIBITORS

Carbonic anhydrase inhibitors such as acetazolamide (Diamox) reduce the hydrogen and bicarbonate ions and have a diuretic effect. Acetazolamide (Diamox) is administered orally, in the treatment of open-angle glaucoma, or short-term preoperatively, to reduce intraocular pressure in angle-closure glaucoma, and is given with miotics or epinephrine products.

Side effects, infrequent and usually dose related, can include:

Nausea, vomiting, diarrhea, and constipation
Thirst and dry mouth
Drowsiness, fatigue, and vertigo
Numbness, muscular weakness, and tingling with high doses
Blood dyscrasias
Hepatic and renal disorders

Contraindications or caution applies to:

Chronic obstructive pulmonary disease (COPD)
Diabetes
Hepatic and renal disorders
Pregnancy

Interactions are frequent because of increasing or decreasing excretion of other drugs and can include:

Decreased effects of lithium, phenobarbital, salicylates, and oral antidiabetics
Increased effects of procaine, quinidine, amphetamines, and other diuretics
Hypokalemia with thiazides and corticosteroids

PATIENT EDUCATION

Patients being treated with carbonic anhydrase inhibitors should be instructed regarding:

Reporting side effects and response to the physician for appropriate dosage regulation.
Importance of follow-up with the physician.
Checking with the physician regarding dosage before taking any other medication.

MIOTICS

Miotics are medications that cause the pupil to contract. Miotics reduce intraocular pressure by increasing the aqueous outflow. They act by contracting the ciliary muscle. Miotics (e.g., pilocarpine) are used in the treatment of open-angle glaucoma or in short-term treatment of angle-closure glaucoma before surgery. Pilocarpine is also used after ophthalmic examinations in glaucoma patients to *constrict the pupil* and counteract the *mydriatic* (pupil-dilating) effect. Myotics are usually administered with acetazolamide, dipivefrin, and/or timolol. Because of their increased duration of effect and less frequent administration, pilocarpine hydrochloride gel or pilocarpine ocular systems may provide some advantages over ophthalmic solutions, especially long term with noncompliant patients.

Side effects of pilocarpine, usually dose related, can include:

Blurred vision and myopia
Twitching, stinging, and burning
Ocular pain and headache
Photophobia and poor vision in dim light
Aggravation of inflammatory processes

Systemic effects with frequent or prolonged use or high doses, especially in children, can include:

Nausea, vomiting, and diarrhea
Increased lacrimation and salivation

Contraindications or caution applies to:

Angle-closure glaucoma
History of retinal detachment or retinal degeneration
Acute inflammatory processes
Soft lenses in place
Corneal abrasion

Interactions may occur with:

Topical epinephrine, timolol, and acetazolamide which, potentiate effectiveness
Some anesthetics, which are potentiated by some miotics

PATIENT EDUCATION

Patients being treated with miotics should be instructed regarding:

Following directions carefully regarding time and amount.
Administration by closing tear duct after instillation (See Figure 18.2).
Reporting side effects to the physician for possible dosage adjustment.
Administration at bedtime to reduce side effects.
Not driving at night.

BETA-ADRENERGIC BLOCKERS

Timolol (Timoptic) acts as a beta-adrenergic blocker. It is used topically to lower intraocular pressure in open-angle glaucoma. Other beta blockers are also used topically to reduce IOP.

Side effects are infrequent but may include:

Ocular irritation, conjunctivitis, or diplopia
Aggravation of *preexisting* cardiovascular or pulmonary disorders, which may cause bradycardia, hypotension, and vertigo, or bronchospasm

Contraindications or extreme caution applies to:

Bradycardia and heart block
Patients receiving oral beta-blocker drugs
Asthma and COPD
Children, pregnancy, and lactation

Interactions may occur with:

Other antiglaucoma drugs to help lower intraocular pressure
Oral beta-blockers to increase chances of hypotension, bradycardia, and heart block

---

PATIENT EDUCATION

Patients being treated with beta-adrenergic blockers should be instructed regarding:

Administration by closing tear duct after instillation to reduce systemic effects (See Figure 18.2).

Caution in patients with cardiac or pulmonary disorders or who are taking oral beta-blockers.

Importance of regular eye examinations.

Continuous use of medications for glaucoma.

When administering more than one ophthalmic medication, allowing time interval (at least 5 min) between medications.

SYMPATHOMIMETICS

Epinephrine has a mydriatic effect in patients with open-angle glaucoma but is ineffective as a mydriatic in normal eyes, except during surgery. Epinephrine is sometimes combined with miotics in the treatment of open-angle glaucoma (not for angle-closure glaucoma). Epinephrine augments the action of miotics.

Because of the frequent adverse side effects of epinephrine, a *prodrug* of epinephrine, dipivefrin (Propine), is used more frequently to reduce elevated intraocular pressure (IOP) in the treatment of chronic open-angle glaucoma. A prodrug is a newly developed group of chemicals that exhibit their pharmacologic activity after biotransformation. Therefore, less of the drug is required and side effects occur less frequently and are milder with dipivefrin than with epinephrine. It is usually combined with one or more other antiglaucoma drugs.

Side effects, frequent with topical application of epinephrine, and milder with dipivefrin, include:

Burning, stinging, pain, and headache

Blurred vision and photophobia

Allergic reactions (e.g., dermatitis and edema)

Systemic effects, including palpitation, tachycardia, and tremor

Contraindications or extreme caution applies to:

Cardiac disorders and hypertension

Diabetes

Thyroid disorders

Cerebral arteriosclerosis

See Table 18.2 for a summary of antiglaucoma agents.

TABLE 18.2. ANTIGLAUCOMA AGENTS

Generic Name	Trade Name	Dosage
Carbonic Anhydrase Inhibitor		
acetazolamide	Diamox	Cap, tab, IV 250–500 mg bid or q4h
Miotics[a]		
pilocarpine HCl	Isopto E-Pilo	Ophthalmic sol, 0.25–6%[b], dose varies
pilocarpine gel	Isopto Carpine	Ophthalmic gel 4% hs
pilocarpine	Ocular System	40 mg/hr for 1 week
Beta-Adrenergic Blocker		
timolol	Timoptic	Ophthalmic sol, 0.1%
Sympathomimetic		
dipivefrin	Propine	Opthalmic sol, 0.1%

[a]Contract the pupil
[b]Wide variation in strengths available. Check carefully for correct percentage.

PATIENT EDUCATION

Patients being treated with sympathomimetics should be instructed regarding reporting side effects to the physician immediately.

Mydriatics

Mydriatics (e.g., atropine) are used topically to *dilate the pupil* for ophthalmic examinations. Atropine also acts as a *cycloplegic* (paralyzes the muscles of accommodation). It is the drug of choice in eye examinations for children. However, other mydriatics, for example, cyclopentolate, are more often used for adults because of faster action and faster recovery time.

Side effects of mydriatics, more likely in geriatric patients, may include:

Increased intraocular pressure
Local irritation, burning sensation transient
Blurred vision common
Flushing, dryness of skin, and fever
Confusion

Contraindications apply to:

Angle-closure glaucoma
Infants

TABLE 18.3. MYDRIATICS AND LOCAL ANESTHETICS FOR THE EYE

Generic Name	Trade Name	Dosage	Comments
Mydriatics[a]			
atropine	Atropine	Oint, sol 0.5–1%[b]	Administered 40–60 minutes before exam
cyclopentolate	Cyclogyl	Ophthalmic sol, 1–2%[b]	
Local Anesthetics			
tetracaine	Pontocaine	Oint or sol, 0.5%	Apply eye patch

[a]Dilate the pupil.
[b]Wide variations in strengths available. Check carefully for correct percentage.

PATIENT EDUCATION

Patients being treated with mydriatics should be instructed regarding:

Administration by closing tear duct after instillation (See Figure 18.2).
Aseptic technique to prevent contamination of medicine.
Blurred vision to be expected .

See Table 18.3 for a summary of the mydriatics.

Local Anesthetics

Local ophthalmic anesthetics, such as tetracaine *(Pontocaine),* are applied topically to the eye for minor surgical procedures, removal of foreign bodies, or painful injury.

Side effects are rare except with prolonged use but may include hypersensitivity reactions such as anaphylaxis in those allergic to the "-caine" local anesthetics.

Contraindicated for prolonged use because of the danger of corneal erosions.

PATIENT EDUCATION

Patients given local opthalmic anesthetics should be instructed regarding:

Necessity of wearing an eye patch after use of Pontocaine because of loss of blink reflex.
Avoidance of touching or rubbing the eye until the anesthesia has worn off.

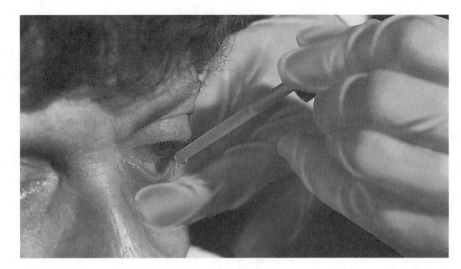

Figure 18.1 Instilling eye medication. Ophthalmic solution is dropped inside the lower eyelid.

PATIENT EDUCATION

Patients taking ophthalmic medications should be instructed regarding:

Making certain the correct medication and correct percent solution are used as prescribed.

Proper aseptic technique to prevent contamination of the other eye, the dropper, or the ointment tube.

Instillation of the *correct number of drops* or amount of ointment into the conjunctival sac (see Figure 18.1).

Closing the eye gently so as not to squeeze the medication out.

Applying gentle pressure to inner canthus after instillation to minimize systemic effects (see Figure 18.2).

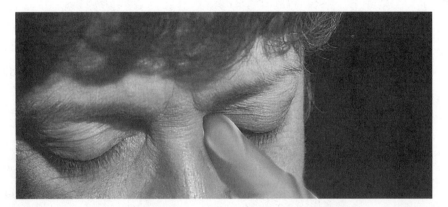

Figure 18.2 Gentle pressure on the inner canthus following administration of ophthalmic medications. Systemic absorption is thus minimized with medications such as corticosteroids, miotics, and mydriatics.

Worksheet for Chapter 18

EYE MEDICATIONS

List the drugs according to category and complete all columns. Learn generic or trade names as specified by instructor.

Classifications and Drugs	Purpose	Side Effects	Contraindications or Cautions	Patient Education
Anti-inflammatory 1.				
Antiglaucoma Carbonic Inhibitor 1.				
Miotics 1. 2.				
Beta-Adrenergic Blocker 1.				
Sympathomimetic 1.				
Mydriatics 1. 2.				
Local Anesthetic 1.				

A. Case Study for Eye Medications

Ida Lake, age 35, has been using corticosteroid eye drops for one week for "blood-shot eyes." She now has a purulent drainage from the left eye. She needs the following information.

1. Corticosteroid ophthalmic drops are used to treat all of the following EXCEPT
   a. Inflammation
   b. Allergies
   c. Infection
   d. Burns
2. Eye infections can be treated with all of the following EXCEPT
   a. Vira-A
   b. Prednisolone
   c. Gentamycin
   d. Polymixin B
3. The choice of antibiotic product would include consideration of the following EXCEPT
   a. Allergies
   b. Resistance
   c. Sensitivity of organism
   d. Age of the patient
4. Side effects of corticosteroid products could include the following EXCEPT
   a. Increased IOP
   b. Stinging
   c. Premature healing
   d. Fungal infections
5. Administration of antibiotic drops would include the following instruction EXCEPT
   a. Wash hands first
   b. Instill in inner canthus
   c. Avoid contaminating tip
   d. Discontinue with itching

B. Case Study for Eye Medications

Frank Frisbey, age 70, has been diagnosed with open-angle glaucoma. He will need the following information.

1. Treatment could include all of the following EXCEPT
   a. Isopto Carpine
   b. Timoptic
   c. Atropine
   d. Propine
2. The purpose of antiglaucoma drugs can include all of the following EXCEPT
   a. reduce IOP
   b. dilate pupil
   c. reduce aqueous formation
   d. increase aqueous outflow
3. The following statements are true of Diamox EXCEPT
   a. Diuretic effect
   b. Given PO
   c. Reduces IOP
   d. Given alone
4. Side effects of pilocarpine could include all of the following EXCEPT
   a. Photophobia
   b. Headache
   c. Urinary retention
   d. Blurred vision

5. Side effects of Timoptic can include all of the following EXCEPT
   a. Palpitations
   b. Bronchospasm
   c. Hypotension
   d. Vertigo

CHAPTER 19

Analgesics, Sedatives, and Hypnotics

OBJECTIVES

Upon completion of this chapter, the student should be able to:

1. Define analgesic, sedative, hypnotic, subjective, objective, placebo, endorphin, endogenous, narcotic, antipyretic, tinnitus, paradoxical, REM, tolerance, and dependence.
2. Compare and contrast the purpose and action of nonopioid, opioid, and adjuvant analgesics, sedatives, and hypnotics.
3. List the side effects of the major analgesics, sedatives, and hypnotics.
4. Describe the necessary information for patient education regarding interactions and cautions.
5. Explain the contraindications to administration of the CNS depressants in this chapter.

Analgesics, sedatives, and hypnotics depress central nervous system action to varying degrees. Some drugs can be classified in more than one category, depending on the dosage.

Analgesics are given for the purpose of relieving pain.

Sedatives are given to calm, soothe, or produce sedation.

Hypnotics are given to produce sleep.

Analgesics

Pain is subjective (i.e., it can be experienced or perceived only by the individual subject). Health care workers can view the patient's pain only in an objective way (i.e., observing the patient's reaction to pain in terms of vital signs, position, and emotional response). Pain has both psychological and physiological components.

Some persons have a higher pain threshold than others because of conditioning, ethnic background, sensitivity, or physiological factors (e.g., endorphin release).

Endorphins are endogenous analgesics (produced within the brain) as a reaction to severe pain or intense exercise (e.g., "runner's high"). Endorphins block the transmission of pain. Endorphin release may be responsible for a placebo effect: relief from pain as the result of suggestion without the administration of an analgesic.

OPIOID ANALGESICS

Analgesics can be classified as opioid, nonopioid, and adjuvant. Opioids are classified as full or pure agonists, partial agonists, or mixed agonist-antagonists depending on the specific receptors they bind to and their activity at the receptor. Full agonists are commonly used because their action is similar to that of opium in altering the perception of pain, and they do not have a ceiling to analgesic effects, that is, medication level where there is no enhanced analgesia. These opioids (e.g., morphine, hydromorphone, meperidine, oxycodone, and fentanyl) will not reverse analgesia like the other classes (e.g., pentazocine, butorphanol, and nalbuphine). Opioids are listed under the controlled substance schedule and include both the natural opium alkaloids (morphine and codeine) and the synthetics (e.g., meperidine). Opioids tend to cause tolerance (i.e., a larger dose of opioid is needed to achieve the same level of analgesia) and physiological dependence (i.e., physical adaptation of the body to the opioid and withdrawal symptoms after abrupt drug discontinuation) with chronic use.

Addiction or psychological dependence is not a problem for patients who require opioids for pain management. The majority of people stop taking opioids when their pain stops. Because of tolerance, the potential for developing dependence, and the potential for developing undesirable side effects, opioids are not used for extended periods except to relieve chronic pain, for example, cancer pain, terminal illness, and selected patients with nonmalignant pain who do not benefit from other pain relief methods. Adequate pain control is important for the terminally ill. Dependence is irrelevant for dying patients and should not be a consideration. More effective pain control can be achieved by combining opioids with nonopioid and adjuvant drugs. Analgesics should be given to the terminally ill patients around the clock, with additional "as needed" doses, and dosages adjusted to achieve pain relief with an acceptable level of side effects. Around-the-clock dosing prevents pain.

Chronic pain therapy, for example, for back pain, sometimes includes the addition of a tricyclic antidepressant or anticonvulsant to the analgesic regimen. These drugs that enhance analgesic effects are called adjuvant analgesics and are explained later in this chapter. This addition can reduce the dosage of opioids.

Side effects of opioids can include:

Sedation
Confusion, euphoria, restlessness, and agitation
Headache and dizziness
Hypotension and bradycardia
Nausea, vomiting, and constipation

Urinary retention
Respiratory depression
Physical and/or emotional dependence
Blurred vision
Convulsions with large doses
Flushing and rash

Contraindications or extreme caution with opioids applies to:

Head injury (i.e., conditions associated with increased intracranial pressure)
CNS depression
Hepatic and renal disease
Hypothyroidism
COPD
Pregnancy, lactation, and pediatrics
Elderly and debilitated
Addiction prone, suicidal, and alcoholic
Hypersensitivity

Interactions include potentiation of effect with all CNS depressants, including:

Psychotropics
Alcohol
Sedatives and hypnotics
Muscle relaxants
Antihistamines
Antiemetics
Antiarrhythmics or antihypertensives

Meperidine is frequently combined with Phenergan postoperatively to potentiate analgesic effect.

Morphine is chemically incompatible with solutions containing many other drugs and, therefore, should *not* be mixed with other medications in the same syringe or IV tubing.

See Table 19.1 for a summary of the opioid analgesics.

Opioid antagonists are used in the treatment of opioid overdoses and in the delivery room and newborn nursery for opiate-induced respiratory depression. Two opiate antagonists are naloxone and naltrexone.

Generic Name	Trade Name	Comments
naloxone	Narcan	For all conditions listed above
naltrexone	ReVia	To treat opiate and alcohol dependence

Caution: Naltrexone is used only *after* withdrawal from opiates, such as heroin and morphine, to help avoid relapses. It acts by robbing the drugs of their pleasurable effects. If given to someone currently dependent on opiates, it can send the addict *instantly into severe life-threatening withdrawal.*

TABLE 19.1. OPIOID ANALGESICS[a]

Generic Name	Trade Name	Dosage	Comments
butorphanol	Stadol	1–4 mg IM, or 0.5–2 mg IV, or 1 mg (one spray) nasal spray q 3–4h PRN	Not recommended for patients with cancer pain or chronic pain, for moderate to severe acute pain, i.e., migraine
codeine	Codeine[b]	15–60 mg PO/IM/ IV/SC q 4h PRN;	For mild to moderate acute, chronic, and cancer pain
		10–30 mg PO/IM/IV/SC q 4–6h PRN	Antitussive
hydrocodone with acetaminophen	Lorcet[c] Lortab Vicodin	5–10 mg PO q 4–6h PRN	For mild to moderate acute, chronic, or cancer pain, or antitussive
meperidine	Demerol	50–150 mg PO/IM/SC, 25–100 mg slow IV q3–4h PRN	For mild to moderate acute pain, not for chronic pain
oxycodone with aspirin	Roxicodone Percodan[d]	1–2 tab or 5–10 ml PO q 4-6h PRN	For mild to severe acute, chronic, or cancer pain
oxycodone with acetaminophen	Tylox, Percocet		
propoxyphene HCl with acetaminophen	Darvon Darvocet	65–100 mg PO q 4h PRN	For mild to moderate acute, chronic, or cancer pain Overdose can cause convulsions
methadone	Dolophine	2.5–10 mg IM/SC/PO initially q 3–4h PRN; 5–20 mg PO maint. q 6–8h PRN	For moderate to severe acute, chronic, and cancer pain Also used for narcotic withdrawal
morphine sulfate	Morphine, MS, MS Contin, (sustained-release) MSIR (immediate release)	10–60 mg PO or 10–20 mg R q 4h PRN; 15–100 mg PO SR q 8–12h; 2.5–15 mg slow IV over 4–5 min; 2.5–20 mg IV/SC q 4h PRN	For moderate to severe acute, chronic, or cancer pain
fentanyl citrate	Fentanyl	200–400 μg PO q 4–6h PRN; or 25–100 μg IV/IM; or transdermal q 72h	For moderate to severe acute, chronic, or cancer pain
pentazocine	Talwin	50–100 mg PO q 3–4h PRN; 15–30 mg IV, or 30–60 mg IM/SC q 3–4h PRN	For mild to moderate, acute, or chronic pain
sufentanil citrate	Sufenta	10–30 μg IV/IM; or 1.5–3.0 μg/kg intranasally	For moderate to severe acute, chronic, or cancer pain

[a]Watch closely for side effects. Check for allergies, especially aspirin combinations.
[b]Each Tylenol #2 tablet contains 300 mg acetaminophen plus codeine, codeine 15 mg; #3, codeine 30 mg; and #4, codeine 60 mg. Each Tylenol with codeine elixir contains codeine 12 mg/5 ml and acetaminophen 120 mg/5 ml. Each Empirin #2 tablet contains (325 mg) aspirin plus codeine 15 mg (0.25 g); #3, codeine 30 mg 0.5 g); and #4, codeine 60 mg.
[c]Each Lorcet, Lortab or Vicodin contains 500 mg acetaminophen and hydrocodone 5 mg. Each Lortab 7.5 mg/500 tablet contains 500 mg acetaminophen and hydrocodone 7.5 mg. Each Lorcet Plus tablet contains 650 mg acetaminophen and hydrocodone 7.5 mg. Each Vicodin ES tablet contains 750 mg acetaminophen and hydrocodone 7.5 mg. Each 5 ml of Lortab liquid contains 120 mg acetaminophen and hydrocodone 2.5 mg.
[d]Each Percodan Codoxy, or Roxiprin, contains aspirin 325 mg and oxycodone 5 mg. Each Percocet, Roxicet, or Oxycet contains acetaminophen 325 mg and oxycodone 5 mg. Each Tylox or Roxilox contains 500 mg acetaminophen and oxycodone 5 mg.

NONOPIOID ANALGESICS

Nonopioid analgesics, many of which are available without prescription as over-the-counter medications, are very popular in this nation of "pill poppers." Therefore, it is extremely important that the health care worker be informed and responsible for patient education in this very important area of public health. The lay public needs to become aware of the dangers of self-medication, overdosage, side effects, and interactions, as well as the grave danger of poisoning to children and the elderly by inappropriate use of these readily available drugs.

The nonopioids are given for the purposes of relieving mild to moderate pain, fever, and anti-inflammatory conditions, for example, arthritis. This group of analgesics is also used as a *coanalgesic* in severe acute or chronic pain requiring opioids. The salicylates (aspirin, salsalate, choline magnesium trisalicylate) are most commonly used for their analgesic and antipyretic properties, as well as for their anti-inflammatory action. Other anti-inflammatory drugs, for example, ibuprofen, are also used for their analgesic properties. The nonsteroidal anti-inflammatory drugs (NSAIDs) are discussed in Chapter 21. Acetaminophen has analgesic and anti-pyretic properties but very little effect on inflammation. Aspirin and acetaminophen are frequently combined with opioids (see Table 19.1) or with other drugs for more effective analgesic action. See Table 19.2 for a representative sample of nonopioid analgesics and antipyretics. There are many other combination analgesic products available over the counter. Patients should be instructed to check all ingredients in these combination products because of potentially serious adverse side effects, for example, aspirin allergy or acetaminophen contraindications.

TABLE 19.2. NONOPIOID ANALGESICS AND ANTIPYRETICS

Generic Name	Trade Name	Dosage	Comments
acetylsalicyclic acid[a]	Aspirin, ASA, Empirin, Ascriptin, Bufferin	5–10 gr PO or rectal supp q4h PRN; large doses for arthritis	Give with milk or food
acetaminophen	Tylenol, Datril, Tempra	325–650 mg PO or rectal supp q4h PRN	No anti-inflammatory action
combinations[b] ASA and caffeine	Anacin		
ASA and meprobamate plus ethoheptazine citrate	Equagesic		
ASA and acetaminophen and caffeine	Excedrin		
chlorzoxazone and acetaminophen	Parafon Forte		Can cause liver toxicity
tramadol	Ultram	500–100 mg	Qd q 4–6h Not to exceed 400 mg

[a]Other nonsteroidal anti-inflammatory drugs with analgesic action are listed in Table 21.2.
[b]Representative sample.

SALICYLATES

Salicylate analgesic and anti-inflammatory actions are associated primarily with preventing the formation of prostaglandins. The salicylates, for example, aspirin (ASA), are also discussed in Chapter 21.

Side effects of salicylates and other NSAIDs, especially with prolonged use and/or high dosages, can include:

Prolonged bleeding time

Bleeding and frequent bruising

Gastric distress, ulceration, and bleeding (which may be silent)

Tinnitus (ringing or roaring in the ears) and hearing loss with overdose

Hepatic dysfunction

Renal insufficiency, decreased urine output with sodium and water retention, renal failure

Drowsiness, dizziness, headache, sweating, euphoria, depression

Rash

Coma, respiratory failure, or anaphylaxis, which can result from hypersensitivity or overdosage, especially with children

GI symptoms, which can be minimized by administration with food, milk, or by using an aspirin buffered with antacids or in enteric-coated form

Poisoning—keep out of reach of children (especially flavored children's aspirin)

Contraindications for salicylates and other NSAIDs include:

GI ulcer and bleeding

Bleeding disorders and patients taking anticoagulants

Asthma

Children with influenza-like illness (because of the danger of Reye's syndrome)

Pregnancy

Lactation

Vitamin K deficiency

Caution in use of salicylates and other NSAIDs with the following:

Anemia

Hepatic disease

Renal disease

Hodgkin's disease

Pre/postoperatively

Interactions may occur with NSAIDs and the following:

Alcohol (may increase potential for ulceration and bleeding)

Anticoagulants (potentiation)

Corticosteroids (gastric ulcer)

Antacids (decreased effect)

Cimetidine (potentiation)

Insulin (increased effects)

Methotrexate (increased effects)

Sulfonylamides (decreased effects)

Probenecid (decreased effects)

PABA (toxic effects)

Furosemide (toxic effects)

Carbonic anhydrase inhibitors (toxic effects)—for example, Diamox

ACETAMINOPHEN

Acetaminophen (Tylenol) is used extensively in the treatment of mild to moderate pain and fever. It has very little effect on inflammation. However, acetaminophen has fewer adverse side effects than the salicylates (e.g., does not cause gastric irritation or precipitate bleeding). Therefore, it is sometimes used only for its analgesic properties in treating the chronic pain of arthritis so that the salicylate dosage may be reduced to safer levels with fewer side effects in these patients.

Side effects are rare, but large doses can cause:

Severe liver toxicity

Renal insufficiency (decreased urine output)

Rash or urticaria

Caution must be used with frequent acetaminophen use and alcohol ingestion because of potential liver damage. Caution also with pregnancy.

Contraindicated for repeated administration with anemia, cardiac or pulmonary conditions, renal or hepatic disease.

TRAMADOL

Tramadol (Ultram) is a centrally acting synthetic analgesic compound similar in effect to the opioids, but is chemically unrelated. It is nonopioid and is not a controlled substance. It produces analgesia by inhibiting the reuptake of norepinephrine and serotonin.

Side effects of Ultram can include:

Dizziness, somnolence, malaise, headache

Nausea, constipation

Sweating and pruritis

Orthostatic hypotension

Anxiety, confusion

Contraindications with Ultram include:

Increased intracranial pressure or head injury

Renal and hepatic disease
Seizure disorders
Pregnant or nursing women
Children under 16

Caution in the elderly and with anyone driving or operating machinery. May impair mental or physical abilities.

Interactions with:

MAO inhibitors or neuroleptics—may increase seizure risk
Carbamazepine (Tegretol) antagonizes Ultram action

See Table 19.2 for a summary of the nonopioid analgesics and antipyretics.

ADJUVANT ANALGESICS

These drugs were originally intended for treatment of conditions other than pain. Adjuvant analgesics may enhance analgesic effect with opioids and nonopioids, produce analgesia alone, or reduce the side effects of analgesics. Two classes commonly used for analgesia include anticonvulsants and tricyclic antidepressants. See Table 19.3 for a summary of adjuvant analgesics.

TRICYCLIC ANTIDEPRESSANTS

Tricyclic antidepressants are used in the treatment of nerve pain associated with herpes, arthritis, diabetes, and cancer, migraine or tension headaches, insomnia, and depression. Often, the patient will describe the pain as "burning." Tricyclic antidepressant actions are associated with increasing available serotonin, which blocks pain transmission. Drugs used commonly for pain include Elavil, Pamelor, and Tofranil.

TABLE 19.3. ADJUVANT ANALGESICS

Generic Name	Trade Name	Dosage	Comments
Tricyclic Antidepressants			
amitripytyline	Elavil	10–25 mg qhs	Cautious increase with concurrent opioids
nortriptyline	Pamelor	50–100 mg qhs	
imipramine	Tofranil	50–100 mg qhs	
Anticonvulsants			
carbamazepine	Tegretol	200 mg PO BID–QID	Initiate at low dose and gradually increase for maintenance dose
phenytoin sodium	Dilantin	100–200 mg TID	Begin with oral loading dose of 1,000 mg in 1st 24 hours, then 300–500 mg/day

Side effects of tricyclic antidepressants can include:

Dry mouth, urinary retention, delirium, constipation
Sedation
Orthostatic hypotension
Tachyarrhythmias
Heart block in cardiac patients

The degree of side effects varies with each antidepressant. Side effects may be additive with opioids (e.g., increased constipation, sedation, etc.).

Caution must be used with prostatic hypertrophy, urinary retention, increased intraocular pressure, and glaucoma.

Contraindications with hypersensitivity and recovery phase of myocardial infarction.

ANTICONVULSANTS

Anticonvulsants (i.e., Dilantin and Tegretol), like tricyclic antidepressants, are commonly used for the management of nerve pain associated with neuralgia, herpes, and cancer. Anticonvulsant therapy is implemented when the patient describes the pain as "sharp," "shooting," "shocklike pain," or "lightening-like."

Side effects of anticonvulsants can include the following:

Sedation, dizziness, and confusion
Nausea, vomiting, constipation, and anorexia
Hypotension and unsteadiness
Hepatitis
Rash, Steven-Johnson syndrome
Bone marrow suppression
Nystagmus, diplopia (double vision), and blurred vision

Caution must be used with allergies, hepatitis, cardiac disease, and renal disease.

Contraindications include:

Hypersensitivity
Psychiatric condition
Pregnancy
Bradycardia
SA (sinoatrial) and (atrioventricular) AV block
Stokes-Adams syndrome
Bone marrow suppression

Interactions occur with:

Alcohol (decreased effects)

Antihistamines (decreased effects)

Antacids (decreased effects)

Antineoplastics (decreased effects)

CNS depressants (decreased effects)

Folic acid (decreased effects)

Incompatible (Dilantin) with any drug in solution or syringe

Sedatives and Hypnotics

Sedatives and hypnotics are controlled substances used to promote sedation in smaller doses and to promote sleep in larger doses. In addition, phenobarbital is used prophylactically with febrile children who are seizure prone or in the treatment of seizure disorders, frequently combined with phenytoin (see Chapter 22). Pentobarbital is also used IV or IM to control status epilepticus or preoperatively (see Chapter 27). Some of the psychotropic drugs are also used as sedative-hypnotics and are discussed in Chapter 20.

The sedative-hypnotics are classified as barbiturates and nonbarbiturates. None of these medications should be used for extended periods of time except under close medical supervision, as in the treatment of epilepsy, because of the potential for psychological and physical dependence. In addition, these medications depress the REM (rapid eye movement, or dream) phase of sleep, and withdrawal after prolonged use can result in a severe rebound effect with nightmares and hallucinations. The nonbarbiturates depress REM sleep to a lesser degree than the barbiturates. Abrupt withdrawal of hypnotics, even after short-term therapy, for example, 1 week, may result in rebound insomnia. Therefore, gradual reduction of dosage is indicated. Additionally, avoidance of caffeine and alcohol should be stressed. Alcohol may help to initiate sleep but results in early awakening.

BARBITURATES

Barbiturates have been implicated in many suicides and fatalities due to accidental overdoses, especially when combined with other CNS depressants or alcohol. They are particularly dangerous because they are slowly metabolized and excreted, that is, they have an extended half-life, remaining in the system longer.

Children or the elderly may manifest paradoxical reactions to the barbiturates, such as hyperexcitability, confusion, or hallucinations. Because of slower metabolism and impaired circulation and memory, the elderly or debilitated patient is particularly susceptible to ill effects and overdose, and should be encouraged to use more natural methods of combating insomnia, such as exercise during the day, avoiding heavy meals near bedtime, warm milk, back rubs, soft music, and other calming influences.

Side effects of the barbiturates can include:

"Hangover effect" including lethargy, incoordination, depression, and headache

Nausea, vomiting, diarrhea, or constipation

Rash

Angioedema

Confusion and delirium

Respiratory depression—IV administration may cause apnea or bronchospasm

Coma

Fatal overdoses

Interactions of barbiturates with the following:

Alcohol (increased CNS depression)

Monoamine oxidase inhibitors (increased CNS depression)

Sedatives (increased CNS depression)

Analgesics (increased CNS depression)

Oral contraceptives (decreased contraceptive effect)

Corticosteroids (decreased corticosteroid effect)

Oral anticoagulants (decreased anticoagulant effect)

Theophyline (decreased theophyline effect)

NONBARBITURATES

Nonbarbiturates have been proclaimed as safer and having less potential for abuse than the barbiturates. However, recent statistics indicate growing misuse of these drugs with potentially fatal results as well. Only short-term use of any hypnotic is recommended.

Older nonbarbiturate hypnotics include the bromides and chloral hydrate. Newer drugs in this category include the benzodiazepines, for example, temazepam (Restoril), and miscellaneous hypnotics like glutethimide and zolpidem tartrate (Ambien).

Side effects of the bromides and chloral hydrate include:

Nausea, vomiting, diarrhea

Rash

Dizziness

Ataxia

Side effects of benzodiazepines can include:

Leukopenia with prolonged use.

Daytime sedation, confusion, and headache—hangover effect

Amnesia, hallucinations, and bizarre behavior may occur more often with triazolam (Halcion) than with other benzodiazepines

Contraindications for all the sedative-hypnotics include:

Hypersensitivity

Severe liver impairment

Severe renal impairment

Porphyria

Caution with all sedative hypnotics for the following:

Elderly

Debilitated

Addiction prone

Renal impairment

Liver impairment

Depressed and mentally unstable

Suicidal individuals

Pregnancy and lactation

Children

TABLE 19.4. SEDATIVES AND HYPNOTICS (USE HYPNOTICS SHORT TERM ONLY)

Generic Name	Trade Name	Dosage	Comments
Barbiturates			
amobarbital	Amytal	65–200 mg PO or IM hs	For insomnia
		30–50 mg PO BID–QID, up to 120 mg/day	For sedation
pentobarbital	Nembutal	100–200 mg PO hs	Do not mix with other drugs in same syringe,
		150–200 mg IM hs	
		30–60 mg R hs	IV only with resuscitative equipment available
secobarbital	Seconal	100–200 PO/IM hs	For insomnia or sedation
talbutal	Lotusate	120 mg PO hs	Short-term treatment of insomnia
Nonbarbiturates			
chloral hydrate	Noctec	500 mg–1 g PO/rectally 1/2 h before hs	Short-term treatment of insomnia only
ethclorvynol	Placidyl	500 mg–1 g PO 1/2 h before hs	For insomnia
		100–200 PO BID or TID	For sedation
flurazepam	Dalmane	15–30 mg PO h5	Long elimination half-life
temazepam	Restoril	15–30 mg PO hs	
triazolam	Halcion	0.125–0.5 mg PO hs	Can cause amnesia, hallucinations, bizarre behavior, long half-life
glutethimide	Glutethimide	250–500 mg PO hs	Try after other measures for sleep
zolpidem tartrate	Ambien	10 mg PO × 7–10 days	May take 2 nights for benefits to be observed
			Rapid induction 30 min
			Short half-life (less than 3 h)

Interactions of all the sedative hypnotics with the following drugs can be dangerous and potentially fatal:

Psychotropic drugs

Alcohol

Muscle relaxants

Antiemetics

Antihistamines

Analgesics

See Table 19.4 for a summary of the sedatives and hypnotics.

PATIENT EDUCATION

Patients taking analgesics, sedatives, or hypnotics should be instructed regarding:

Potential for physical and psychological dependence and tolerance with opioids, sedatives, and hypnotics.

Taking only limited doses for short periods of time, *except* to relieve pain in terminal illness (in terminal cases, analgesics should be given on a regular basis around the clock to prevent or control pain).

Caution with interactions; *not* taking any medications (except under close medical supervision) that potentiate CNS depression (e.g., psychotropics, *alcohol*, muscle relaxants, antihistamines, antiemetics, cardiac medications, and antihypertensives).

Serious potential side effects with prolonged use or overdose of opioids, sedatives, and hypnotics (e.g., oversedation, dizziness, headache, confusion, agitation, nausea, constipation, urinary retention, and *potentially fatal* respiratory depression, bradycardia, or hypotension).

Tolerance effect with prolonged use, with increasingly larger doses required to achieve the same effect.

Potential for overdose of sedatives or hypnotics and paradoxical reactions with the elderly (e.g., confusion, agitation, hallucinations, and hyperexcitability).

Withdrawal after prolonged use of sedatives and hypnotics possibly leading to rebound effects with nightmares, hallucinations, and/or insomnia.

Mental alertness and physical coordination impairment causing accidents or falls.

Caution regarding OTC analgesic combinations and checking ingredients on the label; being aware of possible side effects with those containing aspirin (e.g., gastric distress or bleeding).

Worksheet for Chapter 19

ANALGESICS, SEDATIVES, AND HYPNOTICS

Note the drugs listed according to category and complete all columns. Learn generic or trade names as specified by instructor.

Classifications and Drugs	Purpose	Side Effects	Contraindications or Cautions	Patient Education
Opioids				
1. codeine				
2. hydrocodone (Lorcet)				
3. meperidine (Demerol)				
4. morphine				
5. oxycodone (Percodan)				
6. Talwin				
7. Darvon				
Opioid Antagonist				
1. Narcan				

Worksheet for Chapter 19

ANALGESICS, SEDATIVES, AND HYPNOTICS

Note the drugs listed according to category and complete all columns. See note on Table 14.1 regarding names of drugs.

Classifications and Drugs	Purpose	Side Effects	Contraindications or Cautions	Patient Education
Nonopioid Analgesics				
1. aspirin				
2. acetaminophen (Tylenol)				
3. tramadol (Ultram)				
Sedative-Hypnotic Barbiturates				
1. pentobarbital (Nembutal)				
2. secobarbital (Seconal)				
Sedative-Hypnotic Nonbarbiturates				
1. chloral hydrate (Noctec)				
2. flurazepam (Dalmane)				
3. temazepam (Restoril)				
4. zolpidem (Ambien)				

A. Case Study for Analgesics

Sarah Payne, a 45-year-old terminal cancer patient, is discharged from the hospital to her home with hospice care. Her husband is concerned that she be pain-free, but worries that she will become "addicted" to her pain medicines. He needs the following information.

1. Opioids, for example, morphine, are given regularly with all of the following conditions EXCEPT
   a. Cancer pain
   b. Arthritis pain
   c. Short-term acute pain
   d. Terminally ill

2. Morphine is frequently combined with other drugs to enhance pain relief. Which one would NOT potentiate effect?
   a. Ibuprofen
   b. Tofranil
   c. Narcan
   d. Dilantin

3. Analgesics are *most* effective when given
   a. As necessary
   b. During waking hours
   c. Before meals
   d. Around-the-clock

4. Side effects of opioids can include all of the following EXCEPT
   a. Dizziness
   b. Diarrhea
   c. Nausea
   d. Confusion

5. Opioids are frequently given with nonopioids for better analgesic action. Which one is NOT considered a coanalgesic?
   a. Acetaminophen
   b. Aspirin
   c. Elavil
   d. Ambien

B. Case Study for Hypnotics

Freda Stone, a 70-year-old patient with arthritis pain, has been taking Restoril for sleep for years. She wants to change to Halcion now. She needs the following information.

1. Which statement is generally true of most hypnotics?
   a. Rapid elimination usual
   b. Safe for the elderly
   c. Effective long term
   d. Side effects common

2. Halcion can have all of the following side effects EXCEPT
   a. Amnesia
   b. Hallucinations
   c. Short half-life
   d. Bizarre behavior

3. Which of the following would be LEAST susceptible to ill effects?
   a. Children
   b. Debilitated
   c. Obese
   d. Elderly

4. Common side effects of many hypnotics can include all of the following EXCEPT
   a. Dizziness
   b. Diuresis
   c. Confusion
   d. Hangover

5. Hypnotic interactions can be potentially dangerous with all of the following EXCEPT
   a. Alcohol
   b. Antidepressants
   c. Analgesics
   d. Antacids

CHAPTER **20**

Psychotropic Medications, Alcohol, and Drug Abuse

OBJECTIVES

Upon completion of this chapter, the student should be able to:

1. Define psychotropic, tranquilizer, phenothiazine, tricyclic, neurotransmitter, tardive dyskinesia, ataxia, paradoxical effect, and bipolar disorders.
2. Categorize the most commonly used psychotropic medications according to the following four classifications: CNS stimulants, antidepressants, anxiolytics, and antipsychotic medications.
3. List the purpose, action, side effects, interactions, and contraindications for psychotropic medications in common use.
4. Describe the physiological effects of prolonged alcohol use.
5. Explain treatment of acute and chronic alcoholism.
6. Compare and contrast drug addiction and habituation.
7. Describe the effects of three commonly used illegal drugs.
9. List the responsibilities of the health care worker in combating drug abuse.

Psychotropic refers to any substance that acts on the mind. Psychotropic medications are drugs that can exert a therapeutic effect on a person's mental processes, emotions, or behavior. Drugs used for other purposes can have psychotropic effects. Examples of other medications that affect mental functioning are anesthetics, analgesics, sedatives, hypnotics, and antiemetics, which are discussed in other chapters.

Psychotropic medications can be classified according to the purpose for administration. The four classes are CNS stimulants, antidepressants, anxiolytics, and antipsychotic medications.

Psychotropic medications are frequently prescribed concurrently with psychotherapy or professional counseling.

333

CNS Stimulants

CNS (central nervous system) stimulant medications are given for the purpose of promoting central nervous system functioning. One drug in this category, caffeine citrate, has been used in the treatment of neonatal apnea.

Prolonged, high intake of caffeine in any form may produce tolerance, habituation, and psychological dependence. Physical signs of withdrawal such as headaches, irritation, nervousness, anxiety, and dizziness may occur upon abrupt discontinuation of the stimulant.

Since caffeine crosses the placenta and is also distributed into the milk of nursing women, most clinicians recommend that those who are pregnant or nursing avoid or limit their consumption of foods, beverages, and drugs containing caffeine, for example, over-the-counter (OTC) analgesics or decongestants.

Other CNS stimulant drugs include the amphetamines and methylphenidate (Ritalin), which are used to treat hyperkinetic syndrome or attention deficit disorder in children over 6, and for narcolepsy. Ritalin is also occasionally used in the treatment of senile apathy. The use of amphetamines to reduce appetite in the treatment of obesity is *not* recommended because tolerance develops rapidly and physical or psychic dependence may develop within a few weeks. *These drugs have a high potential for abuse and should be used only under medical supervision for diagnosed medical disorders.*

Side effects of the amphetamines and methylphenidate can include:

Nervousness, insomnia, and irritability, or psychosis from overdose
Tachycardia, palpitations, hypertension, hypotension, and cardiac arrhythmias
Dizziness, headache, and blurred vision (dilated pupils with photophobia)
GI disturbances, including anorexia, nausea, vomiting, and abdominal pain
Habituation and dependence possible with prolonged use

Contraindications or caution applies to:

Treatment for obesity (never more than 2 weeks)—withdrawal causes depression
Patients with anxiety or agitation or history of seizures
History of drug dependence or alcoholism
Hyperthyroidism
Diabetes and renal disorders
Cardiovascular disorders
Glaucoma
Pregnant or nursing women

Pediatric precautions: Prolonged administration of CNS stimulants to children with attention deficit disorder has been reported to cause at least a temporary suppression of normal weight and/or height patterns in some patients, and therefore close monitoring is required. CNS stimulants, including amphetamines, have been reported to exacerbate motor and vocal tics and Tourette's disorder, and clinical

TABLE 20.1. CENTRAL NERVOUS SYSTEM STIMULANTS

Generic Name	Trade Name	Dosage	Comments
caffeine citrate			For neonatal apnea (currently questioned by FDA)
amphetamines	Biphetamine, Dexedrine	5 mg bid or tid	For narcolepsy or attention deficit disorder
methylphenidate	Ritalin	5–10 mg tid	For narcolepsy, attention deficit disorder, or senile apathy

evaluation for these disorders in children and their families should precede use of the drugs. Children should also be observed carefully for development of tics while receiving these drugs.

Abuse of amphetamines: Signs and symptoms of chronic amphetamine abuse and acute toxicity are discussed later in this chapter in the section entitled Drug Abuse. Treatment of acute toxicity is also described in that section.

PATIENT EDUCATION

Patients receiving amphetamines or Ritalin should be warned about the potential side effects.

They should be cautioned about the potential for abuse and should take them only according to physician's orders.

Medication should be taken early in the day to reduce insomnia.

Abrupt withdrawal may result in depression, irritability, fatigue, agitation, and disturbed sleep.

Parents of children receiving these drugs should watch for signs of tics, gastric disturbance, insomnia, weight loss, or nervousness and report to the physician.

Geriatric patients should be warned particularly about dangerous cardiovascular side effects.

See Table 20.1 for a summary of the CNS stimulants.

Antidepressants

Depression is frequently described as a chemical imbalance. In many depressed patients, certain chemicals in the brain may be in short supply. Chemicals in the brain, like serotonin and norepinephrine are known as *neurotransmitters*. Substances that travel across the synapse (contact point of two neurons) transmit messages between nerve cells. If these neurotransmitters are reabsorbed by one nerve ending before they have had a chance to make contact with the next nerve cell, they cannot perform their function. In depression there may be a shortage of the neurotransmitters serotonin or norepinephrine.

Antidepressant medications, sometimes called mood elevators, are used primarily to treat patients with various types of depression. The three categories in general use are the tricyclic antidepressants, the monamine oxidase inhibitors (MAOIs), and the selective serotonin reuptake inhibitors (SSRIs).

TRICYCLICS

The precise mechanism of antidepressant action of the tricyclics is unclear. The pharmacology is complex and includes strong anticholinergic activity that could affect certain neurotransmitters.

The tricyclics have delayed action, elevating the mood and increasing alertness after 10–30 days. They are frequently given at bedtime because of a mild sedative effect. They are used more frequently than the MAOIs because of milder and fewer side effects, except with the elderly.

Side effects of the tricyclics, such as imipramine (Tofranil), are anticholinergic in action and can include:

Dryness of the mouth
Increased appetite and weight gain
Drowsiness and dizziness
Blurred vision
Constipation and urinary retention
Postural hypotension, cardiac arrhythmias, and palpitation
Confusion, especially in the elderly

Contraindications or extreme caution applies to:

Cardiac, renal, and liver disorders
Elderly
Glaucoma
Obesity

Interactions may occur with other CNS drugs and alcohol.

MAO INHIBITORS

MAO inhibitors (MAOIs) were discovered as part of research with isoniazid (INH), an antitubercular drug. The precise mechanism of antidepressant action of MAO is unclear.

The MAOIs such as phenelzine (Nardil), have potentially very serious side effects and cannot be given until 2 weeks after the tricyclics have been discontinued.

Side effects are adrenergic in action and can include:

Nervousness, agitation, and insomnia
Headache

Hypertension or hypertensive crisis (can be fatal)

Tachycardia, palpitation, and chest pain

Nausea, vomiting, and diarrhea

Blurred vision

Contraindications apply to patients with cardiac and liver disease.

Interactions of the MAOIs with some drugs and foods can cause *hypertensive crisis*, manifested by severe headache, palpitation, sweating, chest pain, possible intracranial hemorrhage, and even death. Interactions may occur with:

Adrenergic drugs, diuretics, insulin, and levodopa

Tricyclics, resulting in seizures, fever, hypertension, and confusion

CNS depressants, resulting in circulatory collapse

Foods containing tryamine, tryptamine, or tryptophan, such as yogurt, sour cream, all cheeses, liver (especially chicken), pickled herring, figs, raisins, bananas, pineapple, avocados, broad beans (Chinese pea pods), meat tenderizers, and *alcoholic beverages* (especially red wine and beer), and all fermented or aged foods (e.g., corned beef, salami, and pepperoni)

SELECTIVE SEROTONIN REUPTAKE INHIBITORS

The antidepressants in this category selectively block the reabsorption of the neurotransmitter serotonin, thus helping to restore the brain's chemical balance. Drugs in this newest class of antidepressants include fluoxetine (Prozac) and sertraline (Zoloft). Therapy may be required for several months or longer. Symptomatic relief may require 1–4 weeks and there is prolonged elimination of the drug.

Side effects of the SSRIs may include:

Nausea, anorexia

Diarrhea, sweating

Insomnia, anxiety, nervousness, tremor, drowsiness, fatigue, dizziness, headache

Other side effects have been reported in less than 1% to 3% of patients receiving them.

Caution applies to patients with the following conditions:

Liver or renal impairment

Suicide prone

Diabetes

Bipolar disorders—may precipitate manic attacks

Underweight

Interactions possible with:

Other CNS drugs—not confirmed clinically

MAOIs—never take concurrently

Other SSRIs, different in structure but similar in action, enhancing serotonin and norepinephrine, include paroxetine (Paxil), venlafaxine (Effexor), and trazodone (Desyrel).

Side effects and cautions for Paxil and Effexor are similar to other SSRIs.

Side effects of Desyrel can include:

Drowsiness—common

Insomnia

Urinary flow dysfunction

Priapism or impotence—discontinue the drug

Interactions with other CNS depressants, including alcohol, may potentiate sedation. Food will increase drug absorption and decrease incidence of lightheadedness.

Caution applies to:

Suicide prone

Seizure disorder

Diabetes or liver disorders

Interactions possible with:

Other CNS drugs

Antidiabetic agents

Antimanic Agent

LITHIUM

Lithium salts are antimanic agents, not recommended for depression alone. Bipolar disorders (manic-depressive) are treated *long term* with lithium salts. A maintenance dose is established by monitoring blood levels. Daily serum levels are checked initially and every few months thereafter to maintain a level of 1–1.5 mEq/L. Patients must be monitored and alerted for signs of toxicity.

Side effects of lithium can include:

GI distress (usual initially and resolves)—take medicine with meals.

Cardiac arrhythmias and hypotension

Polyuria (dehydration may cause acute toxicity)

Tremors—can be treated with propranolol

Signs of lithium toxicity can include:

Drowsiness, confusion, blurred vision, and photophobia

Seizures, coma, and cardiovascular collapse

TABLE 20.2.   ANTIDEPRESSANTS AND ANTIMANIC AGENTS

Generic Name	Trade Name	Dosage	Comments
Tricyclics[a]			
amitriptyline	Elavil	75–250 mg qd	All of these drugs interact with CNS drugs
desipramine	Norpramin	75–100 mg qd	
doxepin	Sinequan, Adapin	75–100 mg qd	
imipramine	Tofranil	75–300 mg qd	Also effective for enuresis
nortriptyline	Aventyl, Pamelor	30–75 mg qd	Geriatric and adolescent patients need lower dose
protriptyline	Vivactil	20–60 mg qd	
MAOIs			
isocarboxazid	Marplan	10–30 mg qd	All of these drugs interact with many foods and other drugs in serious reactions
phenelzine	Nardil	15–75 mg qd	
tranylcypromine	Parnate	20–30 mg qd	
SSRIs			
fluoxetine	Prozac	5–20 mg qd	Delayed reaction, prolonged elimination; take in AM
paroxetine	Paxil	20–50 mg qd	Geriatric patient ½ average dose
sertraline	Zoloft	50–200 mg qd	Take in AM
trazodone	Desyrel	150 mg div. doses	Take PC or hs, sedation common
venlafaxine	Effexor	75–150 mg div. doses	Take PC to lessen nausea
Antimanic Agent			
lithium	Lithobid, Eskalith	Dosage varies	For bipolar disorders; take with meals

Note: All of these tricyclics have a delayed action and mild tranquilizing effect. SSRIs also have delayed actions.

Caution must be used with:

Cardiovascular and kidney disorders
Elderly and debilitated patients

Interactions with CNS drugs and diuretics.

See Table 20.2 for a summary of antidepressants and antimanic agents.

Anxiolytics

Antianxiety medications (e.g., benzodiazepines) are sometimes referred to as anxiolytics or minor tranquilizers. They are useful for the *short*-term treatment of (1) anxiety disorders, (2) neurosis while making the patient amenable to psychotherapy, (3) some psychosomatic disorders and insomnia, and (4) nausea and vomiting. Benzodiazepines, such as Valium, are also used as muscle relaxants, anticonvulsants or preoperatively. Anxiolytics, when given in small doses, can reduce anxiety and promote relaxation without causing sedation. Larger doses are sometimes prescribed at bedtime for their sedative effect. Minor tranquilizers should *not* be taken for prolonged periods of time because *tolerance and physical and psychological dependence* may develop. *Sudden withdrawal after prolonged use may result in seizures, agitation, psychosis, insomnia, and gastric distress.*

Side effects of the benzodiazepines may include:

Depression, hallucinations, confusion, agitation, bizarre behavior, amnesia
Drowsiness, lethargy, and headache
Ataxia, tremor, and extrapyramidal reactions
Rash and itching
Sensitivity to sunlight

Contraindications or extreme caution applies to:

Mental depression
Suicidal tendencies
Depressed vital signs
Pregnancy, lactation, and children
Liver and kidney dysfunction
Elderly and debilitated patients (paradoxical reactions), prolonged elimination time
Persons operating machinery

Interactions of benzodizepines with potentiation of effect may occur with:

CNS depressants (e.g., analgesics, anesthetics, sedative hypnotics, other muscle relaxants, antihistamines, and alcohol)
Anticoagulants, corticosteroids, digitalis, and phenytoin

Other anxiolytics,, not related to the benzodiazepines, include buspirone (Buspar). Unlike the benzodiazepines, it has no anticonvulsant or muscle relaxant activity, does not substantially impair psychomotor function, and has little sedative effect. Limited evidence suggests that buspirone may be more effective for cognitive and interpersonal problems, including anger and hostility, associated with anxiety, whereas the benzodiazepines may be more effective for somatic symptoms of anxiety.

Buspirone has a slower onset of action than most anxiolytics (2–4 weeks for optimum effect). It has little potential for tolerance or dependence and has been used without unusual adverse effects or decreased efficiency for as long as a year.

Side effects of buspirone (fewer and less severe) may include:

Dizziness, drowsiness, and headache
GI effects (e.g, nausea)

Caution applies to renal and hepatic impairment.

Another short-term anxiolytic, chemically different from the benzodiazepines, is meprobamate.

TABLE 20.3. ANTIANXIETY MEDICATIONS (ANXIOLYTICS)

Generic Name	Trade Name	Dosage	Comments
Benzodiazepines (short term only)			
alprazolam	Xanax	0.25–0.5 mg tid	Abrupt withdrawal may cause severe side effects
chlordiazepoxide	Librium	5–10 mg qid	Larger doses IV with severe anxiety
chlorazepate	Tranxene	15–60 mg qd 7.5–15 mg qd	For elderly patients no more than 15 mg qd
diazepam	Valium	2–10 mg qid	Do not mix in syringe with other medications, also used as muscle relaxant or IV in status epilepticus
lorazepam	Ativan	2–3 mg qid PO or IM	For elderly who are agitated
oxazepam	Serax	10–15 mg tid or qid	For elderly who are agitated
Other Anxiolytics			
buspirone	Buspar	15–30 mg qd div. doses	Slow onset of action, may be used long term
meprobamate	Equanil, Miltown	400–800 mg bid	Withdraw slowly to prevent severe side effects; short term only
hydroxyzine (antihistamine)	Atarax, Vistaril	25–100 mg qid PO or 25–100 mg deep IM	Antiemetic, antipruritic, or preoperative

Side effects of meprobamate may include:

Drowsiness, ataxia, dizziness
Allergic reactions, itching, urticaria

Caution applies to:

Renal, hepatic, seizure disorders
Withdrawal—gradually tapered over 1–2 weeks to prevent severe side effects (see benzodiazepine withdrawal above)

See Table 20.3 for a summary of antianxiety medications.

Antipsychotic Medications/Major Tranquilizers

Antipsychotic medications, or major tranquilizers, such as haloperidol (Haldol), are sometimes called *neuroleptics*. They are useful in three major areas:

Relieving symptoms of psychoses or severe neuroses, including delusion, hallucinations, agitation, and combativeness

Relieving nausea and vomiting, for example, chlorpromazine (see Chapter 16)
Potentiation of analgesics, for example, promethazine (see Chapter 27)

Many of the antipsychotics are classified chemically as phenothiazines, for example, chlorpromazine (Thorazine). Dosage can be regulated to modify disturbed behavior and relieve severe anxiety in many cases without profound impairment of consciousness. Tranquilizers, such as promethazine (Phenergan), are sometimes combined with other drugs for potentiation of sedative or antiemetic action.

A newer antipsychotic, risperidone, chemically different from the phenothiazines, blocks both serotonin and dopamine receptors. It has been approved for *short*-term management of psychoses and depression, withdrawal, and apathy associated with schizophrenia. Side effects are similar to all of those listed below, including extrapyramidal symptoms, and additionally, can cause nausea and rhinitis.

Side effects of the antipsychotics may include:

Postural hypotension, tachycardia, bradycardia, and vertigo
Insomnia, agitation, depression, headaches, seizures
Dry mouth, blurred vision, and fever
Jaundice, rash, photosensitivity or hypersensitivity reactions
Confusion, drowsiness, restlessness, and weakness
Constipation, urinary retention, and anorexia

Extrapyramidal reactions, severe CNS adverse effects, include:

Parkinsonian symptoms, for example, tremors, drooling, dysphagia—more common in the elderly
Tardive dyskinesia (involuntary movements such as tics)—more common in the elderly, especially females
Dystonic reactions (spasms of the head, neck, or tongue)—more frequent in children
Akathisia (motor restlessness)—more common in children

Note: Parkinsonian symptoms and tardive dyskinesia may become permanent and irreversible. Therefore, patients receiving antipsychotic agents should be assessed frequently for these conditions. Dosage should not be terminated abruptly in those receiving high doses for prolonged periods of time.

Treatment of parkinsonian symptoms includes concomitant administration of an anticholinergic antiparkinsonian agent, for example, Artane or Cogentin (see Chapter 22). Prophylactic administration of these drugs will not prevent extrapyramidal symptoms. These drugs will not alleviate symptoms of tardive dyskinesia and can make them worse. Dystonic reactions usually appear early in therapy and usually subside rapidly when the antipsychotic drug is discontinued. Artane, Cogentin or Diphenhydramine are used to treat dystonic reactions. Patients receiving antipsychotic medication should be assessed for tardive dyskinesia (T.D.) *at least* every 6 months with the Abnormal Involuntary Movement Scale (AIMS) (see Fig. 20.1 and Fig. 20.2), or Dyskinesia Identification System: Condensed User Scale (DISCUS), available from SANDOZ Pharmaceuticals Corporation.

INSTRUCTIONS: Complete Examination Procedure (reverse side) before making ratings.

Code: 0 = None, 1 = Minimal, may be extreme normal, 2 = Mild, 3 = Moderate, 4 = Severe

	1. Muscles of Facial Expression	(CIRCLE ONE)
FACIAL AND ORAL MOVEMENTS:	e.g., movements of forehead, eyebrows, periorbital area, cheeks; include frowning, blinking, smiling, grimacing	0 1 2 3 4
	2. Lips and Perioral Area e.g., puckering, pouting, smacking	0 1 2 3 4
	3. Jaw e.g., biting, clenching, mouth opening, lateral movement	0 1 2 3 4
	4. Tongue Rate only increase in movement both in and out of mouth, NOT inability to sustain movement	0 1 2 3 4
EXTREMITY MOVEMENTS:	**5. Upper (arms, wrists, hands, fingers)** Include choreic movements (i.e., rapid, objectively purposeless, irregular, spontaneous), athetoid movements (i.e., slow, irregular, complex, serpentine). Do NOT include tremor (i.e., repetitive, regular, rhythmic)	0 1 2 3 4
	6. Lower (legs, knees, ankles, toes) e.g., lateral knee movement, foot tapping, heel dropping, foot squirming, inversion and eversion of foot	0 1 2 3 4
TRUNK MOVEMENTS:	**7. Neck, shoulders, hips** e.g., rocking, twisting, squirming, pelvic gyrations	0 1 2 3 4
GLOBAL JUDGEMENTS:	**8. Severity of abnormal movements**	0 1 2 3 4
	9. Incapacitation due to abnormal movements	0 1 2 3 4
	10. Patient's awareness of abnormal movements Rate only patient's report	No awareness 0 Aware, no distress 1 Aware, mild distress 2 Aware, moderate distress 3 Aware, severe distress 4
DENTAL STATUS:	**11. Current problems with teeth and/or dentures**	No = 0 Yes = 1
	12. Does patient usually wear dentures?	No = 0 Yes = 1

It is always preferable to perform the entire AIMS Examination. This establishes consistent testing conditions and allows test results to be compared. Nonambulatory residents may be observed informally for abnormal involuntary movements while in bed or in a wheelchair. Uncooperative residents should be observed during normal activities.

You must check one of these boxes: ☐ Full examination conducted and scored
                                        ☐ Scores from informal observations—Resident was:
                                                    ☐ Not ambulatory—observed in   ☐ bed   ☐ wheelchair
                                                    ☐ Not cooperative

RATER	DATE:	PATIENT	Resident #

Figure 20.1 Abnormal Involuntary Movement Scale (AIMS). This test, or a comparable one, is performed every 3 to 6 months with all patients receiving antipsychotic medication to identify any signs of tardive dyskinesia.

EXAMINATION PROCEDURE

Either before or after completing the examination procedure observe the patient unobtrusively, at rest (e.g., in waiting room).

The chair to be used in this examination should be a hard, firm one without arms.

1. Ask patient whether there is anything in his/her mouth (i.e. gum, candy, etc.) and if there is, to remove it.
2. Ask patient about the *current* condition of his/her teeth. Ask patient if he/she wears dentures. Do teeth or dentures bother patient *now*?
3. Ask patient whether he/she notices any movements in mouth, face, hands, or feet. If yes, ask to describe and to what extent they *currently* bother patient or interfere with his/her activities.
4. Have patient sit in chair with hands on knees, legs slightly apart, and feet flat on floor. (Look at entire body for movements while in this position.)
5. Ask patient to sit with hands hanging unsupported. If male, between legs, if female and wearing a dress, hanging over knees. (Observe hands and other body areas.)
6. Ask patient to open mouth. (Observe tongue at rest within mouth.) Do this twice.
7. Ask patient to protrude the tongue. (Observe abnormalities of tongue movement.)
◆ 8. Ask patient to tap thumb, with each finger, as rapidly as possible for 10–15 seconds; separately with right hand, then with left hand. (Observe facial and leg movements.)
9. Flex and extend patient's left and right arms (one at a time). (Note any rigidity and rate on DOTES.)
10. Ask patient to stand up. (Observe in profile. Observe all body areas again, hips included.)
◆ 11. Ask patient to extend both arms outstretched in front with palms down. (Observe trunk, legs, and mouth.)
◆ 12. Have patient walk a few paces, turn, and walk back to the chair. (Observe hands and gait.) Do this twice.

◆ Activated movement, some practitioners score these movements differently.

INTERPRETATION OF THE AIMS SCORE

- Individuals with no single score exceeding 1 are at very low risk of having a movement disorder.
- A score of 2 in only one of the seven body areas is borderline and the patient should be monitored closely.
- A patient with a score of 2 in two or more of the seven body areas should be referred for a complete neurological examination.
- A score of 3 or 4 in only one body area warrants referring the patient for a complete neurological examination.

Figure 20.2 Abnormal Involuntary Movement Scale (AIMS). Examination procedure.

Contraindications for antipsychotics include:

Seizure disorders
Parkinsonian syndrome
Severe depression
Pregnancy

Caution with the elderly, children, hepatic or renal disease, or prostatic hypertrophy.

Interactions of the antipsychotics may include:

Potentiation with CNS depressants
Antagonism with anticonvulsants (seizure activity may increase)

See Table 20.4 for a summary of the antipsychotic medications. See Figure 20.3 for a summary of psychotropic drugs.

There is no "ideal" psychotropic medication. All have side effects, and prolonged use often leads to addiction or habituation. However, research indicates a chemical component in many forms of mental illness. By altering abnormal levels

TABLE 20.4. ANTIPSYCHOTIC MEDICATIONS/MAJOR TRANQUILIZERS

Generic Name	Trade Name	Dosage[a]	Comments
chlorpromazine	Thorazine	200–500 mg qd, also R, deep IM or IV	Primarily for severe anxiety; also for nausea and vomiting and severe behavior problems
haloperidol	Haldol	1–20 mg qd PO or IM	For agitation, especially with schizophrenia and delusions in the elderly
prochlorperazine	Compazine	PO, supp, or IM	For agitation; primarily for nausea and vomiting in adults
promethazine	Phenergan	12.5–25 mg qid, PO, supp, or IM	Primarily for nausea and vomiting pre- and postoperatively, and sedation
thioridazine	Mellaril	10–100 mg qid	For psychoneurosis, agitation, or combativeness
trifluoperazine	Stelazine	1 mg tab bid	Tranquilizer for psychotic disorders
thiothixene	Navane	2–10 mg tid PO or IM	For chronic schizophrenic or behavioral management of withdrawn patients
fluphenazine HCl	Prolixin	1–10 mg qd div. doses	For geriatrics, reduce dose to ½ or ¼
perphenazine	Trilafon	4–8 mg tid	For psychosis, nausea and vomiting in adults
risperidone	Risperdal	1–3 mg bid	Atypical. Cardiovascular side effects. Reduce geriatric dose to ½.

[a]Varies with condition.

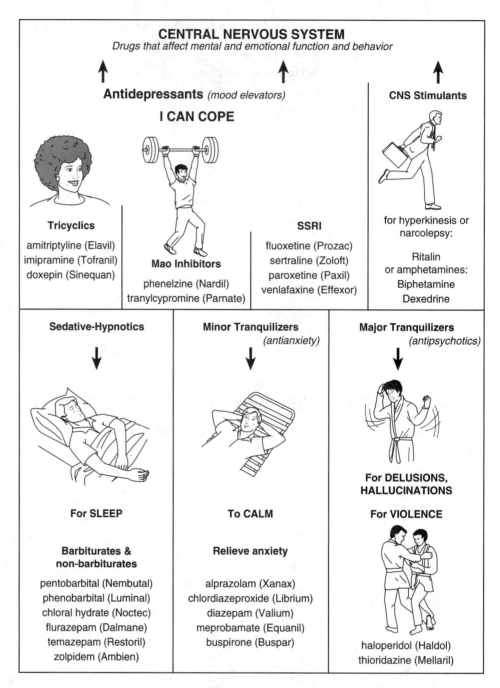

Figure 20.3 Summary of psychotropic drugs.

of certain chemicals in the brain, such as serotonin, norepinephrine, or dopamine, many patients with mental or emotional illness have been helped. Psychiatric hospitalization has decreased since the advent of psychotropic medications.

PATIENT EDUCATION

Patients taking psychotropic drugs should be instructed regarding:

Potential for psychological and/or physical dependence with prolonged use.

Caution in taking medication only in prescribed dosage and for limited period of time under medical supervision to reduce possibility of serious side effects from overdose or prolonged use.

Reporting adverse side effects to physician at once (e.g., dizziness, blurred vision, nervousness, palpitations and other cardiac symptoms, urinary retention, GI symptoms, adverse mental changes, and extrapyramidal reactions).

Avoiding chemical abuse (e.g., alcohol or drugs) and obtaining professional treatment when these conditions exist.

Possible severe withdrawal reactions (e.g., seizures) after prolonged use of psychotropic medications (withdrawal should never be abrupt, and medical supervision is indicated for prolonged administration of any of the psychotropic drugs).

Caution with interactions; *not* taking any other medications (except under close medical supervision) that can potentiate CNS depression (e.g., analgesics, *alcohol*, muscle relaxants, antihistamines, antiemetics, cardiac medications, or antihypertensives).

Geriatric patients are more at risk for the side effects mentioned above because of slowed metabolism and cardiovascular, kidney, liver, and visual impairment. They should be issued the following cautions:

Rise slowly because of potential for hypotension.

Avoid operating machinery or driving while taking these drugs. Report to the physician immediately any side effects, especially dizziness, confusion, sleep disturbances, or weakness.

Avoid taking any OTC drugs or alcohol.

Tell the prescribing physician about all other medicines you are taking, including eyedrops.

Alcohol

Alcohol can be classified as a psychotropic drug and a CNS depressant. It is the number one drug problem in the United States.

Alcohol is a fast-acting depressant, pharmacologically similar to ether. The body reacts to both drugs with excitement, sedation, and finally anesthesia. Large amounts of alcohol can result in alcoholic stupor, cerebral edema, and depressed respiration.

Alcohol is rapidly absorbed from the GI tract into the bloodstream. Alcohol depresses primitive areas of the cortex first and then decreases control over judgment, memory, and other intellectual and emotional functioning. Within a few hours, motor areas are affected, producing unsteady gait, slurred speech, and incoordination. Prolonged use can cause permanent CNS damage and result in peripheral neuritis, convulsive disorders, Wernicke's syndrome, and Korsakoff's psychosis with mental deterioration, memory loss, and ataxia.

Prolonged alcohol use affects almost all organs of the body. Chronic drinking causes liver damage and pancreatitis. Alcohol irritates the mucosa of the digestive system, leading to possible esophageal varices, gastritis, ulceration, and hemorrhage. Alcohol can also lead to malabsorption of nutrients and malnutrition.

Cardiovascular effects include peripheral vasodilation (producing the flushing and sweating seen with intoxication) and vasoconstriction of the coronary arteries. Alcohol increases the heart rate and, with chronic use, can cause cardiac myopathy, either directly or through metabolic and electrolyte imbalances. Potassium deficiency can cause cardiac arrhythmias.

ALCOHOL POISONING

Symptoms of acute alcoholic poisoning include cold, clammy skin, stupor, slow, noisy respirations, and alcoholic breath.

Treatment includes close observation for:

Respiratory problems. Establish and maintain airway.

Vomiting. Gastric lavage if indicated.

Convulsions. Phenytoin sometimes given prophylactically to decrease seizure activity.

Cerebral edema. Diuretics sometimes required (e.g., mannitol).

Electrolyte imbalance. IV fluids with high doses of vitamin B complex and vitamin C added.

Delirium tremens. Chlordiazepoxide (Librium) sometimes given.

CHRONIC ALCOHOLISM

Symptoms of chronic alcoholism include:

Frequent falls and accidents

Blackouts and memory loss

Dulling of mental faculties

Neuritis and muscular weakness

Irritability

Tremors

Conjunctivitis

Gastroenteritis

Neglect of personal appearance and responsibilities

Treatment of chronic alcoholism can include an intensive in-house rehabilitation program in a special facility for a period of 28 days. Treatment frequently includes:

Megadoses of vitamin B complex and vitamin C IM or PO.

Low-carbohydrate and high-protein diet to combat hypoglycemia.

Elimination of caffeine (in coffee, tea, chocolate, and soft drinks).

Reeducation of the patient, with intensive individual, group, and family counseling, including Alcoholics Anonymous techniques.

Sometimes disulfiram (Antabuse) is used, with patient cooperation, as part of *behavior modification*. Patients receive daily doses of disulfiram and are taught to expect a very unpleasant reaction if even a small amount of alcohol is ingested.

Disulfiram-alcohol reactions can include:

Flushing and throbbing headache

Nausea and vomiting

Sweating and dyspnea

Palpitation, tachycardia, and hypotension

Vertigo and blurred vision

Anxiety and confusion

PATIENT EDUCATION

Patients taking disulfiram should be instructed regarding:

Avoidance of cough syrups, sauces, vinegars, elixirs, and other preparations containing alcohol.

Caution with external applications of liniments, lotions, aftershave, or perfume.

Signs of disulfiram-alcohol reaction.

Reporting to emergency facility if effects do not subside or with severe reaction

Carrying identification card noting therapy.

Avoiding other medications that may interact with disulfiram (e.g., anticoagulants and phenytoin).

A newer treatment for alcoholism includes the use of daily maintenance doses of naltrexone (ReVia), as part of counseling programs, to *keep* alcoholics sober after detoxification. Naltrexone acts by blocking the pleasurable sensations associated with alcohol, and therefore stops the desire or craving to drink.

Naltrexone is also used in treatment programs for opiate addicts (e.g., heroin and morphine). *After* withdrawal from the drugs, it helps to prevent relapses. It acts by robbing the drugs of their pleasurable effects.

Caution: If naltrexone is given to someone currently dependent on opiates, it can send the addict *instantly into severe life-threatening* withdrawal.

Side effects of naltrexone are usually minor and include:

Nausea and joint pains

Liver damage can occur with doses larger than recommended dose of 50 mg daily

Drug Abuse

Drug abuse can be defined as the use of a drug for other than therapeutic purposes. Drug *addiction* consists of the combination of all four of the following side effects: tolerance, psychological dependence, physical dependence, and withdrawal reaction with physiological effects. *Habituation* consists of psychological dependence only. *Chemical dependency* is the term in common usage today to describe a condition in which alcohol or drugs have taken control of an individual's life and affect normal functioning.

Health care workers have ready access to many prescription drugs and, therefore, sometimes become involved in illegal misuse of psychotropic drugs. Drugs most often abused by medical personnel are the *downers* such as sedatives, hypnotics, tranquilizers, or narcotic analgesics. Counteractive measures include accurate record keeping of all controlled substances and recognition of the side effects and symptoms associated with drug abuse. (See Chapter 19 for descriptions of narcotic analgesics, sedatives, and hypnotics, and for treatment of overdose and the use of narcotic antagonists.) Report suspected abuse to the one in authority.

This section describes four types of drugs that can be produced illegally: marijuana, cocaine, the hallucinogens (LSD and PCP), and the amphetamines.

AMPHETAMINES

There has been a steady increase in the illegal use of *uppers*, such as the amphetamines ("speed") or cocaine. While amphetamines can be produced and prescribed legally, they are also produced in illegal labs as well. At normal dosage levels, administration of an amphetamine may produce tolerance within a few weeks. However, in hypersensitive individuals, psychotic syndrome may occur within 36–48 hours of a single large dose of amphetamine. Some emotionally unstable individuals come to depend on the pleasant mental stimulation the drugs offer.

Symptoms of chronic abuse of amphetamines include:

Emotional lability, irritability

Anorexia

Mental impairment, confusion

Occupational deterioration, social withdrawal

Continuous chewing or teeth grinding resulting in trauma or ulcers of the tongue and lip

Photophobia—frequently wear sunglasses indoors

Paranoid syndrome with hallucinations with prolonged use of high doses

Symptoms of acute toxicity can include:

Cardiovascular symptoms, including flushing or pallor, palpitation, tachypnea, tremor, extreme fluctuations of pulse and blood pressure, cardiac arrhythmias, chest pain, circulatory collapse

Dilated pupils, diaphoresis, and hyperpyrexia

Mental disturbances such as confusion, delirium, belligerence, combativeness, restlessness, paranoia, and suicidal or homicidal tendencies

Fatigue and depression usually follow CNS stimulation

Treatment: There is no specific antidote for amphetamine overdosage. Treatment of overdose is symptomatic and includes administration of sedative drugs, preferably short-acting barbiturates, and isolation of the patient to avoid possible external stimuli. General physiologic supportive measures include treatment for shock or cardiac irregularities as appropriate. Emesis or gastric lavage may help if applied soon enough. Hypothermic measures or drugs to reduce intracranial pressure may be employed if appropriate.

Abrupt withdrawal of amphetamines may unmask mental problems. Therefore, patients require careful supervision during withdrawal and long-term follow-up may be required since some manifestations (e.g., depression) may persist for prolonged periods.

MARIJUANA

Tetrahydrocannabinol (THC) is commonly known as marijuana. Although classified technically as a CNS depressant, it also possesses properties of a euphoriant, sedative, and hallucinogen. Marijuana is currently under investigation as a possible treatment for glaucoma and also for the vomiting associated with chemotherapy. It is not an approved treatment at this time.

The *Cannabis* plant grows over the entire world, especially in tropical areas. Potency varies considerably from place to place and time to time. Marijuana is much more potent today than a few years ago.

THC, the active ingredient released when marijuana is smoked, is fat soluble and is stored in many fat cells, especially in the brain and reproductive organs. THC metabolizes slowly. A week after a person smokes one marijuana cigarette, 30–50% of the THC remains in the body, and 4–6 weeks are required to eliminate all the THC.

Side effects of marijuana include:

Short-term memory loss, impaired learning, and slowed intellectual performance

Perceptual inaccuracies, impaired reflex reaction (dangerous with driving)

Apathy, lethargy, and decreased motivation

Increased heart rate

Lung irritation and chronic cough

Reduced testosterone level and sperm count

Reduced estrogen level, crossing of placental barrier, and transmission through mother's milk; miscarriage and stillbirth possible

Delayed development of coping mechanisms in children and adolescents

COCAINE

Cocaine use is increasing in the United States. It is a CNS stimulant and produces euphoria and increased expenditure of energy. The only approved medical use is as a local anesthetic, usually for nasal procedures, *applied topically only.*

Cocaine is highly addictive, causing psychic dependence after even short-time use. It is abused by intranasal application (sniffing or snorting), intravenous injection, or by inhalation (smoking "crack"). Nasal application can damage mucous membranes and/or the nasal septum. The effects of intravenous use are extremely rapid and dangerous and can be fatal. Smoking causes the most rapid addiction, sometimes after only one use. Cocaine crosses the placental barrier and has resulted in babies who are irritable, jittery, anorexic, and seizure prone. Cocaine use has caused numerous crimes and deaths. Severe depression can be associated with withdrawal, which is a lengthy and difficult process.

Side effects, which are serious, include:

Euphoria, agitation, and excitation

Hypertension, tachycardia, cardiac arrhythmias or cardiac failure

Anorexia, nausea, and vomiting

Tremor and seizures

Hallucinations and possible psychosis

Possible death from circulatory collapse

Perforated nasal septum from prolonged nasal use

HALLUCINOGENS

Lysergic acid (LSD) and phencyclidine (PCP), an animal tranquilizer, are hallucinogens. They produce bizarre mental reactions and distortion of physical senses. Hallucinations and delusions are common, with confused perceptions of time and space (e.g., the user can walk out of windows because of the impression that he or she can fly). PCP is also an amnesic.

Side effects of both include:

Increased pulse and heart rate and rise in blood pressure and temperature

Possible "flashbacks" months later

Panic or paranoia (lack of control)

Possible psychotic episodes

Possible physical injury to self or others

THE ROLE OF MEDICAL PERSONNEL

The role of medical personnel in combating drug abuse includes:

Thorough knowledge of psychotropic drugs, action, and side effects

Willingness to participate in education of the patient, the patient's family, and others in the community

Giving competent care to those under the influence of drugs in a nonjudgmental way

Recognizing drug abuse and making appropriate referrals

It is the responsibility of all medical personnel not only to recognize drug abuse, but also to report any observed drug abuse to the *proper person in authority*. To look the other way not only enables the individual to continue to harm him- or herself but also endangers those in his or her care.

There are many services available to help medical personnel deal with drug abuse problems. Check with your state licensing agency or certification board for information about programs in your area, such as the Impaired Nurse program. Local mental health clinics or psychiatric facilities can also provide assistance and information. Other agencies that can provide information include:

Department of Health and Human Services
Public Health Service
Alcohol, Drug Abuse, and Mental Health Administration
Washington, D.C. 20402

National Clearinghouse for Drug Abuse Information
P.O. Box 1706
Rockville, MD 20850

Worksheet 1 for Chapter 20

PSYCHOTROPICS

Note the drugs listed according to category and complete all columns. Learn generic or trade names as specified by instructor. Fill in blank spaces in first column with names of other drugs common in your area.

Classifications and Drugs	Purpose	Side Effects	Contraindications or Cautions	Patient Education
CNS Stimulants 1. amphetamines 2. Ritalin				
Tricyclics 1. Elavil 2. Tofranil				
MAOIs 1. Marplan 2. Nardil				
SSRIs 1. sertraline (Zoloft) 2. fluoxetine (Prozac) 3. paroxetine (Paxil)				
Antimanic 1. lithium				

Worksheet 2 for Chapter 20

PSYCHOTROPICS (Continued)

Classifications and Drugs	Purpose	Side Effects	Contraindications or Cautions	Patient Education
Antianxiety Medications 1. Ativan 2. Valium 3. meprobamate 4. Xanax 5. BuSpar				
Antipsychotic Medications 1. Thorazine 2. Haldol 3. Mellaril 4. Navane 5.				
Illegal Drugs 1. marijuana 2. cocaine				

Worksheet 3 for Chapter 20

ALCOHOL

Complete the columns including medications and cautions under treatment.

Diagnosis	Signs and Symptoms	Possible Effects on the Body	Treatment
Chronic Alcoholism			
Acute Alcohol Poisoning			

A. Case Study for Psychotropic Medications

Miss Blue, a 25-year-old secretary, presents in the physician's office with a history of depression for 1 month. She complains of crying frequently, loss of appetite, and insomnia. The physician prescribes Tofranil. The patient should be given the following information:

1. She should expect to feel better
   - a. In a few days
   - b. In a few weeks
   - c. 1 hour after taking medicine
   - d. 1 day after taking medicine
2. The medicine should be taken
   - a. Before meals
   - b. With meals
   - c. In the morning
   - d. At bedtime
3. She can expect all of the following side effects EXCEPT
   - a. Increased appetite
   - b. Improved sleep
   - c. Weight loss
   - d. Dry mouth
4. She should be told to report any of the following side effects EXCEPT
   - a. Dizziness
   - b. Palpitations
   - c. Blurred vision
   - d. Increased thirst

B. Case Study for Psychotropic Medications

Mr. Elzware, a 90-year-old nursing home resident with Alzheimer's, Parkinson's, and enlarged prostate, has been pacing the hall talking loudly in a confused way. He is wringing his hands. The nurse calls the physician's office and requests Haldol "to calm him down." Both the nurse in the nursing home and the medical assistant in the physician's office should be aware of the following facts about Haldol.

1. Haldol is only an appropriate medication for which condition listed below?
   - a. Nervousness
   - b. Confusion
   - c. Uncooperativeness
   - d. Combativeness
2. Haldol is appropriate in which of the following conditions?
   - a. Seizure disorder
   - b. Parkinson's disease
   - c. Prostatic hypertrophy
   - d. Paranoid psychosis
   - e. Depression
3. Agitation can be caused by all of the following EXCEPT
   - a. Pain
   - b. Constipation
   - c. Senility
   - d. Urinary retention
4. Geriatric patients receiving antipsychotic medication are at increased risk of having extrapyramidal reactions including all of the following EXCEPT
   - a. Dystonia
   - b. Diaphoresis
   - c. Tardive dyskinesia
   - d. Parkinsonian syndrome

5. The following statements are true of tardive dykinesia EXCEPT
   a. Can be permanent   c. Assessed with AIMS test
   b. Cured with medicine   d. Manifested by tics
6. Side effects of antipsychotics, like Haldol, can include all of the following EXCEPT
   a. Depression   c. Blurred vision
   b. Weakness   d. Increased appetite

CHAPTER 21

Musculoskeletal and Anti-Inflammatory Drugs

OBJECTIVES

Upon completion of this chapter, the student should be able to:

1. Identify commonly used skeletal muscle relaxants.
2. Describe the side effects to be expected with muscle relaxants.
3. List the drugs that can interact with the muscle relaxants and cause serious potentiation of effect.
4. Differentiate between the anti-inflammatory drugs, antirheumatic drugs, and drugs used to treat acute episodes of gout.
5. Explain the serious side effects of NSAIDs.
6. List drug interactions with NSAIDs.
7. Explain appropriate patient education for those taking skeletal muscle relaxants and NSAIDs.
8. Describe the new medication for osteoporosis.

Disorders of the musculoskeletal system are rather common. Drugs used to treat such conditions may be classified in two broad categories: skeletal muscle relaxants and nonsteroidal anti-inflammatory drugs (NSAIDs). Corticosteroid therapy for inflammatory conditions is discussed in Chapter 23.

Skeletal Muscle Relaxants

Some disorders of the musculoskeletal system can be attributed to structural defects (e.g., ruptured disks) that may require surgical intervention rather than medication. However, many disorders associated with pain, spasm, abnormal contraction, or impaired mobility do respond to medications classified as skeletal muscle relaxants. Acute, painful musculoskeletal conditions, such as backache or neck strain, are treated with a combination of muscle relaxants, rest, physical therapy (e.g., hot or cold packs), and mild analgesics (e.g., NSAIDs). Muscle relaxants are given only on a short-term basis, and, after the acute pain subsides, exercises are usually prescribed by the physician to strengthen the weak muscles.

Muscle relaxant drugs can affect the spinal cord and brain, as well as acting on the peripheral areas. The resulting action not only reduces muscle spasm but produces a sedative effect, promoting rest and relaxation of the affected part. Drugs used to treat acute, painful musculoskeletal conditions include diazepam (Valium) and methocarbamol (Robaxin). See Table 21.1 for others.

A different type of muscle relaxant, dantrolene, causes a direct effect on skeletal muscles and is used in the management of spasticity resulting from upper motor neuron disorders such as multiple sclerosis or cerebral palsy. This medication is ineffective for amyotrophic lateral sclerosis and is not indicated for the treatment of muscle spasms resulting from rheumatic disorders or musculoskeletal trauma.

Another type of muscle relaxant includes neuromuscular blocking agents such as succinylcholine or tubocurarine, used during surgical, endoscopic, or orthopedic procedures. These drugs are potentially very dangerous and can result in respiratory arrest. Neuromuscular blocking agents are administered only by anesthesiologists or specially trained personnel skilled in intubation and cardiopulmonary resuscitation.

Muscle relaxants must be used with caution because of possible serious CNS problems such as respiratory arrest and allergic reactions. Antidotes such as neostigmine (Prostigmin) or edrophonium (Tensilon) may be indicated. Prostigmin may also be used in the treatment of myasthenia gravis and Tensilon in the diagnosis of myasthenia gravis. See Chapter 13 for cholinergic drugs.

TABLE 21.1. SKELETAL MUSCLE RELAXANTS

Generic Name	Trade Name	Dosage	Comments
carisoprodol	Soma	350 mg PO qid	Caution with asthma
cyclobenzaprine	Flexeril	30–60 mg PO qid in div. doses	For acute painful musculoskeletal conditions
chlorzoxazone	Parafon Forte	250 mg PO tid or qid	For acute conditions; can cause serious liver toxicity
diazepam	Valium	2–10 mg PO qid IM IV 2–20 mg q3–4h	Abrupt withdrawal after prolonged use may cause seizures
methocarbamol	Robaxin	1.2–8 g PO qid also IM, IV	For acute painful musculoskeletal conditions
dantrolene	Dantrium	25–100 mg PO qid	For multiple sclerosis and cerebral palsy, not for trauma or rheumatic disorders

Side effects can include:

Drowsiness, dizziness, or dry mouth
Weakness, tremor, ataxia
Headache
Confusion and nervousness
Slurred speech
Blurred vision
Hypotension
GI symptoms including nausea, vomiting, diarrhea, or constipation
Urinary problems, including enuresis, frequency, or retention
Hypersensitivity reactions including severe liver toxicity with chlorzoxazone
Respiratory depression

Contraindications are:

Muscular dystrophy
Myasthenia gravis
Pregnancy or lactation
Children under 12 years old

Caution should be used with:

History of drug abuse
Impaired kidney function
Liver disorders
Blood dyscrasias
Asthma
Cardiac disorders
Elderly

Interactions with possible potentiation of effect may occur with:

Alcohol
Analgesics
Psychotropic medications
Antihistamines

PATIENT EDUCATION

Patients taking skeletal muscle relaxants should be instructed regarding:

Potential side effects (e.g., drowsiness, dizziness, weakness, tremor, blurred vision, hypotension, respiratory distress, or GI disorders). Care with driving.

Avoidance of other CNS depressants at the same time (e.g., tranquilizers, antihistamines, or alcohol), which can cause serious CNS depression, and care with analgesics, only as prescribed by a physician.

Importance of following the physician's orders regarding rest and physical therapy (e.g., heat and firm mattress or bed board with back problems) and exercises as prescribed (after the acute pain subsides) to strengthen the weak muscles.

The acronym, RICE (rest, ice, compression [elastic bandage], elevation), represents appropriate care for musculoskeletal injuries to extremities.

Taking the medication only as long as absolutely necessary and observing caution regarding prolonged use, which could lead to physical or psychological dependence and withdrawal symptoms (e.g., seizures from Valium withdrawal after prolonged use).

See Table 21.1 for a summary of the skeletal muscle relaxants.

Anti-Inflammatory Drugs

Anti-inflammatory drugs are used to treat disorders in which the musculoskeletal system is not functioning properly due to inflammation. Such conditions as arthritis, bursitis, spondylitis, gout, and muscle strains and sprains can cause swelling, redness, heat, pain, and limited mobility. Analgesics and corticosteroids are used at times for acute stages of these disorders and are discussed in Chapters 19 and 23. The corticosteroids are not used for extended periods of time because of serious side effects. However, nonsteroidal anti-inflammatory drugs (NSAIDs) are frequently given for lengthy time periods in maintenance doses as low as possible for effectiveness.

NONSTEROIDAL ANTI-INFLAMMATORY DRUGS

NSAIDs inhibit synthesis of prostaglandins, substances responsible for producing much of the inflammation and pain of rheumatic conditions, sprains, and menstrual cramps. No cure has been found for rheumatic disorders but many medications are used to alleviate the pain and crippling effects. Because of lower metabolic rates and other complications, the elderly are particularly susceptible to side effects from NSAIDs and should be cautioned to report any untoward signs or symptoms to their doctor without delay.

The salicylates are the oldest drug in this category with analgesic, anti-inflammatory, and antipyretic effects. Many newer NSAIDs are on the market and some are tolerated better than aspirin by some patients, especially as short-term analgesics. However, with large doses and/or long term, they all share many of the same side effects and interactions to a greater or lesser degree. Patients on prolonged therapy with any of the NSAIDs should be monitored carefully. Those at risk of gastric ulcer, for example, the elderly or those with ulcer history, are sometimes treated with drugs to inhibit gastric acid, for example, misoprostol (Cytotec). (See Chapter 16.) Elderly or debilitated patients seem to tolerate ulceration or bleeding (which can be silent) less well than other individuals, and most reports of fatal GI events are in these populations.

Side effects of NSAIDs frequently include:

GI ulceration and bleeding—may not be preceded by warning signs or symptoms

Epigastric pain, nausea, and heartburn

Constipation

Tinnitus and hearing loss

Headache or dizziness

Visual disturbances

Hematuria and albuminuria

Rash, hypersensitivity reactions, bronchospasm (especially with aspirin)

Blood dyscrasias, especially prolonged bleeding time

Liver toxicity—may be severe, without symptoms, and even fatal, especially with phenylbutazone (Butazolidin) and diclofenac (Voltaren)

Contraindications or extreme caution with NSAIDs applies to:

Asthma—may manifest aspirin sensitivity as bronchospasm

Cardiovascular disorders—see Chapter 25 for aspirin therapy for these conditions

Kidney disease

Liver dysfunction

History of GI ulcer or inflammatory bowel disease

Blood dyscrasias, especially clotting disorders or anemia

Thyroid disease

Children with viral infections (danger of Reye's syndrome)

Gastroesophageal reflux disorder (GERD)

These medications should be given with meals or milk to reduce GI side effects. Enteric-coated, timed-release capsules or buffered aspirin are sometimes also recommended to reduce gastric irritation.

Interactions (especially of salicylates) are many, but the most important clinically occur with:

Alcohol, which potentiates possibility of GI bleeding

Anticoagulants, which potentiate possibility of bleeding

Sulfonylureas (oral hypoglycemics), which potentiate hypoglycemia
Corticosteroids, which potentiate salicylate absorption and toxicity
Methotrexate, with potentiation and increased risk of methotrexate toxicity
Uricosurics (Benemid or Anturane), whose action is antagonized by salicylates
Triamterene—can cause renal impairment
Ascorbic acid supplements—tissue stores of the vitamin inhibited

See Table 21.2 for a summary of the nonsteroidal anti-inflammatory drugs.

GOUT MEDICATIONS

Gout is a metabolic disorder characterized by accumulation of uric acid crystals in various joints, especially the big toe, ankle, knee, and elbow, with resultant pain and swelling. Colchicine is a specific drug that is used to relieve inflammation in acute gouty arthritis. It is also used as a prophylaxis in persons prone to this condition.

Side effects can include:

Rash
GI upset
Blood disorders

Always encourage large fluid intake to facilitate excretion of uric acid crystals. Other medications for chronic gout are discussed in Chapter 15. They act in a different way and are not effective against inflammation in acute cases of gout or gouty arthritis.

TABLE 21.2. NONSTEROIDAL ANTI-INFLAMMATORY DRUGS AND GOUT MEDICATION

Generic Name	Trade Name	Dosage
diclofenac	Voltaren	150–200 mg qd in div. doses
ibuprofen	Motrin, Advil (OTC), Nuprin (OTC)	300–600 mg PO qid
indomethacin	Indocin	Up to 200 mg qd PO in div. doses
ketorolac	Toradol	15–30 mg q6h PO or IM, PRN
oxaprozin	Daypro	600 mg once daily
mefenamicacid	Ponstel	250 mg q4h PRN
naproxen	Naprosyn, Anaprox, Aleve (OTC)	250–500 mg PO bid, q12h
phenylbutazone	Butazolidin	100–200 mg PO qid
piroxicam	Feldene	20 mg PO qd
sulindac	Clinoril	150–200 mg PO bid
Gout medication		
colchicine	Colchicine	0.5–1.8 mg PO qd

Note: Other NSAIDs are available. This is a representative list.

PATIENT EDUCATION

Patients taking NSAIDs should be instructed regarding:

Administration with food to reduce gastric irritation.

Caution with dosage (follow physician's directions carefully regarding amount of drug to reduce chance of overdose).

Discontinuing drug and reporting to physician any sign of abnormal bleeding (gums, stool, urine, and bruising), epigastric pain or nausea, ringing in the ears or hearing loss, visual disturbances, weight gain or edema, and skin rash.

Avoiding taking any other drugs, either prescribed or OTC, without checking first with a physician or pharmacist regarding possible interactions.

When taking gout medications (e.g., colchicine), always taking large amounts of fluids.

Avoiding taking large amounts of aspirin or other NSAIDs with kidney, liver, or heart disease or with history of GI ulcer (with these conditions, take only under medical supervision). Patients with asthma may manifest sensitivity to aspirin and other NSAIDs.

The danger that GI ulceration and bleeding can occur without previous warning signs or symptoms.

Osteoporosis Therapy

Alendronate (Fosamax) is the first nonhormonal treatment approved for osteoporosis. It is a biophosphate that inhibits bone resorption, thereby increasing bone mineral density. Fosamax 10 mg q AM ac is indicated in the treatment of osteoporosis in postmenopausal women and for Paget's disease of the bone.

Side effects, rare and mild, can include:

GI distress

Muscle pain

Contraindicated with renal insufficiency

Caution with active upper GI problems, for example, dysphagia, GERD, gastritis, or ulcers

PATIENT EDUCATION

Patients taking Fosamax should be instructed regarding:

The importance of taking the medicine with a full glass of water (6–8 oz) at least 30 minutes before the first food, beverage, or medication of the day,

Not lying down for at least 30 minutes to speed delivery to the stomach and avoid esophageal irritation.

Taking supplemental calcium and vitamin D.

Weight-bearing exercises.

Modification of cigarette smoking and alcohol consumption, if these factors exist.

Worksheet for Chapter 21

MUSCULOSKELETAL AND ANTI-INFLAMMATORY DRUGS

Note the drugs listed and complete all columns. Learn generic or trade names as specified by instructor.

Classifications and Drugs	Purpose	Side Effects	Contraindications or Cautions	Patient Education
Skeletal Muscle Relaxants 1. Flexeril 2. Valium 3. Robaxin 4. Soma				
NSAIDs 1. ibuprofen OTC 2. Indocin 3. Naprosyn 4. Toradol 5. Daypro				
Gout Medication (Anti-Inflammatory)				
Osteoporosis Therapy				

A. Case Study for Musculoskeletal Drugs

Truly Hardy, a 35-year-old construction worker, is diagnosed with muscle strain of the lumbar spine. Valium 5 mg q4h PRN is prescribed. His discharge instructions should contain the following information.

1. Muscle relaxants are only appropriate for which condition?
   a. Chronic pain
   b. Muscle weakness
   c. As prophylactic
   d. Acute muscle spasm
2. Muscle relaxants are *contraindicated* in some cases. Which one below would be appropriate for use?
   a. Muscular dystrophy
   b. Myasthenia gravis
   c. Backache
   d. For children
3. Caution must be used with all of the conditions below EXCEPT
   a. Asthma
   b. Herpes
   c. Nephritis
   d. Cirrhosis
4. All of the following side effects are possible EXCEPT
   a. Dizziness
   b. Insomnia
   c. Urinary retention
   d. Blurred vision
5. Interactions with possible potentiation of effect can occur with all of the following EXCEPT
   a. Alcohol
   b. Analgesics
   c. Antihistamines
   d. Antacids

B. Case Study for Anti-Inflammatory Drugs

Rita Robbins, age 65, comes into the physician's office with complaints of knee pain. The physician prescribes naproxen 500 mg q12h for arthritis. She should be given the following information.

1. How should the drug be administered?
   a. Before meals
   b. With fruit juice
   c. With meals
   d. With alcohol
2. Which of the following statements is true of NSAIDs?
   a. Rapidly effective
   b. Cure arthritis
   c. Contraindicated with elderly
   d. May be used long term
3. Side effects of NSAIDs can include all of the following EXCEPT
   a. Gastric bleeding
   b. Blurred vision
   c. Anxiety
   d. Heartburn
4. NSAIDs are contraindicated in all of the following conditions EXCEPT
   a. Asthma
   b. Spondylitis
   c. Gastroesophageal reflux
   d. Inflammatory bowel disease

5. There are possible serious side effects from interactions of NSAIDs with all of the following EXCEPT
   a. Alcohol
   b. Antacids
   c. Anticoagulants
   d. Oral hypoglycemics

CHAPTER 22

Anticonvulsants and Antiparkinsonian Drugs

OBJECTIVES

Upon completion of this chapter, the student should be able to:

1. Compare and contrast different types of seizures.
2. List the medications used for each type of epilepsy, and common side effects.
3. List the drugs used for parkinsonism and common side effects.
4. Describe the patient education appropriate for those receiving anticonvulsants and antiparkinsonian drugs.

Anticonvulsants

Anticonvulsants are used to reduce the number and/or severity of seizures in patients with epilepsy. Epilepsy is defined as a *recurrent* paroxysmal disorder of brain function characterized by sudden attacks of altered consciousness, motor activity, or sensory impairment. Treatment is based on type, severity, and cause of seizures. Although most epilepsy is idiopathic (unknown cause), it may sometimes be associated with cerebral trauma, intracranial infection or fever, brain tumor, intoxication, or chemical imbalance. Sometimes the underlying disorder can be corrected and anticonvulsive medicine is not indicated, for example, fever, hypoglycemia, or electrolyte imbalance.

The International Classification of Epileptic Seizures currently classifies seizure disorders into four main categories:

1. *Generalized* seizures—bilaterally symmetrical and without local onset
2. *Partial* seizures—complex symptomatology (temporal lobe or psychomotor seizures)

3. *Unilateral* seizures—predominantly one-sided
4. *Unclassified*—insufficient data to classify

GENERALIZED SEIZURES

Generalized seizures include *grand mal* and *absence (petit mal)* seizures. They are bilaterally symmetrical and without local onset.

Grand mal seizures are characterized by loss of consciousness, falling, and generalized tonic, followed by clonic contractions of the muscles. The attack usually lasts 2–5 minutes and urinary and fecal incontinence may occur.

Initial treatment consists *only* of preventing injury by removing any objects that could cause trauma, cushioning the head and turning it to the side, and loosening tight clothing, especially collars and belts. Do not try to open the mouth or force anything between the teeth.

If seizures are so frequent that the patient does not regain consciousness between seizures, the condition is known as status epilepticus. The treatment of choice is IV diazepam (Valium) administered slowly. Sometimes IV phenytoin is also given.

Drugs for Petit Mal Epilepsy

Petit mal, or *absence,* epilepsy is so called because of the absence of convulsions. It is characterized by a 10–30-second loss of consciousness with no falling.

The drug of choice for management of petit mal epilepsy is ethosuximide (Zarontin), which is effective only for this type of epilepsy. Other drugs sometimes used in the treatment of absence seizures, when Zarontin is ineffective, include clonazepam (Klonopin) and valproic acid (Depakene).

Side effects of the drugs for petit mal epilepsy can include:

Sedation, dizziness, or irritability
GI distress including anorexia, nausea, vomiting, diarrhea
Rash, leukopenia

Extreme caution should be used with:

Hepatic or renal disease
Pregnancy and lactation

Drugs for Grand Mal and Psychomotor Epilepsy

Psychomotor (or temporal lobe) seizures are also called *partial seizures with complex symptomology.* They are caused by a lesion in the temporal lobe of the brain. Complex symptoms can include confusion, impaired understanding and judgment, staggering, purposeless movements, bizarre behavior, and unintelligible sounds, but no convulsions.

TABLE 22.1. ANTICONVULSANTS

Generic Name	Trade Name	Dosage	Comments
carbamazepine	Tegretol	400 mg–1.2 g PO qd in div. doses susp, tabs	For psychomotor (partial or mixed seizures); serious side effects
phenytoin	Dilantin	PO 300–600 mg qd in div. doses IM 100–200 mg q4h IV 150–250 mg	For grand mal, psychomotor, and focal seizures; frequently combined with phenobarbital
primidone	Mysoline	PO 0.75–2 qd in div. doses	Few toxic side effects, used mainly for psychomotor
ethosuximide	Zarontin	PO 250 mg–1.5 g qd in div. doses	For petit mal seizures
clonazepam	Klonopin	Varies	For petit mal seizures
valproic acid	Depakene, Depakote	15–60 mg/kg qd. in div. doses	For petit mal seizures

Unilateral seizures affect only one side of the body. Some patients may have mixed seizure patterns combining more than one type. It is important to observe and report type and length of seizures and general responsiveness to medications.

Prophylactic treatment of *grand mal* and *psychomotor* epilepsy usually consists of phenytoin (Dilantin), frequently combined with phenobarbital, administered orally. The aim of therapy is to prevent seizures without oversedation, and the dosage will be adjusted according to the individual patient's response.

Side effects of phenytoin (Dilantin), which frequently decrease with continued treatment, can include:

Sedation, ataxia, dizziness, and headache

Blurred vision, nystagmus, and diplopia

Gingivitis (inflamed gums)

GI distress, including nausea, vomiting, anorexia, constipation, or diarrhea

Rash and dermatitis

Megaloblastic anemia (treated with folic acid)

Osteomalacia (bone softening, treated with vitamin D)

Contraindications or extreme caution with Dilantin applies to:

Kidney or liver disease

Diabetes

Congestive heart failure, bradycardia, heart block, and hypotension

Pregnancy and lactation

Another medicine sometimes used for partial, generalized, or mixed seizures is carbamazepine (Tegretol), which can cause many dangerous, very serious adverse side effects, especially cardiac, kidney, and liver complications.

An alternative medication in treatment of grand mal and psychomotor epilepsy is primidone (Mysoline), which has fewer side effects than phenytoin.

Febrile convulsions in children are frequently treated with phenobarbital alone. However, long-term use of phenobarbital in prophylaxis alone, when the child is afebrile, is now questionable because of cognitive impairment. There is increasing evidence that anticonvulsant therapy may have adverse effects on behavior and cognition in children, especially phenobarbital, phenytoin, and carbamazepine. Close observation and monitoring of children in this area is essential as well as reporting of adverse changes to the physician for possible dosage reduction or substitution of an alternative anticonvulsant.

See Table 22.1 for a summary of the anticonvulsants.

PATIENT EDUCATION

Patients taking any anticonvulsant medication should be instructed regarding:

Caution with driving or operating machinery, until regulated with the medication, because of drowsiness or dizziness.

Reporting of any side effects, such as rash or eye problems, staggering, slurred speech, and any other symptoms.

Careful oral hygiene until tenderness of the gums subsides as treatment progresses.

Always taking medication on time and *never* omitting dosage (abrupt withdrawal of medication can lead to status epilepticus).

Wearing Medic-Alert tag or bracelet at all times in case of accident or injury.

Taking medication with food or milk to lessen stomach upset.

Parents and teachers should be cautioned to observe and report changes in cognitive function, mood, and behavior in children receiving anticonvulsants.

Antiparkinsonian Drugs

Antiparkinsonian drugs are usually given for Parkinson's disease, a chronic neurologic disorder characterized by fine, slowly spreading muscle tremors, rigidity and weakness of muscles, and shuffling gait. There is no cure for Parkinson's disease, and the treatment goal is to relieve symptoms and maintain mobility.

LEVODOPA

Levodopa (L-dopa) is the drug of choice for long-term treatment. Sinemet (a combination of levodopa and carbidopa, is most often used. Young robust patients frequently respond better than do older, frail patients.

Side effects, which are numerous and frequent, can include:

Dyskinesias (involuntary movements of many parts of the body)
Nausea, vomiting, and anorexia

Behavioral changes, anxiety, agitation, confusion, depression, psychosis

Hypotension, dizziness, syncope

Note: Side effects may be severe, requiring dosage reduction or withdrawal of the drug.

Contraindications include:

Bronchial asthma, or emphysema

Cardiac disease or hypotension

Active peptic ulcer

Diabetes, renal or hepatic disease

Glaucoma

Psychoses

Pregnant, postpartum, or nursing women

Interactions may occur with:

Antihypertensives, which may potentiate hypotensive effect

Phenytoin, which antagonizes levodopa

Vitamin B_6 (pyridoxine), which antagonizes levodopa alone but does not affect action of Sinemet

MAOIs, which may cause hypertensive crisis

Patients receiving levodopa for prolonged periods of time may develop a tolerance, resulting in ineffectiveness of the drug, called "wearing off." To prevent or treat this late failure of levodopa, a semisynthetic drug, bromocriptine (Parlodel), has sometimes been added to the treatment regimen for parkinsonian syndrome. Addition of bromocriptine allows a gradual reduction in the dosage of levodopa. Bromocriptine is not generally used alone in treatment because of a high incidence of adverse side effects.

Side effects of bromocriptine can include:

Psychosis, hallucinations, and confusion

Hypotension

Nausea

Selegiline (Eldepryl), an MAO type B inhibitor, is another drug sometimes prescribed after levodopa has been used for several years and begins to "wear off," or become less effective. Levodopa and selegiline are used *concurrently,* and the levodopa dosage is then reduced by 10–30 % to lessen chance of side effects. Selegiline is not given alone.

Contraindicated with the following drugs, which can interact, resulting in *severe* CNS toxicity, hyperpyrexia, hypertensive crisis, and even death. Do *not* use selegiline with:

Meperidine (Demerol)

Tricyclic antidepressants

Selective serotonin reuptake inhibitors (SSRIs)

When given at the recommended dosage of 10 mg daily in divided doses, there is not the danger of hypertensive crisis associated with interactions of other MAOIs and certain foods (the "cheese reaction"). See Chapter 20 for a description of this reaction, which can occur if the recommended dosage is exceeded. No dietary restrictions are recommended for selegiline at the recommended dose.

ANTICHOLINERGIC AGENTS

Drugs with anticholinergic and antihistaminic actions were the first to be used for parkinsonism and are still useful in mild forms of the disease and for drug-induced parkinsonism. The anticholinergics include synthetic atropinelike drugs, such as benztropine (Artane) and trihexyphenidyl (Cogentin), which are used to prevent or treat parkinsonlike tremors associated with long-term use of the major tranquilizers or for other forms of parkinsonian syndrome.

Side effects of the anticholinergic agents are:

Dry mouth

Dizziness and drowsiness

Blurred vision

Constipation or urinary retention

Confusion

Depression

Nausea

Tachycardia

AMANTADINE

Another drug unrelated to the other antiparkinsonian agents is amantadine (Symmetrel). It is used to treat parkinsonism (extrapyramidal reactions) associated with prolonged use of phenothiazines, carbon monoxide poisoning, or cerebral arteriosclerosis in the elderly.

Side effects of Symmetrel, usually dose related and reversible, can include:

Psychic disturbances, including depression, confusion, hallucinations, anxiety, irritability, nervousness, and dizziness

Headache, weakness, and insomnia

Congestive heart failure, edema, and hypotension

GI distress, constipation, and urinary retention

Contraindications or extreme caution applies to:

Liver and kidney disease

Cardiac disorders

Psychosis, neurosis, and mental depression

Epilepsy

Patients taking CNS drugs

PATIENT EDUCATION

Patients taking antiparkinsonian drugs should be instructed regarding:

Administration on a regular schedule as prescribed, with food to lessen GI distress.

Avoiding abrupt withdrawal of medication, which may greatly increase parkinsonian symptoms.

Several weeks sometimes required before benefit is apparent.

Caution with CNS drugs, alcohol, or antihypertensives (not taking other medicines including vitamins, without physician approval).

Caution with driving or operation of machinery; drugs may cause drowsiness, dizziness, or lightheadedness.

Reporting adverse side effects to the physician (e.g., involuntary movements, blurred vision, constipation, urinary retention, GI symptoms, palpitations, and mental changes).

Reporting any signs that the drug is no longer effective after prolonged use (sometimes after months or years, the dosage may need to be increased or another drug substituted by the physician); avoiding any dosage changes without medical supervision.

Maintaining physical activity, self-care, and social interaction, an essential part of therapy for Parkinson's disease.

Rising slowly.

See Table 22.2 for a summary of the antiparkinsonian drugs.

TABLE 22.2. ANTIPARKINSONIAN DRUGS

Generic Name	Trade Name	Dosage	Comments
levodopa	L-dopa	PO 3–8 g qd pc	**Most effective** for nondrug-induced parkinsonism; delayed onset of action
levodopa and carbidopa	Sinemet	25–250 mg given in div. doses pc	Terminate levodopa at least 8 h before Sinemet
bromocriptine	Parlodel	1.25–2.5 mg bid	Used with levodopa, dosage gradually increased to optimum maintenance dose
Anticholinergics			
benztropine	Cogentin	PO, IM, or IV 1–4 mg qd in one or div. doses	For drug-induced parkinsonism and other forms of parkinsonian syndrome
trihexyphenidyl	Artane	PO 1–15 mg qd in div. doses	For drug-induced parkinsonism and other forms of parkinsonian syndrome
Other Drugs			
amantadine	Symmetrel	100–300 mg qd div. doses	Also for viral upper respiratory infection and drug-induced parkinsonism
selegiline	Eldepryl	5 mg bid	Used with levodopa after years; levodopa dosage decreased

Worksheet for Chapter 22

ANTICONVULSANTS AND ANTIPARKINSONIAN DRUGS

List the drugs according to category and complete all columns.

Classifications and Drugs	Purpose	Side Effects	Contraindications or Cautions	Patient Education
Anticonvulsants 1. 2. 3.				
Antiparkinsonian Drugs with Levodopa 1. L-dopa 2. Sinemet				
Anticholinergics for Parkinson's 1. 2.				
Other Drugs Symmetrel				
Eldepryl				

A. Case Study for Anticonvulsants

Sandy, age 5, has been diagnosed with epilepsy. She has been placed on Dilantin and phenobarbital elixir. Her mother will need all of the following information.

1. Dilantin can have all of the following side effects EXCEPT
   - a. Sore gums
   - b. Staggering
   - c. Insomnia
   - d. Nausea

2. All of the following should be reported to the physician EXCEPT
   - a. Slurred speech
   - b. Increased appetite
   - c. Rash
   - d. Double vision

3. Children's teachers should be alerted to watch for and report all of the following EXCEPT
   - a. Behavior changes
   - b. Drowsiness
   - c. Hyperactivity
   - d. Inattention

4. The mother should do all of the following EXCEPT
   - a. Give medicine with food
   - b. Give medicine on time
   - c. Stress oral hygiene
   - d. Stop medicine if no seizures

5. Which of the following statements is NOT true?
   - a. Doctor may reduce dosage
   - b. Children outgrow epilepsy
   - c. Side effects often subside
   - d. Other drugs sometimes used

B. Case Study for Antiparkinsonian Drugs

Sam Snow, age 70, has Parkinson's disease and has been taking levodopa (L-dopa) for 5 years. He wants to discontinue the drug because he says it's not helping him anymore. He needs the following information.

1. He should be told the following EXCEPT
   - a. Tolerance can develop
   - b. He can increase the dose
   - c. M.D. may change medicine
   - d. Withdrawal increases symptoms

2. When L-dopa loses effectiveness, other drugs can be combined with it for better effect. Which is *not* a drug combination with L-dopa?
   - a. Eldepryl
   - b. Sinemet
   - c. Tegretol
   - d. Parlodel

3. All of the following can be side effects of L-dopa EXCEPT
   - a. Dizziness
   - b. Constipation
   - c. Involuntary movements
   - d. Agitated confusion

4. All of the following may antagonize L-dopa or potentiate side effects EXCEPT
   - a. Antihypertensives
   - b. Vitamin B_6
   - c. Phenytoin
   - d. Aspirin

5. Selegiline is sometimes combined with levodopa. There are serious interactions with selegiline and the following medications EXCEPT
   a. Meperidine
   b. Amantadine
   c. Tricyclics
   d. SSRIs

CHAPTER 23

Endocrine System Drugs

OBJECTIVES

Upon completion of this chapter, the student should be able to:

1. Identify the hormones secreted by these four endocrine glands: pituitary, adrenals, thyroid, and islets of Langerhans.
2. Describe at least five conditions that can be treated with corticosteroids.
3. Explain administration practice important to corticosteroid therapy.
4. List at least four serious potential side effects of long-term steroid therapy.
5. Compare and contrast medications given for hypothyroidism and hyperthyroidism.
6. Describe side effects of thyroid and antithyroid agents.
7. Explain uses and side effects of oral antidiabetics.
8. Compare and contrast insulins according to action (rapid, intermediate, and long acting), naming onset, peak, and duration of each category.
9. Identify the symptoms of hypoglycemia and hyperglycemia, and appropriate interventions.
10. Explain appropriate patient education for those receiving endocrine system drugs.

Endocrine system drugs include natural hormones secreted by the ductless glands or synthetic substitutes. Hormones that affect the reproductive system are discussed in Chapter 24. This chapter covers four categories: pituitary hormones, adrenal corticosteroids, thyroid agents, and antidiabetic agents.

Pituitary Hormones

The pituitary gland, located at the base of the brain, is called the master gland because it regulates the function of the other glands. It secretes four hormones:

somatotropin, adrenocorticotropic hormone (ACTH), thyroid-stimulating hormone (TSH), and gonadotropic hormones (FSH, LH, and LTH; see Chapter 24). The two pituitary hormones discussed in this chapter are somatotropin and ACTH.

The anterior pituitary lobe hormone, somatotropin, is called human growth hormone (HGH). It regulates growth. Insufficient production of HGH will result in growth abnormalities, which should be treated only by an endocrinologist.

Adrenocorticotropic hormone (ACTH) is available only for parenteral use as corticotropin. It is used mainly for diagnosis of adrenocortical insufficiency. Treatment of associated disorders is usually reserved for the corticosteroids in which dosage is more easily regulated and which are available in oral form as well.

Adrenal Corticosteroids

The adrenal glands, located adjacent to the kidneys, secrete hormones called *corticosteroids*, which act by *suppressing the body's response to infection or trauma*. They *relieve inflammation, reduce swelling,* and *suppress symptoms* in acute conditions. Corticosteroid use can be subdivided into two broad categories: (1) as replacement therapy when secretions of the pituitary or adrenal glands are deficient and (2) for their anti-inflammatory and immunosuppressant properties.

Corticosteroid therapy is *not curative*, but is used as *supportive therapy with other medications*. Some conditions treated on a *short-term* basis with corticosteroids include:

Allergic reactions (e.g., to insect bites, poison plants, chemicals or other medications), in which there are symptoms of rash, hives, or anaphylaxis.

Acute flare-ups of rheumatic or collagen disorders, especially where only a few inflamed joints can be injected with corticosteroids to decrease crippling, or in life-threatening situations, such as rheumatic carditis or lupus.

Acute flare-ups of severe skin conditions that do not respond to conservative therapy; topical applications are preferable to systemic therapy, when possible, to minimize side effects.

Acute respiratory disorders, such as status asthmaticus (oral inhalations preferable), sarcoidosis, or to prevent hyaline membrane disease in prematures by administering IM to mother at least 24 hours before delivery.

Malignancies (e.g., leukemia, lymphoma, and Hodgkin's disease), in which corticosteroids (e.g., prednisone) are used with other antineoplastic drugs as part of the chemotherapy regimen.

Cerebral edema associated with brain tumor or neurosurgery.

Organ transplant, in which corticosteroids are used with other immunosuppressive drugs to prevent rejection of transplanted organs.

Life-threatening shock due to adrenocortical insufficiency. Treatment of other forms of shock controversial.

Acute flare-ups of ulcerative colitis. Short-term only to avoid hemorrhage.

Prolonged administration of corticosteroids can cause suppression of the pituitary gland with adrenocortical atrophy, and the body no longer produces its own hormone. To minimize this effect, corticosteroids are given by alternate-day therapy when they are required for extended time periods. Withdrawal of corticosteroids following long-term therapy should always be gradual with step- down (i.e., tapering) dosage. Abrupt withdrawal can lead to acute adrenal insufficiency, shock, and even death.

Because of potentially serious side effects, corticosteroids are administered for as short a time as possible and *locally if possible* to reduce systemic effects (e.g., in ointment, intra-articular injections, ophthalmic drops, and respiratory aerosol inhalants).

Side effects of the corticosteroids, used for longer than very brief periods, can be quite serious and possibly include:

Adrenocortical insufficiency, adrenocortical atrophy

Delayed wound healing and *increased susceptibility to infection*

Fluid and electrolyte imbalance, possibly resulting in edema, potassium loss, hypertension, and congestive heart failure

Muscle pain or weakness

Osteoporosis with fractures, especially in elderly women

Stunting of growth in children (premature closure of bone ends)

Increased intraocular pressure or cataracts

Endocrine disorders, including cushingoid state, amenorrhea, and *hyperglycemia*

Nausea, vomiting, diarrhea, or constipation

Gastric or esophageal irritation, ulceration, or hemorrhage

CNS effects including headache, vertigo, insomnia, euphoria, psychosis, or anxiety

Petechiae, easy bruising, skin thinning and tearing

Contraindications or extreme caution applies to:

Long-term use (regulated carefully)

Viral or bacterial infections (used only in life-threatening situations along with appropriate anti-infectives)

Fungal infections (only if specific therapy concurrent)

Hypothyroidism or cirrhosis (exaggerated response to corticosteroids)

Hypertension or congestive heart failure

Psychotic patients or emotional instability

Diabetes (drugs increase hyperglycemia)

Glaucoma (drugs may increase intraocular pressure)

History of gastric or esophageal irritation (may precipitate ulcers)

Children (drugs may retard growth)

Pregnancy and lactation

History of thromboembolic disorders, seizures or immunosuppression

Interactions may occur with:

Barbiturates, phenytoin (Dilantin), and rifampin—require dosage adjustment

Estrogen may potentiate corticosteroids

Nonsteroidal anti-inflammatory agents (e.g., aspirin may increase risk of GI ulceration)

Diuretics, which potentiate potassium depletion, for example, thiazides, furosemide

Vaccines and toxoids (corticosteroids inhibit antibody response)

PATIENT EDUCATION

Patients taking corticosteroids should be instructed regarding:

Following exact dosage and administration orders (never taking longer than indicated and *never stopping medicine abruptly*).

Notifying physician of any signs of infection or trauma *while taking corticosteroids or within 12 months after long-term therapy is discontinued* and similarly notifying surgeon, dentist, or anesthesiologist if required.

Taking oral corticosteroids during or immediately after meals to decrease gastric irritation.

Avoiding any other drugs at same time (including OTC drugs, e.g., aspirin) without physician's approval. Antacids or other antiulcer drugs sometimes prescribed.

Side effects to expect with long-term therapy (e.g., fluid retention and edema).

Dangers of infection, delayed wound healing, osteoporosis, mental disorders.

Reporting any side effects to physician immediately.

See Table 23.1 for a summary of the pituitary and adrenal corticosteroids.

TABLE 23.1. PITUITARY AND ADRENAL CORTICOSTEROID DRUGS

Generic Name	Trade Name	Dosage[a]
Pituitary Drug		
corticotropin	Acthar, ACTH	IM sol, gel for diagnosis
Adrenal Corticosteroids[a]		
cortisone acetate	Cortisone, Cortone	PO for replacement
dexamethasone	Decadron	PO, IV, IM, inhalation
hydrocortisone	Cortef or Solu-Cortef	PO, IV, deep IM
methylprednisolone	Medrol or Solu-Medrol	PO, IV, deep IM
prednisone	Prednisone, Deltasone	PO tabs or sol

Note: Many other products available. Representative list only. Note also oral inhalation products in Chapter 26.

[a]Dosage varies greatly, depending on the condition treated; massive doses are given for acute conditions on a short-term basis; long-term therapy is usually alternative-day, and dosage is reduced gradually.

Thyroid Agents

Thyroid agents can be natural (Thyroid) or synthetic (e.g., Synthroid). Thyroid preparations are used in replacement therapy for hypothyroidism caused by diminished or absent thyroid function. Levothyroxine (Synthroid) is generally preferred because its hormonal content is standardized and its effect is therefore predictable. Hypothyroid conditions requiring replacement therapy include *cretinism* (congenital; requires immediate treatment to prevent mental retardation) and *myxedema* or adult hypothyroidism due to simple goiter, Hashimoto's thyroiditis, or other thyroid disorders, pituitary disorders, and thyroid destruction from surgery or radiation. Hypothyroidism causes slowed metabolism with symptoms ranging from fatigue, dry skin, weight gain, sensitivity to cold, and irregular menses to mental deterioration if untreated.

Hypothyroidism is diagnosed by blood tests (e.g., RT3U and FTI) before medication is given. The use of thyroid agents in weight reduction programs to increase metabolism when thyroid function is normal (euthyroid) is *contraindicated,* ineffective, and dangerous, leading to decrease in normal thyroid function and possible life-threatening cardiac arrhythmias.

Transient hypothyroidism is rare, and thyroid replacement therapy for true hypothyroidism must be continued for life, although dosage adjustments may be required. Monitoring for toxic effects and periodic lab tests are recommended.

Toxic effects are the result of overdosage of thyroid and are manifested in the signs of *hyperthyroidism:*

Palpitations, tachycardia, cardiac arrhythmias, and increased blood pressure
Nervousness, tremor, headache, and insomnia
Weight loss, diarrhea, and abdominal cramps
Intolerance to heat, fever, and excessive sweating
Menstrual irregularities

Contraindications or extreme caution applies to:

Cardiovascular disease, including angina pectoris and hypertension
Elderly persons (may precipitate dormant cardiac pathology)
Adrenal insufficiency—corticosteroids required first
Diabetes—close monitoring of blood glucose required
Euthyroid persons

Interactions of thyroid may occur with:

Potentiation of oral anticoagulant effects
Insulin and oral hypoglycemics (dosage adjustment necessary)
Potentiation of adrenergic effect (e.g., epinephrine)—watch closely!

PATIENT EDUCATION

Patients being treated with thyroid medication should be instructed regarding:

Importance of taking the prescribed dosage of thyroid medication consistently every day.

Importance of reporting any symptoms of overdose (e.g., palpitations, nervousness, excessive sweating, and unexplained weight loss).

Periodic laboratory tests to determine effectiveness and proper dosage.

Antithyroid Agents

Antithyroid agents (e.g., Tapazole and Propylthiouracil) are used *to relieve the symptoms of hyperthyroidism* in preparation for surgical or radioactive iodine therapy.

Side effects are rare and may include:

Rash, urticaria, and pruritus
Blood dyscrasias (especially agranulocytosis)

Contraindications or caution applies to:

Prolonged therapy (seldom used)
Patients older than 40 years old
Pregnancy and lactation
Hepatic disorders

Interactions with other drugs causing agranulocytosis are potentiated.

PATIENT EDUCATION

Patients being treated with antithyroid medication should be instructed to notify the physician immediately of signs of illness (e.g., chills, fever, rash, sore throat, malaise, and jaundice).

See Table 23.2 for a summary of thyroid and antithyroid agents.

TABLE 23.2. THYROID AND ANTITHYROID AGENTS

Generic Name	Trade Name	Dosage
Thyroid Agents		
levothyroxine	Synthroid, Levothroid	100–200 µg qd
thyroid	Thyroid	60–180 mg qd
Antithyroid Agents		
methimazole	Tapazole	Tabs, 5–30 mg qd
propylthiouracil	Propylthiouracil	Tabs, 100-150 mg qd

Antidiabetic Agents

Antidiabetic agents are administered to *lower blood glucose levels* in those with impaired metabolism of carbohydrates, fats, and proteins. Diabetes mellitus is classified as insulin dependent (type I, IDDM) or non-insulin dependent (type II, NIDDM). Type II diabetes was formerly described as maturity-onset diabetes because it is only found in adults over 40 years of age. However, adults can also develop type I diabetes and require insulin.

INSULIN

Insulin is required as replacement therapy for type I diabetics with insufficient production of insulin from the islets of Langerhans in the pancreas. Insulin is also required in patients with type II (NIDDM) who have failed to maintain satisfactory concentrations of blood glucose with therapy including dietary regulation and oral antidiabetic agents. Insulin is also indicated for stable type II (NIDDM) at the time of surgery, fever, severe trauma, infection, serious renal or hepatic dysfunction, endocrine dysfunction, gangrene, or pregnancy. Insulin (regular) is used in the emergency treatment of diabetic ketoacidosis or coma.

Insulin must be administered parenterally because it is destroyed in the GI tract. In the past, insulins were prepared only from beef or pork pancreas. These forms are still used. However, another *different* form is now also available. Called *insulin human* because its structure is identical to human insulin, it is prepared *in the laboratory* in one of two ways:

1. *Biosynthetic* preparation includes a complex series of scientific steps in which cultures of *Escherichia coli* are modified by a process known as *recombinant DNA technology* to produce such insulins as Humulin R (regular) and Humulin N (isophane).
2. Semisynthetic preparation involves purifying or modifying pork or beef insulin to produce such insulins as Iletin II Purified (Regular) and Iletin II Purified NPH (isophane).

Biosynthetic insulin human (Humulin) is preferred to insulins from animal sources in patients with systemic allergic reactions, in some patients who are very difficult to regulate, or during pregnancy. Insulin human tends to peak sooner than the animal insulins, and therefore smaller amounts are required by some patients. Closer monitoring for hypoglycemia is also required at first.

Most of the insulin used today is U-100, which means that there are 100 units of insulin in each milliliter. The insulin syringe *must be marked U-100* to match the insulin used. Remember that on the 100 U (1 ml) insulin syringe each line represents 2 Units. If a smaller 50 U (1/2 ml) syringe is used, each line represents 1 unit of insulin. See Chapters 4 and 9 for details. Always have someone else compare the insulin in the syringe with the dosage ordered to prevent errors, which could have serious consequences.

Insulin preparations differ mainly in their onset, peak, and duration of action (Table 23.3). *Regular* insulin is rapid acting and of short duration. *Regular* insulin is the *only* type that may be given intravenously as well as subcutaneously. The other insulins, which can *only* be given subcutaneously, include *isophane* (NPH) or Lente, which are intermediate acting; and Ultralente, which is long acting.

Regular insulin is sometimes combined with isophane or zinc insulin in the same syringe. When two insulins are ordered at the same time, the *regular insulin should be drawn into the syringe first*.

Regular insulin is sometimes ordered on a *sliding scale*. This means that the blood is tested for sugar and a specific amount of regular insulin is administered SC based on the glucose level shown by the test.

For example, the physician might write an order to give regular insulin SC according to the following blood glucose levels:

> 350	call physician for dosage
301–350	12 U
251–300	8 U
200–250	5 U
< 200	No insulin

TABLE 23.3. INSULINS

Beef or Pork	Synthetics	Action	Onset (h)	Peak Hours	Duration (h)
Regular	Humulin R, Novolin R, Iletin II Purified (Regular)	Rapid acting	1/2–1	2–3	5–7
Isophane (NPH)	Humulin N, Novolin N	Intermediate acting	1–2	6–12	18–24
Lente	Iletin II Purified NPH				
Ultralente	Humulin U	Long acting	4–8	10–30	36

Note: This is a representative list. Other insulin products are also available. Dosage varies. Before giving insulin, always check expiration date on the vial, and be sure that regular insulins are clear, and isophane and zinc insulins are cloudy. Only regular insulins may be administered IV. Isophane and zinc insulins are administered only SC, never IV. Opened vials may be stored at room temperature.

This is just an *example* of a possible prescription for a *sliding scale*. The actual dose prescribed by the physician will vary with the individual patient. Be sure to check the medication order *carefully* and have someone else verify the amount of insulin drawn into the syringe. Verification of insulin dosage is important to prevent one of the most common and most dangerous medication errors.

Hyperglycemia, or elevated blood glucose, may result from:

Undiagnosed diabetes
Insulin dose insufficient
Infections
Surgical or other trauma
Emotional stress
Other endocrine disorders
Pregnancy

Symptoms of hyperglycemia may include:

Dehydration and excessive thirst
Anorexia and unexplained weight loss in persons under 40 years old
Polyuria (frequent urination)
Fruity breath
Lethargy, weakness, flu symptoms, and coma if untreated
Vision problems
Ketoacidosis—can be determined by testing urine for acetone

Treatment of acute hyperglycemia includes:

IV fluids to correct electrolyte imbalance
Regular insulin added to IV fluids

Interactions: Insulin action is antagonized by corticosteroids or epinephrine, necessitating increased insulin dosage. Oral contraceptives may also increase insulin requirements. Propranolol with insulin poses risks of hypoglycemia or hyperglycemia.

Interactions of insulin with *potentiation* of *hypoglycemic* effect include:

Alcohol
MAOIs
Salicylates
Anabolic steroids

Hypoglycemia, or lowered blood glucose, may result from:

Overdose of insulin
Delayed or insufficient food intake (e.g., dieting)
Excessive or unusual exercise
Change in type of insulin, for example, from pork or beef to human insulin

Symptoms of hypoglycemia may develop suddenly, and are manifested usually at peak of insulin action, including:

Increased perspiration

Irritability, confusion, or bizarre behavior

Tremor, weakness, headache, or tingling of the fingers

Blurred or double vision

Loss of consciousness and convulsions if untreated

Hypoglycemic reactions in elderly diabetics may mimic a CVA (cerebrovascular accident)

Treatment of hypoglycemia includes:

If conscious, administration of 4 oz orange juice, candy, honey, or syrup (especially sublingual).

If comatose, administration of 10–30 ml of 50% dextrose solution IV or administration of 0.5–1 U of glucagon (1 mg) IM or IV—follow with carbohydrate snack when patient awakens to prevent secondary hypoglycemia.

Avoid giving excessive amounts of sugar or frequent overdoses of insulin, which can result in rebound hyperglycemia (Somogyi effect) from an accelerated release of glucagon. Treatment of rebound hyperglycemia involves reduction of insulin dosage with continuous monitoring of blood glucose.

ORAL ANTIDIABETIC AGENTS, (SULFONYLUREAs)

Patients with type II, non-insulin-dependent diabetes may sometimes be treated with diet alone or a combination of a low-calorie, low-fat, sugar-free diet and oral antidiabetic agents (e.g., Diabinese, Tolinase, or Glucotrol), structurally known as sulfonylureas. Oral antidiabetic agents may be administered as a single daily dose before breakfast, or 2 divided doses daily, before morning and evening meals. These medications are not a substitute for dietary management. Weight reduction and modified diet are still considered the principal therapy for the management of type II diabetes.

Symptoms of type II diabetes may include:

Excessive weight gain after age 40

Excessive thirst (polydipsia)

Excessive urination (polyuria)

Excessive weakness, poor circulation, and slow healing

Visual problems

Side effects of oral antidiabetic agents may include:

GI distress (may subside with dosage regulation)

Dermatologic effects, including pruritus, rash, urticaria, or photosensitivity

Hepatic dysfunction, including jaundice (rare)

Weakness, fatigue, lethargy, vertigo, and headache

Blood dyscrasias, including anemia

Hypoglycemia

Possible increased risk of cardiovascular death—controversial

Contraindications or extreme caution applies to:

Debilitated or malnourished patients.

Impaired liver and kidney function.

Unstable diabetes or type I diabetes.

Major surgery, severe infection, and severe trauma.

Contraindicated with the elderly—Diabinese, which has a longer half-life, greater chance of hypoglycemia, and also a risk of inappropriate antidiuretic hormone secretion (water intoxication).

Interactions of sulfonylureas with *potentiation* of hypoglycemic effect can include:

Beta-blockers, MAOIs or probenecid

Alcohol with facial flushing

Cimetidine or miconazole

Salicylates and other nonsteroidal anti-inflammatory agents

Interactions with antagonistic action (larger dose may be required)

Oral anticoagulants

Thiazide and nonthiazide diuretics

Corticosteroids and phenothiazines

Estrogens and oral contraceptives

Calcium blockers

Rifampin and isoniazid

When these agents are administered or discontinued in patients receiving sulfonylureas, the patient should be observed closely for loss of diabetic control.

See Table 23.4 for a summary of the oral hypoglycemics.

TABLE 23.4. ORAL ANTIDIABETIC AGENTS (SULFONYLUREAS)

Generic Name	Trade Name	Usual Dosage
acetohexamide	Dymelor	250 mg–1.5 g qd ac once daily or bid in div. doses
chlorpropamide	Diabinese	250 mg qd ac, contraindicated with elderly
glipizide	Glucotrol	5–25 mg qd 2.5 mg qd geriatrics
glyburide	Micronase, Diabeta	2.5–15 mg qd Lower dose geriatrics
tolazamide	Tolinase	100–250 mg qd with breakfast
tolbutamide	Orinase	250 mg–2q qd, varies greatly, give pc in div. doses

Other products available. This is a representative list.

PATIENT EDUCATION

Both types of diabetics should be instructed regarding:

The importance of control with proper drug and diet therapy.

Early symptoms and treatment of hypoglycemia—carrying ready source of carbohydrate (e.g., lump sugar or candy). Orange juice, 4 oz, is also appropriate.

Properly balanced diet (i.e., restricted calories; avoidance of sugar, sweets, and alcohol; reduced fats, high bulk; and sufficient fluids).

Regular exercise and maintenance of proper body weight; weight reduction if obese.

Importance of reporting to a physician *immediately* if nausea, vomiting, diarrhea, or infections occur (IV fluids may be required to prevent dehydration and acidosis).

Good foot care to reduce chance of infections.

Carrying identification card and wearing identification tag.

Taking medication (oral or insulin) at approximately the same time each day.

Checking urine or blood glucose as directed by the physician, especially with hypoglycemia or stress.

For type I diabetics (those requiring insulin), the foregoing instructions are important, as well as these additional rules:

Rotate injection sites (Fig. 23.1). Insulin is absorbed more rapidly in arm or thigh, especially with exercise. Inject insulin into abdomen if possible for most consistent absorption.

Maintain aseptic technique with injections.

Have someone check the amount of insulin in the syringe before injection, especially with the elderly or those with vision impairment (retinal problems are common in diabetics).

Check all insulin for expiration date.

Check regular insulin for clearness; do *not* give if cloudy or discolored.

Rotate isophane and zinc insulin vials to mix contents; do *not* give if solution is clear or clumped in appearance after rotation; do not shake the vial; rotate gently between hands (Fig. 23.2).

If regular insulin is to be mixed with NPH or Lente, draw regular insulin into syringe first.

Unopened vials of insulin should be stored at 2–8^{0}C and should not be subjected to freezing. The vial in use may be stored at room temperature. Avoid exposure of insulin to extremes in temperature or direct sunlight. Do not put vial in glove compartment, trunk, or suitcase.

Insulin dosage may sometimes be adjusted slightly, *if the physician agrees,* by following these rules:

Increase insulin with illness, stress, or trauma.

Reduce insulin with more exercise or less food. *Never omit insulin.*

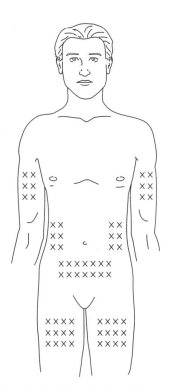

Figure 23.1 Common sites for insulin injection. Sites should be rotated.

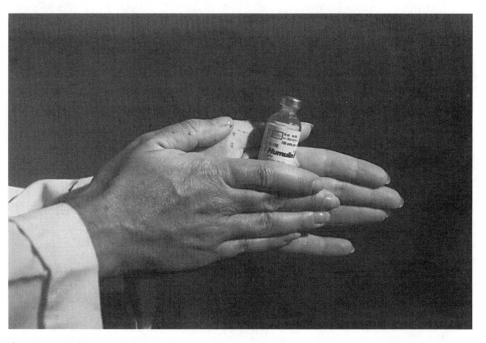

Figure 23.2 Rotate isophane and zinc insulin vials gently to mix contents. Do not shake.

Worksheet 1 for Chapter 23

ENDOCRINE SYSTEM DRUGS

List the drugs according to category and complete all columns. Learn generic or trade names as specified by instructor.

Classifications and Drugs	Purpose	Side Effects	Contraindications or Cautions	Patient Education
Corticosteroids 1. Decadron 2. Solu-Medrol 3. prednisone				
Thyroid Agents 1. Synthroid 2. Thyroid				
Antithyroid Agents 1. Tapazole 2. Propylthiouracil				
Oral Antidiabetic Agents 1. Diabinese 2. Dymelor 3. Glucotrol 4. Micronase 5. Tolinase 6. Orinase				

Worksheet 2 for Chapter 23

INSULINS

Fill in the blanks and complete all columns.

Regular, Humulin R: rapid acting, peak _____ h

NPH, Lente, Humulin N: intermediate acting, peak _____ h

PZI, Ultralente, Humulin U: long acting, peak _____ h

	Causes	Symptoms	Treatment
Hyperglycemia			
Hypoglycemia			

A. Case Study for Endocrine System Drugs

Lois Pal, a 65-year-old patient with glaucoma, asks the physician for prednisone tablets to take long term for osteoarthritis in her knees. She needs the following information.

1. Corticosteroids for severe flare-ups of joint pain are usually administered
   a. By mouth
   b. Topically
   c. Intramuscularly
   d. Intra-articularly
2. The *usual* type of administration of corticosteroids include any of the following EXCEPT
   a. Step-down
   b. Ongoing
   c. Alternate-day
   d. Short term
3. The following are possible corticosteroid side effects EXCEPT
   a. Osteoporosis
   b. Decreased intraocular pressure
   c. Fluid retention
   d. Gastric bleeding
4. Other side effects can include all of the following EXCEPT
   a. Headache
   b. Anxiety
   c. Sedation
   d. Slow healing
5. Corticosteroids can be used to treat all of the following EXCEPT
   a. Asthma attack
   b. Poison ivy
   c. Organ transplant
   d. Fungal infection

B. Case Study for Antidiabetic Agents

Vicky Craft, a 70-year-old type II diabetic, has been taking Orinase for 6 years. Her blood sugar is now elevated and the physician plans to start her on insulin. She will need the following information.

1. The following is true of NPH insulin EXCEPT
   a. Peaks in 6–12 hours
   b. Can be Humulin N
   c. Used for sliding scale
   d. Acts in 1–2 hours
2. Signs of hypoglycemia can include the following EXCEPT
   a. Tremor
   b. Dehydration
   c. Confusion
   d. Blurred vision
3. Treatment of hypoglycemia could include any of the following EXCEPT
   a. 4 oz orange juice
   b. Candy
   c. Diet cola
   d. Glucagon IM
4. If vomiting and diarrhea occur, the following might be necessary EXCEPT
   a. Decrease insulin
   b. IV fluids
   c. Regular insulin IV
   d. NPH insulin subcu

5. The following is true of regular and NPH insulins EXCEPT
   a. Can be mixed
   b. Rotate injection sites
   c. Keep at room temperature
   d. Both are cloudy

CHAPTER **24**

Reproductive System Drugs

OBJECTIVES

Upon completion of this chapter, the student should be able to:

1. Identify the uses, side effects, and precautions for the androgens.
2. List the uses, side effects, and contraindications for the estrogens and progestins.
3. Compare and contrast contraceptives.
4. Describe the use of oxytocics and the precautions to be observed.
5. Explain the uses of Ritodrine, Brethine, Prostaglandin, and magnesium sulfate.
6. Describe the uses of GnRH analogs.
7. Explain drug therapy for infertility.
8. Present appropriate patient education for all drugs in this section.

Hormones that regulate the functions of the reproductive systems include *endogenous* chemical substances, which originate within different areas of the body. For the purpose of simplification, we will divide the reproductive hormones into four main categories: gonadotropic, androgens, estrogens, and progestins.

The pituitary gland is located at the base of the brain. The anterior lobe secretes four hormones. Those affecting growth, thyroid function, and adrenocorticosteroid production are discussed in Chapter 23. This chapter includes the gonadotropic hormones, which are secreted by the anterior and posterior pituitary lobes.

The gonadotropic hormones include (1) follicle-stimulating hormone (FSH), which stimulates development of ovarian follicles in the female and sperm production in the testes of the male; (2) luteinizing hormone (LH), which works in conjunction with FSH to induce secretion of estrogen, ovulation, and development of corpus luteum; and (3) luteotropic hormone (LTH), which stimulates the secretion of progesterone by the corpus luteum and secretion of milk by the mammary gland, hence the term lactogenic hormone.

Androgens

Androgens, the male hormones, are secreted mainly in the interstitial tissue of the testes in the male and secondarily in the adrenal glands of both sexes. Androgens, which stimulate the development of male characteristics (masculinization), include testosterone and andosterone. Inadequate production of androgens in the male may be due to pituitary malfunction; or atrophy, injury to, or removal of the testicles (castration), resulting in eunuchism or eunuchoidism. Eunuchoid characteristics include retarded development of sex organs, absence of beard and bodily hair, high-pitched voice, and lack of muscular development. Hypogonadism may also result in impotence or deficient sperm production (oligospermia).

Uses of androgens include:

Replacement in cases of diminished testicular hormone (e.g., impotence or oligospermia) with testosterone

Congenital hypogonadism (e.g., cryptorchidism or undescended testicles) or delayed puberty in the male

Acquired hypogonadism (e.g., orchitis, trauma, tumor, radiation, or surgery of the testicles)

Palliative treatment of females with advanced metastatic (skeletal) carcinoma of the breast, for example, methyltestosterone

Endometriosis and fibrocystic breast disease for example, danazol

Side effects of androgens can include:

Edema (diuretics may be indicated)

Acne, increased oiliness of skin and hair, or alopecia

Oligospermia (deficient sperm production resulting in sterility)

Increased or decreased sexual stimulation or libido, impotence

Gynecomastia in males (enlarged breast tissue)

Hirsutism, deepening of voice, and amenorrhea in females

Jaundice and hepatitis

Nausea and vomiting

Premature closure of bone ends in adolescents, with stunting of growth

Anxiety, depression, headache

Contraindications or caution applies to:

Cardiac, renal, and liver dysfunction (edema common)

Geriatric males (may increase risk of prostatic hypertrophy and carcinoma or overstimulation sexually)

Prepubertal males who have not reached their full growth potential (may stunt growth by premature closure of bone ends)

Diabetes

Interactions may occur with:

Oral anticoagulants (potentiation may cause bleeding)

Decreased blood glucose and decreased insulin requirements in diabetics

TABLE 24.1. ANDROGENS

Generic Name	Trade Name	Dosage	Comments
danazol	Danocrine	PO 100–400 mg bid	For endometriosis, fibrocystic breast disease
methyltestosterone	Android, Testred	PO 10–50 mg qd, buccal 5–25 mg qd	For male hypogonadism
		PO 50-200 mg qd, buccal 25-100mg qd	For advanced breast cancer
testosterone	Depo-Testosterone	Deep IM, dosage varies; pellet implant, SC	For hypogonadism, advanced breast cancer
testosterone in combination with estrogen	Estratest, Premarin with methyltestoterone	PO dose varies	For menopausal symptoms if estrogen alone is insufficient

---

PATIENT EDUCATION

Patients on androgen therapy should be instructed regarding:

Taking only prescribed drugs according to directions.

Side effects to report, especially edema, jaundice, nausea, or vomiting.

Sexual effects for males to report, such as decreased ejaculatory volume and excessive sexual stimulation, especially in geriatric patients beyond cardiovascular capacity.

Sexual effects for females to expect (e.g., hirsutism and voice deepening).

Possibility of stunted growth when administered to adolescent boys before puberty.

Dangers of illegal use of anabolic steroids: Health care personnel have a responsibility to caution athletes, especially adolescents, regarding the hazards of taking illegal synthetic testosterone products to build muscle power or physique. Besides the potentially serious adverse side effects just mentioned, another risk is the development of psychosis with delusions, paranoia, depression, mania, and aggression with violence.

See Table 24.1 for a summary of the androgens.

Estrogens

Estrogens, the female sex hormones, are produced mainly by the ovary and secondarily by the adrenal glands. Estrogens are responsible for the development of female secondary sexual characteristics, including breast enlargement, and during the menstrual cycle they act on the female genitalia to produce an environment suitable for fertilization, implantation, and nutrition of the early embryo. Estrogens also affect the secretion of the hormones FSH and LH from the anterior pituitary gland in a complex way. This results in inhibition of lactation and inhibition of ovulation, the latter process utilized in contraceptive therapy.

Estrogen in combination with testosterone is sometimes used in the management of severe menopausal symptoms that do not respond to estrogen alone.

Uses of estrogen therapy include:

Contraceptives (combined with progestin)—these combination products are also used to treat menstrual irregularities and dysmenorrhea.

Menopausal vasomotor symptom relief (*not* effective against depression or nervous symptoms).

Female hypogonadism due to ovarian pathology or oophorectomy.

Postmenopausal prevention of osteoporosis (calcium depletion) Well-controlled studies show estrogen replacement to be the single most effective treatment for prevention or arrest of bone reabsorption leading to fractures and osteoporosis in postmenopausal women.

Post menopausal estrogen replacement may reduce cardiovascular heart disease in women by 50–70%.

Atrophic vaginitis from decreased secretions—low dose vaginal cream biweekly.

Inhibition of lactation in nonnursing mothers.

Postcoital use after rape or incest (within 24–48 h) of a single large dose to prevent, not terminate, pregnancy.

Palliative treatment for males with advanced, inoperable prostate cancer.

Side effects of estrogen therapy, especially with high doses, can include:

Increased risk of thromboembolic disorders, hypertension, myocardial infarction, and stroke

GI effects, including vomiting, abdominal cramps, bloating, diarrhea or constipation, and weight gain

Skin discolorations (acne may decrease or occasionally increase)

Fluid retention and edema

Increased serum triglyceride levels

Severe hypercalcemia in cancer patients with large doses

Folic acid deficiency (may require folic acid supplements)

Liver function abnormalities, including jaundice, anorexia, and pruritis

Breakthrough or irregular vaginal bleeding

Increased risk of cervical erosion and *Candida vaginitis*

Headache, especially migraine, and depression

Visual disturbances

Breast tenderness, enlargement, and secretion

Increased risk of gallbladder disease

Contraindications and cautions exist because the use of estrogens, especially in large doses, may be associated with increased risk of several serious conditions. Before estrogen therapy is begun, a complete history and physical examination are essential, and yearly physicals during therapy are important. Estrogens are *contraindicated* for anyone with a history of the following conditions, and estrogen therapy should be *discontinued with signs of these conditions:*

Thromboembolus, stroke, and myocardial infarction

Liver dysfunction and gallbladder disease

Visual disturbances, severe headaches, and migraine

Hypertension, shortness of breath, and chest or calf pain

Seizure, asthma, and kidney disorders

Surgery (estrogens should be discontinued 4 weeks before if possible)

Other contraindications include the following:

Prolonged continued use of high-dose estrogens in postmenopausal women, which has shown an increased risk of endometrial cancer in some studies; therefore, cyclic administration at the *lowest* possible dose is recommended with regular physical examinations, including a Pap test every year.

Pregnancy, in which estrogens can cause serious fetal toxicity, congenital anomalies, and vaginal or cervical cancer for the offspring in later life. Estrogens should *never* be used to treat threatened abortions or if there is any possibility of pregnancy. A pregnancy test should be done before initiating therapy.

Nursing mothers should avoid estrogen.

Caution with diabetes and with heavy smokers

Interactions include the following:

Rifampin and isoniazid decrease estrogenic activity, and therefore other forms of contraception should be used with patients receiving rifampin or isoniazid

Corticosteroid effects are potentiated by estrogen

Oral anticoagulant action is decreased by estrogen

Laboratory test interference includes endocrine function tests, decreased glucose tolerance, and thyroid function tests

Anti-infectives may decrease contraceptive action

Anticonvulsants, hypotensives, and oral hypoglycemic actions may be decreased or increased

Progestins

Progesterone is a hormone secreted by the corpus luteum and adrenal glands. It is responsible for changes in uterine endometrium in the second half of the menstrual cycle in preparation for implantation of the fertilized ovum, development of maternal placenta after implantation, and development of mammary glands. Synthetic drugs that exert progesterone-like activity are called progestins.

Uses of synthetic progestins include:

Treatment of amenorrhea and abnormal uterine bleeding caused by hormonal imbalance

Contraception, either combined with estrogen or used alone

Postmenopausal—sometimes combined with estrogen in replacement cyclical therapy

Adjunctive and palliative therapy for advanced and metastatic endometrial or renal cancer

Depo-Provera, 100-500 mg IM weekly to monthly has been used in the management of paraphilia (sexual deviancy in males) especially for pedophilia and sexual sadism. The drug has been shown to decrease erotic cravings, but sexual deviance usually returns following discontinuance of the drug.

Side effects of continuous progestin use can include:

Menstrual irregularity and amenorrhea, breakthrough bleeding and spotting

Edema and weight gain

Nausea

Breast tenderness, enlargement, and secretion

Jaundice, rash, and pruritis

Headache and migraine

Mental depression

Cervical erosion

Thromboembolic disorders

Vision disorders

Possible decrease in bone density with prolonged use

Contraindications and cautions with progestin (similar to cautions with estrogen) apply to:

Any condition that might be aggravated by fluid retention (e.g., asthma, seizures, migraine, and cardiac or renal dysfunction)

History of mental depression

History of thromboembolic disorders

History of cerebrovascular accident

Liver disorders

Undiagnosed vaginal bleeding

Pregnancy (progestins are no longer used to treat threatened abortion because of the potential adverse effects to the fetus)

See Table 24.2 for a summary of the estrogens and progestins.

CONTRACEPTIVE AGENTS

The use of estrogen-progestin combined hormones as a safe and effective method of birth control has been well established. They act by suppressing release of the pituitary hormones, follicle-stimulating hormone (FSH) and luteinizing hormone (LH), thus resulting in the prevention of ovulation. Additional methods of action have been suggested, that is, changes in the cervical mucus to prevent sperm pen-

TABLE 24.2. ESTROGENS, PROGESTINS, AND CONTRACEPTIVE AGENTS

Generic Name	Trade Name	Dosage	Comments
Estrogens			
chlorotrianisene	TACE	PO; dose varies with condition	For female hypogonadism, breast engorgement, prostate cancer
diethylstilbestrol	DES	PO, intravaginal; dose varies with condition	For female hypogonadism, breast engorgement, prostate cancer
estradiol	Estraderm Estrace Depo-estradiol	Transdermal, PO tabs IM, intravaginal, dose varies	For menopause, prostate cancer, breast engorgement
conjugated estrogens	Premarin	PO, vaginal cream, parenteral; dose varies with condition	For female hypogonadism, breast engorgement, prostate cancer, menopausal symptoms
Progestins			
medroxyprogesterone	Provera Cycrin	Parenteral, PO, IM, dose varies	For abnormal uterine bleeding, menopausal symptoms, contraception
synthetic progestins			See contraceptives
Contraception Agents[a]			
monophasic preparations contain the same amount of estrogen and progesterone in each tablet. 50 µg. estrogen	Ovral Ovcon 50 Ortho-novum 1/50	PO	
35 µg estrogen	Norinyl 1/35 Demulen 1/35 Ortho-cyclen	PO	
30 µg estrogen	LoOvral Desogen/Ortho-cept	PO	
20 µg estrogen	LoEstrin 1/20	PO	
Biphasic Preparations—2 parts progestin/1 part estrogen			
35 µg estrogen	Ortho-novum 10/11 Janest	PO	
Triphasic Preparations—3 parts progestin/1 part estrogen			
	Triphasil/Tri-levlen Tri-norinyl Tri-cyclen	PO, dose varies	
Progestin-Only Preparations			
	Micronor/Ovrette Depo-Provera Norplant Progestasert	PO IM, 150 mg Subdermal implants In IUD	
Postcoital Contraception	Ovral	PO, 2 tabs q12h. for total of 4 tablets (must be administered within 72 hours)	
	Danocrine IUD RU 486	IM, dose varies Still under study, FDA approval not yet available	

Note: Because of adverse side effects, estrogen and progestin products should be administered at the lowest possible dose for effectiveness.

[a]List of trade names is not all-inclusive as the number of available oral contraceptives are too numerous to mention.

etration and changes in the endometrium or lining to the uterus to discourage implantation and cell growth.

The *progestin-only* contraceptives prevent pregnancy by inhibiting ovulation, changing the amount or thickness of cervical mucus, thus inhibiting sperm transport, and creating a thin, atrophic endometrium not conducive to sustaining the fertilized ovum. The progestin-only preparations may be indicated for women who cannot tolerate estrogenic side effects or for whom estrogen is contraindicated. Examples would be estrogen-related headaches, hypertension, or history of thrombophlebitis or thromboembolic complications. Other indications include breast-feeding women, since progestin has no effect on lactation or nursing infants. Young women who have a history of noncompliance on oral contraceptives might benefit from injections or implants. The failure rate for progestin-only preparations ranges from 0.1% to 0.3% for injections and implants, and 2–3% for uses of oral progestin-only pills and progestin-containing IUDs (intrauterine devices).

Uses of *combined* or *progestin-only* contraceptives include:

Prevention of pregnancy

Treatment and/or improvement of other medical conditions, such as endometriosis, painful, heavy periods, irregular cycles, and acne

Other medical benefits of oral contraceptives include decreased incidence of ovarian cysts, ovarian or endometrial cancer, benign breast disease, and ectopic pregnancy. There is also a protective effect against pelvic inflammatory disease.

Minor side effects of contraceptives include:

Nausea
Increased breast size
Fluid retention
Weight gain or loss
Bleeding between periods, break-through bleeding (BTB)
Scanty menstrual flow (considered a benefit)
Changes in libido
Mood changes

Serious side effects of estrogen can include:

Migraine headaches or headaches increasing in frequency and severity
Severe depression
Blurred vision or loss of vision

Absolute contraindications for estrogen products include:

Thrombophlebitis or thromboembolic disorder or history thereof
History of cerebrovascular accident
Coronary artery heart disease

Known or suspected history of breast cancer or other estrogen-dependent malignancy

Pregnancy

History of liver disease or impaired liver function

In addition to the above contraindications, estrogen-progestin contraceptives should be used with caution in the following conditions:

Women over 35 and currently smoking 15 or more cigarettes a day

Migraine headaches that start after initiating oral contraceptives

Hypertension with resting diastolic above 90 or systolic above 140

Diabetes mellitus

Undiagnosed vaginal bleeding

Confirmed sickle-cell disease

Lactation

Oral contraceptives may accelerate development of gallbladder disease in women already susceptible

Interactions: Many drugs may interact with oral contraceptives and alter the effectiveness, including pain relievers, alcohol, anticoagulants, antidepressants, tranquilizers or barbiturates, corticosteroids, antibiotics, asthma drugs, beta-blockers, anticonvulsants, oral hypoglycemic drugs, and vitamin C.

PATIENT EDUCATION

Women taking oral contraceptives should be instructed regarding the use of back-up contraception for the first month on oral contraceptives, and for the first 2 weeks with Depo-Provera.

Taking the contraceptive at the same time every day. If oral contraceptives are missed, the general instruction is that the pill should be doubled up until the patient has caught up, using a back-up method until period begins. If 3 pills or more are missed, the patient is instructed to throw away the pack until she starts her period, and then begin a new pack of pills. Stop oral contraceptives if pregnancy is suspected and stop smoking.

Using back-up contraception when taking other medicines that may alter effectiveness. (See Interactions above.)

Reporting the following symptoms to your health care provider should they occur while on oral contraceptives: chest pain, severe headache, dizziness, weakness, numbness, eye problems, or severe leg pains in the calf or thigh.

Choice of Oral Contraceptives:

Estrogen-progestin oral contraceptives are available in several formulations and varieties of chemical preparations. They are usually classified according to their estrogen content and formulation as follows:

1. Monophasic preparations contain the same amount of estrogen and progestin in each tablet.
2. Biphasic preparations contain two sequences of progestin doses and less than 50 µg estrogen.
3. Triphasic preparations contain three sequences of progestin doses and less than 50 µg estrogen.

Choice of a particular contraceptive will be made after considering the patient's history, hormone-related side effects, prior use, and desired effect. In general, whenever possible, the smallest dose of estrogen and progestin should be used that is compatible with a low failure rate and meets the individual needs of the woman. Broad categories are listed in Table 24.2. Individual oral contraceptives are too numerous to mention in their entirety; however, a few examples in each category are included.

PROGESTIN-ONLY CONTRACEPTIVES

These preparations are recommended for patients who do not tolerate estrogen or in whom it is contraindicated. Choice of method of delivery (i.e., oral tablets, injection, or implants) should be made to appropriately accommodate the patient's needs and compliance.

NORPLANT

The Norplant subdermal implant consists of six Silastic rods containing levonorgestrel, released at a slow, steady rate over a period of 5 years. Its physiologic action is similar to the progestin-only pills but has the added benefit of continuous contraception with no chance of user failure. It provides continuous, long-term contraception, yet when removed, the contraceptive effect wears off quickly.

Insertion of Norplant is a minor surgical procedure in which the rods are placed on the inside of the upper arm, using local anesthesia. Implants are placed under the skin in a fan-shaped configuration with little or no discomfort. At the end of five years, or if a woman should choose to have the implants removed sooner, local anesthesia is again used and the rods are removed through a small, 1 cm incision made at the base of the rods. There is little or no scarring involved.

Side effects: Contraindications and patient education information have been previously discussed concerning progestin-only products. The patient must be well informed of the common side effects, prior to insertion, as well as the more serious warning signals for this type of contraception. Thorough patient education and counseling prior to insertion will ensure that the woman is happy with her choice of a subdermal form of contraception.

PROGESTIN-CONTAINING INTRAUTERINE DEVICE (IUD): PROGESTASERT

An intrauterine device (IUD) containing a reservoir of progesterone is one of the two IUDs available in the United States. It releases small amounts of progesterone daily, providing 1 year of continuous contraception protection. The mechanism of action of the IUD is not fully understood but is generally thought to have an inhibitory effect on sperm migration, change in the ovum transport, and alteration of the endometrium. The progesterone in the IUD is thought to offer support to all of these actions.

Cautions and side effects: There are many considerations, contraindications, and side effects that must be addressed when considering the IUD as a method of contraception. These are too numerous to mention in this text. The purpose of including the IUD here is to inform the reader that it is one of several delivery systems in the use of progestin as a contraceptive drug.

POSTCOITAL CONTRACEPTION

While the use of combined estrogen-progestin contraceptive pills as a means of postcoital contraception is not without risk, it is an available option to women who are exposed to an unintentional risk of pregnancy. This includes such circumstances as a broken condom, rape, defective barrier methods, lost or forgotten oral contraceptives, or any other method that is not available at the time that it is needed. When using postcoital or "morning after" contraception, it is essential that the woman's history is reviewed, that she is informed of the risks and benefits of postcoital contraception, and that she gives informed consent. It must be administered within 72 hours of unprotected intercourse. Typical dosages for oral contraceptives in this instance would be Ovral, 2 tablets taken in 2 doses, 12 hours apart, for a total of 4 tablets, or Lo\Ovral, Nordette, or Triphasil, 4 tablets taken in 2 doses, 12 hours apart. Side effects, which include nausea and vomiting, headache, and breast tenderness, usually subside within 1–2 days after treatment. Again, it must be noted that postcoital contraception must be administered within 72 hours of unprotected intercourse.

Other postcoital options less frequently used due to cost or high incidence of side effects, includes:

Danazol, 8–1200 mg, in 2–3 doses, 12 hours apart.

Progestin-only pills, no appropriate dosage of oral progestin-only pills is available in the United States as it would require the patient to take 16 or more tablets.

Postcoital IUD insertion; within 5–7 days after ovulation, this is an effective but not widely used method due to the cost and risk of concomitant exposure or presence of sexually transmitted diseases.

RU-486; this is an antiprogesterone drug currently available in the United States only under clinical trial for use in effective termination of pregnancy. It has not been approved for use as a postcoital contraceptive. However, it is possible that in the future this drug, in a lower dose, may be tested and established as an alternative postcoital contraceptive.

See Table 24.2 for a summary of estrogens, progestins, and contraceptive agents.

PATIENT EDUCATION

Patients taking estrogen, progesterone, or combinations of the two should be instructed regarding:

Importance of following prescribed schedule with contraceptives

Taking with or after evening meal or at hs, same time every day

Minor adverse effects of contraceptives, for example, edema, weight gain, nausea

Possible serious side effects and the importance of reporting any signs of cardiovascular or kidney disorders, liver or gallbladder dysfunction, rash, jaundice, GI symptoms, visual disturbance, severe headache, breast lumps, irregular vaginal bleeding, shortness of breath, and chest or calf pain

Increased risk of stroke or myocardial infarction (MI) for smokers

Regular breast self-examination

Complete physical examination including Pap test at least yearly

Avoidance of all estrogen or progestin products if pregnant or nursing

---

Drugs for Labor and Delivery

In addition to the hormones secreted by the anterior pituitary gland, there is also a hormone secreted by the posterior pituitary lobe: oxytocin. This hormone stimulates the uterus to contract, thus inducing childbirth. Oxytocin also acts on the mammary gland to stimulate the release of milk. Synthetic chemicals used to stimulate uterine contractions are called oxytocics and include *oxytocin,* prostaglandin E_2, and ergonovine/methylergonovine.

OXYTOCIN

Uses of oxytocin (IV infusion of dilute solutions slowly and at a carefully monitored rate) include:

Induction of labor with at-term or near-term pregnancies associated with hypertension (e.g., preeclampsia, eclampsia, or cardiovascular-renal disease), maternal diabetes, or uterine fetal death at term.

Stimulating uterine contractions during the first or second stages of labor if labor is prolonged or if dysfunctional uterine inertia occurs.

Pelvic adequacy and other maternal and fetal conditions must be evaluated carefully prior to induction of labor. Cesarean section may be preferable and safer in some instances.

Side effects of oxytocin can be serious, resulting even in maternal or fetal death. *Extreme caution* with administration and *constant maternal* and *fetal monitoring* are required to prevent dangerous side effects such as:

Tetanic contractions with risk of uterine rupture

Cervical lacerations

Abruptio placenta

Impaired uterine blood flow

Amniotic fluid embolism

Fetal trauma, including intracranial hemorrhage or brain damage

Fetal cardiac arrhythmias, including bradycardia, tachycardia, and premature ventricular contractions

Fetal death due to asphyxia

With large amounts of oxytocin, watch for:

Severe hypotension

Tachycardia and arrhythmias

Postpartum hemorrhage

Subarachnoid hemorrhage

Hypertensive episodes

Contraindications include:

Elective induction of labor merely for physician or patient convenience, which is *not* a valid indication for oxytocin use

Cephalopelvic disproportion, unfavorable fetal position or presentation

Uterine or cervical scarring from major cervical or uterine surgery

Fetal distress when delivery is not imminent

Placenta previa, prolapsed cord, and multiparity

Prolonged use with severe toxemia

PROSTAGLANDIN E$_2$

Uses (vaginal insertion of dinoprostone suppositories or gel) for:

Therapeutic abortion in the second trimester (beyond the 12th week)

Uterine evacuation in cases of intrauterine fetal death in late pregnancy, benign hydatidiform mole, or fetuses with ancephaly, erythroblastosis fetalis, or other congenital abnormalities incompatible with life

Side effects can be minimized by administration of a prior test dose and symptomatic treatment of such effects as:

GI hypermotility, including nausea, vomiting, diarrhea—decreased by premedication with antiemetics and antidiarrhea agents

Bradycardia, hypotension, hypertension, and arrhythmias

Dizziness, syncope, flushing, and fever

Bronchospasm, including wheezing, dyspnea, chest constriction, and chest pain

Cervical laceration or uterine rupture (less common)

Retained placenta (less common)

Contraindications and precautions include:

Use only by trained physicians in a hospital where intensive care and surgical facilities are available

Contraindicated with history of pelvic surgery, uterine fibroids, cervical stenosis, and acute pelvic inflammatory disease

Caution with asthma, hypertension, cardiovascular or renal disease

ERGONOVINE AND METHYLERGONOVINE

Uses of these ergot alkaloids include prevention and treatment of postpartum and postabortion hemorrhage.

Side effects occur most commonly when administered IV undiluted or too rapidly, or in conjunction with regional anesthesia or vasoconstrictors, and can include:

Nausea and vomiting

Dizziness, headache, diaphoresis, palpitation, dyspnea, and arrhythmias

Hypertension (less common with Methergine)

Numbness and coldness of extremities with overdose

Seizures with overdose

Contraindications include:

When administered during third stage of labor, may lead to retained placenta

Contraindicated with cardiovascular disease, especially hypertension, and with hepatic and renal impairment

TERBUTALINE (BRETHINE)

Terbutaline, although classified as a bronchodilator drug primarily used for pulmonary disorders, is also used with careful monitoring in the management of preterm labor. Its sympathomimetic action inhibits uterine contractions and has the advantage of causing less severe side effects on mother and fetus than ritodrine. Although the manufacturer does not recommend its use for preterm labor at this time, it is widely used for this purpose with careful monitoring, both in the hospital setting and with home uterine monitoring. It is available for oral or subcutaneous administration.

Side effects: nervousness, tremors, increased heart rate, headache, nausea, vomiting, heart palpitations. Side effects tend to be less severe with a subcutaneous pump, rather than PO.

Caution: Watch patient closely for signs of pulmonary edema. Should not be used in patients with hypertension, cardiac disease, hyperthyroidism, diabetes, or history of seizures.

Note: At this time, manufacturer does not recommend terbutaline be used for tocolysis in preterm labor. The safety of use of this drug for this purpose has not been adequately established. Therefore, the expected therapeutic benefit must be weighed against its possible hazards to mother and fetus.

RITODRINE

Ritodrine (Yutopar) is an adrenergic drug used to inhibit uterine contractions in premature labor. Prolongation of gestation may reduce the incidence of neonatal death and respiratory distress syndrome. Ritodrine is used only after a gestation period of 20–36 weeks, with regular contractions every 7–10 min, with amniotic membranes intact, and with cervical dilatation not more than 4 cm.

Side effects of ritodrine are usually dose related and can include:

Increase in maternal and fetal heart rates with palpitations
Elevated blood glucose with glycosuria and ketoacidosis
Tremor, nausea, vomiting, headache, irritability, anxiety, and chest pain

Contraindications or extreme caution applies to:

Cardiac disease and hypertension
Diabetes
Hyperthyroidism

MAGNESIUM SULFATE

Treatment of severe preeclampsia or eclampsia consists of magnesium sulfate ($MgSO_4$) injection for prevention and control of seizures. Magnesium sulfate acts by depressing the CNS and blocking neuromuscular transmission, thus producing anticonvulsant effects. Magnesium sulfate has also been used in the management of uterine tetany associated with the use of oxytocic agents. Magnesium sulfate also acts peripherally, producing vasodilation and lowering the blood pressure. Patients receiving this drug must be monitored closely for vital signs and reflexes.

Side effects, which can be serious and even fatal, can include:

Flaccid paralysis and CNS depression
Circulatory collapse, cardiac depression, and hypotension

TABLE 24.3. DRUGS FOR LABOR AND DELIVERY

Generic Name	Trade Name	Dosage	Comments
Oxytocics[a]			
ergonovine	Ergotrate	PO, IM, IV; dosage varies	For postpartum hemorrhage
methylergonovine	Methergine	PO, IM, IV; dosage varies	For postpartum hemorrhage
oxytocin	Pitocin, Syntocinon	IV, nasal spray	For induction of labor, postpartum hemorrhage, promotion of milk ejection
Prostaglandin E2			
dinoprostone	Prostin E$_2$	Vaginal supp.	For therapeutic abortion
Adrenergic[b]			
ritodrine HCl	Yutopar	IV, PO; dosage varies	For preterm labor
terbutaline	Brethine	Subcu, PO, dose varies	For preterm labor
Treatment for Preeclampsia or Eclampsia			
magnesium sulfate	MgSO$_4$	IV; dosage varies	Watch for respiratory complications

[a]Stimulate uterine contractions.

[b]Inhibit uterine contractions in preterm labor.

Fatal respiratory paralysis

Flushing and sweating

The antidote for overdose of magnesium sulfate (e.g., respiratory depression or heart block) is IV administration of calcium gluconate.

Contraindications or extreme caution applies to:

Impaired renal function

Heart block or myocardial damage

Use more than 24 h before delivery and within 2 h of delivery because of potential respiratory depression in the neonate

See Table 24.3 for a summary of drugs for labor and delivery.

Other Gonadotropic Drugs

Drugs classified as analogs of gonadotropin-releasing hormones (GnRH) act in the pituitary to suppress ovarian and testicular hormone production and inhibit estrogen and androgen synthesis. Leuprolide (Lupron) has been used as an antineoplastic agent to inhibit the growth of hormone-dependent tumors. It has been used to reduce the size of the prostate and inhibit prostatic tumor growth. It has also been used following other therapies, for example, mastectomy, radiation, and/or other antineoplastic drugs, to treat breast cancer. Lupron is sometimes combined with the antiestrogen drug, tamoxifen, in the treatment of breast cancer. (See Chapter 14 for dosage and side effects.)

GnRH analogs that inhibit gonadotropin secretion, for example, Lupron and Synarel, are used in the management of endometriosis. They inhibit ovulation and stop menstruation, thereby providing pain relief and a reduction in endometriotic lesions. Lupron is administered as a monthly IM injection. Synarel is administered as a nasal spray. Treatment with either is limited to 6 months. They appear to be better tolerated than the androgen, danazol, in the treatment of endometriosis.

Lupron is also the drug of choice for precocious puberty in children. Experimental studies indicate other potential uses for Lupron, for example, as a male contraceptive agent, but the long-term safety and contraceptive efficacy of this therapy have not been determined.

Side effects of the GnRH agonists can include:

Hot flashes
Vaginal dryness
Headache
Emotional or mood swings
Weight gain or loss
Nasal congestion
Acne or insomnia

Cautions and contraindications: Not to be considered effective as a contraceptive, patient should use a backup barrier method.

Not safe during pregnancy or lactation
Prolonged use creates a hypoestrogenic state that may lead to an increased risk of loss of bone density

Patients must be fully informed of the benefits and risks of the use of GnRH analog drugs, and generally speaking, the therapeutic values should outweigh any potential risks. Patient compliance is enhanced with adequate patient education, counseling, and support.

Infertility Drugs

CLOMIPHENE CITRATE (CLOMID)

Clomiphene is an orally administered, nonsteroidal agent that may induce ovulation in selected anovulatory women. Its chief action is to stimulate the pituitary gland to release more FSH and LH, resulting in the maturation and release of mature follicles from the ovary.

Side effects: Ovarian enlargement, vasomotor flushes, breast tenderness, nausea and/or vomiting, nervousness, and insomnia. While the incidence of multiple pregnancies increases with use of clomiphene, 90% in one study were single pregnancies, 10% were twins, and less than 1% resulted in triplets.

Cautions: Thorough evaluation to assure that the patient is an appropriate candidate for clomiphene therapy is essential. The drug should not be given to women with a known ovarian cyst, known cancer of the endometrium, pregnant women, undiagnosed vaginal bleeding, or any liver, thyroid, adrenal, or intracranial disorder.

MENOTROPINS FOR INJECTION (PERGONAL)

Pergonal is a purified preparation of gonadotropin containing equal amounts of FSH and LH. It is injected IM to stimulate follicle development in the ovaries. In order to trigger ovulation, human chorionic gonadotropin (CG) is given at the appropriate time to effect release of the mature follicles from the ovary. Pergonal may also be given to men, along with CG, to stimulate spermatogenesis.

Side effects: Ovarian enlargement with or without ovarian cysts, abdominal pain, GI symptoms such as nausea, vomiting or abdominal cramping or dizziness

Cautions and contraindications: Similar to clomiphene. Patients must be thoroughly and appropriately assessed and evaluated to assure that they are candidates for treatment with Pergonal and CG.

CHORIONIC GONADOTROPIN (PROFASI)

Chorionic gonadotropin (CG) is used to induce ovulation in women who have been appropriately treated with menotropins. This drug is given as a single IM dose 1 day following the course of therapy with Pergonal.

Chorionic gonadotropin (CG) has also been used in the treatment of prepubertal cryptorchidism and hypogonadism resulting from pituitary deficiency. Treatment of such conditions should be managed by an endocrinologist.

Side effects of CG: Headache, irritability, restlessness, depression, edema and fatigue.

Contraindications: Any known neoplasm or prior allergic reaction to CG.

UROFOLLITROPIN FOR INJECTION (METRODIN)

Metrodin is a preparation containing FSH extracted from the urine of postmenopausal women. It has little or no LH activity. It is indicated for the induction of ovulation in women with polycystic ovarian disease who have an elevated LH level and a low to normal FSH level, and are unresponsive to clomiphene therapy. Like Pergonal, ovulation is induced following the administration of Metrodin by using an injection of CG. It is administered IM for 7–12 days.

Side effects of Metrodin: Similar to other infertility drugs, that is, ovarian enlargement, nausea, vomiting or abdominal cramping, headache, or breast tenderness.

Caution and contraindications: Metrodin should not be administered to patients who have demonstrated a hypersensitivity to gonadotropins, women with increased levels of FSH that would indicate ovarian failure, abnormal or undiagnosed bleeding, or in pregnancy.

See Table 24.4 for a summary of other gonadotropin associated drugs.

TABLE 24.4. OTHER GONADOTROPIC DRUGS

Generic Name	Trade Name	Dosage	Comments
nafarelin acetate	Synarel	Nasal spray, dose varies	For endometriosis, treatment not to exceed 6 months
leuprolide acetate	Lupron Depot	IM dose varies	For endometriosis, some cases of infertility, treatment not to exceed 6 months; also for prostate cancer (see Antineoplastics)
clomiphene citrate	Clomid, Seraphene	PO dose varies	For treatment of infertility, ovulation induction
menotropins	Pergonal	IM q day for 7–12 days	Treatment of infertility, stimulates follicle development
chorionic gonadotropin (CG)	Profasi	IM single dose, 5–10,000 U	For treatment of infertility, given 1 day after Pergonal, to induce ovulation
urofollitropin	Metrodin	IM q day for 7–12 days	For induction of ovulation in women with polycystic ovaries followed with injections of CG

Worksheet for Chapter 24

REPRODUCTIVE SYSTEM DRUGS

List the drugs according to category and complete all columns. Learn generic or trade names as specified by instructor.

Classifications and Drugs	Purpose	Side Effects	Contraindications or Cautions	Patient Education
Androgens 1. testosterone 2. danazol				
Estrogens 1. TACE 2. diethylstilbestrol (DES) 3. Premarin 4. estradiol 5. Estratest				
Progestins 1. Provera 2. synthetics				

Contraceptives
1. estrogen/progesterone combinations
2. progestin only
    oral
    IM
    Subdermal
    IUD				

Classifications and Drugs	Purpose	Side Effects	Contraindications or Cautions	Patient Education

For Labor and Delivery
1. Oxytocics
   Pitocin
   ergotrate
   prostaglandin E_2
 	
2. Andrenergics
   Ritodrine
   Brethine
 	
3. CNS depressant
   $MgSO_4$				

Other Gonadotropics GnRH analogs 1. Lupron 2. Synarel				
Ovulation Induction 1. Clomid 2. Pergonal 3. Metrodin				
Chorionic gonadotropin CG (Profasi)				

A. Case Study for Reproductive System Drugs

May B., age 38, visits her obstetrician's office for her 6-week postpartum checkup. She smokes. She has a history of thrombophlebitis. She plans to continue nursing her baby. She asks the doctor for a prescription for Ortho-novum for birth control purposes. She needs all of the following information.

1. Ortho-novum falls into which contraceptive category?
   - a. Estrogen only
   - b. Progestin only
   - c. Estrogen-progestin combination
   - d. Postcoital contraceptive

2. Contraceptives containing estrogen are not advised in which conditions?
   - a. History of thrombophlebitis
   - b. Coronary artery disease
   - c. Lactation
   - d. All of the above
   - e. Only (a) and (c)

3. Progestin-only contraceptives are available in all of the following forms EXCEPT
   - a. Pills
   - b. Suppository
   - c. Injection
   - d. Rod implants
   - e. IUD

4. Side effects of estrogen products can include all of the following EXCEPT
   - a. Severe headaches
   - b. Depression
   - c. Heavy menstrual flow
   - d. Fluid retention
   - e. Blurred vision

5. Those more at risk for complications with estrogen therapy include all of the following EXCEPT
   - a. Diabetics
   - b. Smokers
   - c. With pernicious anemia
   - d. With gallbladder problems

6. Those taking combination birth control pills would be wise to avoid all of the following EXCEPT
   - a. Asthma drugs
   - b. Antibiotics
   - c. Antidepressants
   - d. Tobacco
   - e. Sex

B. Case Study for Reproductive System Drugs

I. M. Puny, a 16-year-old male weighing 100 pounds, asks the physician to prescribe some "steroids" to improve his physique and increase the size of his muscles. He needs to be given the following information about androgens (synthetic testosterone).

1. Androgens are used in all of the following conditions EXCEPT
   - a. Delayed puberty in male
   - b. Endometriosis in female
   - c. Testicular malfunction
   - d. Impaired growth

2. Side effects of androgens can include all of the following EXCEPT
   a. Jaundice
   c. Growth spurts
   b. Impotence
   d. Fluid retention

3. Androgens have been known to lead to all of the following EXCEPT
   a. Paranoia
   c. Increased aggression
   b. Delusions
   d. Increased sensitivity

4. Androgens are generally contraindicated in all of the following EXCEPT
   a. Diabetics
   c. Geriatric males
   b. Cryptorchidism
   d. Prepubertal males

Note: Always explain medical information in terms the patient can understand.

CHAPTER 25

Cardiovascular Drugs

OBJECTIVES

Upon completion of this chapter, the student should be able to:

1. Define cardiotonic, digitalization, cardioversion, bradycardia, tachycardia, hypotensive, ischemia, and hypoxia.
2. Describe the action and effects of digitalis and toxic side effects that require reporting.
3. Identify the different types of antiarrhythmics and the side effects of each.
4. Identify the most commonly used antihypertensives and the usual side effects, as well as the exceptions to the rule.
5. Describe the different types of coronary vasodilators with cautions and side effects.
6. Name the two most commonly used vasoconstrictors and their purpose.
7. Compare and contrast heparin and coumarin derivatives in terms of administration, action, and antidotes.
8. Explain appropriate and important patient education for each of the seven categories of cardiovascular drugs.
9. Describe when aspirin therapy is used and appropriate patient education regarding it.

Cardiovascular drugs include medications that affect the heart and blood vessels, as well as the anticoagulants. The drugs in this chapter are divided into seven categories: cardiac glycosides, antiarrhythmic agents, antilipemic agents, antihypertensives, vasodilators, vasoconstrictors, and anticoagulants. Some of the drugs described in this chapter fall into more than one category because of multiple actions and uses (e.g., propranolol, which is used to treat cardiac arrhythmias, hypertension, and angina). Diuretics, which also affect the blood vessels and reduce blood pressure, are discussed in Chapter 15.

Cardiac Glycosides

Cardiac glycosides occur widely in nature or can be prepared synthetically. They have been called *cardiotonic* because they strengthen the heartbeat. These glycosides act directly on the myocardium to increase the force of myocardial contractions. Cardiac glycosides are used primarily in the treatment of congestive heart failure. They are sometimes also used in conjunction with antiarrhythmic agents to *slow* the heart rate in certain types of tachycardia or atrial fibrillation or flutter.

In patients with congestive heart failure, the heart fails to pump adequately to remove excess fluids from the pulmonary circulation, and pulmonary congestion results. The heart increases in size to compensate for the increased work load. Symptoms of congestive heart failure are dyspnea, cyanosis, increased heart rate, cough, and pitting edema.

In patients with congestive heart failure, the cardiac glycosides act by *increasing the force of the cardiac contractions* without increasing oxygen consumption, thereby increasing cardiac output. As a result of increased efficiency, the heart beats slowly, the heart size shrinks, and the diuretic action decreases edema.

The most commonly used cardiac glycosides are digitalis products. Of these, digoxin (Lanoxin) is used most frequently because it can be administered orally and parenterally and has intermediate duration of action. Digitoxin (Crystodigin) has a prolonged action and the effects may persist for weeks.

Digitalization is the process of establishing the correct therapeutic dose of digitalis for maintaining optimal functioning of the heart without toxic effects. There is a very narrow margin between effective therapy and dangerous toxicity. Careful monitoring of cardiac rate and rhythm with EKG (electrocardiogram), cardiac function, side effects, and blood digitalis level is required to determine the therapeutic maintenance dose. Checking the apical pulse before administering digitalis is an important part of this monitoring process. If the apical pulse rate is less than 60, digitalis should be withheld until the physician is consulted. The action taken should be documented.

Modification of dosage is based on individual requirements and response, as determined by general condition, renal function, and cardiac function, monitored by EKG. When changing from tablets or IM therapy to liquid-filled capsules or IV therapy, digoxin dosage must be reduced about 20%.

Toxic side effects of digitalis, which should be reported to the physician immediately, can include:

Anorexia, nausea, and vomiting (early signs of toxicity)
Abdominal cramping, distention, and diarrhea
Headache, fatigue, lethargy, and muscle weakness
Vertigo, restlessness, irritability, tremors, and seizures
Visual disturbances including blurring, diplopia or halos
Cardiac arrhythmias of all kinds, especially bradycardia (rate less than 60)
Electrolyte imbalance
Insomnia, confusion, and mental disorders, especially with the elderly

Treatment of digitalis toxicity includes:

Discontinuing the drug immediately (usually sufficient)

Monitoring electrolytes for hyperkalemia and especially hypokalemia

Drugs such as atropine for severe bradycardia

Antiarrhythmics if indicated

Digoxin immune Fab as antidote in life-threatening toxicity

Contraindications or extreme caution applies to:

Severe pulmonary disease

Hypothyroidism

Acute myocardial infarction, acute myocarditis, severe heart failure

Impaired renal function

Arrhythmias not caused by heart failure

Pregnancy and lactation

Interactions of digitalis may occur with:

Antacids, sulfa, neomycin, and anticholinergics reduce absorption of digitalis (administer far apart)

Diuretics, calcium, and corticosteroids can increase chance of arrhythmias

Antiarrhymics, *especially* quinidine, may potentiate digitalis toxicity

Adrenergics (epinephrine, ephedrine, and isoproterenol) increase the risk of arrhythmias

Phenobarbital or phenytoin reduce digitalis levels

PATIENT EDUCATION

Patients taking digitalis should be instructed regarding:

Recognition and immediate reporting of side effects.

Holding medication, if any side effects occur, until the physician can be consulted.

Avoiding taking any other medication at the same time without physician approval.

Avoiding all OTC medication, especially antacids and cold remedies.

Avoiding abrupt withdrawal after prolonged use; must be reduced gradually under physician supervision.

Antiarrhythmic Agents

Antiarrhythmic agents include a variety of drugs that act in different ways to suppress various types of cardiac arrhythmias, including atrial or ventricular tachycardias, atrial fibrillation or flutter, and arrhythmias that occur with digitalis toxicity or during surgery and anesthesia. The choice of a particular antiarrhythmic agent is based on careful assessment of many factors, including the type of arrhythmia; frequency; cardiac, renal, or other pathologic condition; and current signs and symptoms.

The role of the health care worker is vital in this area in accurate and timely reporting of vital signs and pertinent observations regarding effectiveness of medications and adverse side effects. Adequate knowledge of drug action and effects, and good judgment are essential.

Side effects of the individual medications are discussed separately. However, keep in mind that most of the drugs given to counteract arrhythmias have the potential for lowering blood pressure and slowing heartbeat. Therefore, it is especially important to be alert for signs of *hypotension* and *bradycardia,* which could lead to cardiac arrest. Although the antiarrhythmics commonly slow the heart rate, there are exceptions (e.g., procainamide and quinidine, which may cause *tachycardia*). When other cardiac drugs are administered concomitantly, cardiac effects may be additive or antagonistic. Antiarrhythmic agents can worsen existing arrhythmias or cause new arrhythmias and *careful monitoring is essential.*

Arrhythmia detection and monitoring can include EKG rhythm strips and 24-hour Holter monitoring as indicated. Electrolyte surveillance, especially for hyperkalemia, is very important for patients on antiarrhythmic agents.

ADRENERGIC BLOCKERS

Beta-adrenergic blockers, for example, propranolol (Inderal), combat arrhythmias by inhibiting adrenergic (sympathetic) nerve receptors. The action is complex, and the results can include a membrane-stabilizing effect on the heart. Propranolol (Inderal) is effective in the management of some cardiac arrhythmias and less effective with others. It is also used in the treatment of hypertension and some forms of chronic angina. For additional use of beta-blockers, for example, with migraine, see Chapter 13.

Side effects of propranolol, especially in patients over 60 years old and more commonly with IV administration of the drug, can include:

Hypotension, with vertigo and syncope

Bradycardia, with heart block and cardiac arrest

CNS symptoms (usually with long-term treatment with high doses), including dizziness, irritability, confusion, nightmares, insomnia, visual disturbances, weakness, sleepiness, lassitude, or fatigue

GI symptoms, including nausea, vomiting, and diarrhea or constipation

Rash or hematologic effects (rare or transient)

Bronchospasm, especially with history of asthma

Hypoglycemia

Impotence reported rarely

Contraindications or extreme caution with the beta-blockers applies to:

Withdrawal after prolonged use (should always be gradual)

Major surgery (withdrawal 48 h before surgery usually recommended)

Diabetes—may eause hypoglycemia

Renal and hepatic impairment

Asthma and allergic rhinitis—may cause bronchospasm

Bradycardia, heart block, and congestive heart failure

Pediatric use, pregnancy, and lactation

Chronic obstructive pulmonary disease (COPD)

Interactions include antagonism of propranolol by:

Adrenergics (e.g., epinephrine and isoproterenol)

Anticholinergics

Tricyclic antidepressants

Potentiation of the hypotensive effect of propranolol occurs with:

Diuretics and other antihypertensives, for example, calcium blockers

Phenothiazine and other tranquilizers

Cimetidine (Tagamet), which slows metabolism of drug

Other cardiac drugs, which may potentiate toxic effects

Alcohol, muscle relaxants, and sedatives, which may precipitate hypotension, dizziness, confusion, or sedation

CALCIUM BLOCKERS

Calcium blockers, such as verapamil (Isoptin), counteract arrhythmias by suppressing the action of calcium in contraction of the heart muscle, thereby reducing cardiac excitability and dilating the main coronary arteries. Calcium blockers are also used in the treatment of angina and hypertension.

Side effects of calcium blockers can include:

Hypotension, with vertigo, *headache*

Bradycardia, with heart block

Edema

Constipation, nausea, and abdominal discomfort

Contraindications or extreme caution applies to:

Heart block, heart failure, or angina

Hepatic and renal impairment

Pregnancy and lactation

Children

Interactions of verapamil with other cardiac drugs, for example, digoxin, can potentiate both good and adverse effects. It has antagonistic effects with:

Oral anticoagulants

Salicylates

Sulfonamides

Lithium

Hypotensive effect potentiated with diuretics and ACE (angiotensin-converting enzyme) inhibitors

Contraindicated with quinidine

DISOPYRAMIDE

Another antiarrhythmic, disopyramide (Norpace), is a synthetic agent that decreases myocardial excitability, inhibits conduction, and may depress myocardial contractility. It has anticholinergic properties.

Side effects can include:

Hypotension, dizziness, and chest pain
Edema and weight gain
Anticholinergic effects, including dry mouth, blurred vision, constipation, and urinary retention
Nausea, vomiting, bloating, and gas

Contraindications or extreme caution applies to:

History of angle-closure glaucoma
Heart block and congestive heart failure
Hepatic and renal disorders
Children, pregnancy, and lactation

Interactions of disopyramide occur with potentiation of the effects of:

Other cardiac drugs
Oral anticoagulants

LIDOCAINE

Local anesthetics (e.g., lidocaine) are administered for their antiarrhythmic effects and membrane-stabilizing action. Lidocaine is the drug of choice for premature ventricular contractions (PVC) associated with myocardial infarction.

Newer drugs in this category, for example, flecainide (Tambocor) and tocainide (Tonocard), because of substantial risks, are not recommended for postmyocardial infarction patients. They are reserved for *life-threatening* ventricular arrhythmias.

Side effects of lidocaine are usually of short duration and dose related and can include:

CNS symptoms, including tremors, seizures, dizziness, confusion, and blurred vision.
Hypotension, bradycardia, and heart block.
Dyspnea, respiratory depression, and arrest.
EKG monitoring and availability of resuscitative equipment are necessary during IV administration of lidocaine.

Pulmonary fibrosis, anemia, bone marrow depression possible with tocainide.

Contraindications or extreme caution applies to:

Patients hypersensitive to local anesthetics of this type
Heart block and respiratory depression
Pregnancy, lactation, and children

Interactions with other cardiac drugs may be additive or antagonistic and may potentiate adverse effects. Cimetidine may potentiate effects.

PROCAINAMIDE

Procainamide (Pronestyl) is usually administered orally in antiarrhythmic therapy. It is used primarily as prophylactic therapy to maintain normal rhythm after conversion by other methods. Its action is similar to that of quinidine. It possesses anticholinergic properties.

Side effects of procainamide are numerous and can include:

Hypotension
Tachycardia, conduction defects, asystole
Hypersensitivity reactions, including rash, fever, and weakness
Blood dyscrasias, especially eosinophilia and leukopenia
Nausea and vomiting or diarrhea—more common with large dose

Contraindications include:

Heart block and congestive heart failure
Hypersensitivity to local anesthetics of this type
Myasthenia gravis
Pregnancy
Renal and hepatic disease caution

Interactions may occur with potentiation of:

Muscle relaxants
Anticholinergics
Other cardiac drugs

QUINIDINE

Quinidine (Quinaglute, Cardioquin) is one of the oldest antiarrhythmic agents. It acts by decreasing myocardial excitability and may depress myocardial contractility. Quinidine, like procainamide, is used primarily as prophylactic therapy to maintain normal rhythm after conversion by other methods. It is commonly administered orally in tablets or timed-release capsules. It has anticholinergic properties.

Side effects of quinidine are numerous and may necessitate cessation of treatment. They may include:

Diarrhea, anorexia, nausea, and vomiting, which are common
Tachycardia and syncope
Severe hypotension
Vascular collapse and respiratory arrest
Headache, tinnitus, vertigo, fever, and tremor
Confusion and apprehension
Vision abnormalities or hearing disturbances
Blood dyscrasias, including anemia, clotting deficiencies, and leukopenia
Hepatic disorders
Precipitation of asthmatic attacks
Hypoglycemia

TABLE 25.1. CARDIAC GLYCOSIDE AND ANTIARRHYTHMICS

Generic Name	Trade Name	Dosage	Comments
Cardiac Glycoside			
digoxin	Lanoxin, Lanoxicaps	PO: tablets, liquid-filled capsules, elixir IV, dosage varies	Intermediate duration
Antiarrhythmics			
atenolol[a]	Tenormin	50 mg PO qd 5–10 mg IV	Beta-blocker
propranolol[a]	Inderal	10–30 mg PO qid 0.5–3 mg IV	Beta-blocker
verapamil[a]	Isoptin, Calan	5–10 mg IV 240–480 mg PO qd in div. doses	Calcium blocker
lidocaine	Xylocaine	IM or IV **diluted**	Local anesthetic-type Check IV dilution directions
flecainide	Tambocor	PO, dose varies	Local anesthetic type For **life-threatening** conditions only
tocainide	Tonocard	PO, dose varies	Local anesthetic type For **life-threatening** conditions only
procainamide	Pronestyl, Procan SR	PO, dose varies IV or IM for emergency	Local anesthetic, anticholinergic
quinidine	Quinaglute, Cardioquin	PO tabs, caps, ER, dose varies	Myocardial depressant, anticholinergic
disopyramide	Norpace, Norpace CR	150 mg PO q6h, or 300 mg PO q12h, extended release	Myocardial depressent, anticholinergic properties

Note: Other antiarrhythmics are available. This is a representative sample.

[a]Has other cardiac uses.

Contraindications or extreme caution with quinidine applies to:

Atrioventricular block and conduction defects
Electrolyte imbalance
Digitalis intoxication
Congestive heart failure and hypotension
Myasthenia gravis
Asthma and other respiratory disorders
Hyperthyroidism or diabetes
Children, pregnancy, and lactation
Hepatic or renal disorders

Interactions with increased possibility of quinidine toxicity may occur with:

Muscle relaxants
Anticholinergics
Thiazide diuretics
Antacids or sodium bicarbonate
Anticonvulsants (e.g., phenytoin and phenobarbital)
Other cardiac drugs, especially digitalis and antihypertensives
Anticoagulants, whose action can be potentiated by quinidine

PATIENT EDUCATION

Patients taking antiarrhythmics should be instructed regarding:

Immediate reporting of adverse side effects, especially palpitations, irregular or slow heartbeat, faintness, dizziness, weakness, respiratory distress, and visual disturbances.
Holding medication, if there are side effects, until the physician is contacted.
Rising slowly from reclining position.
Modification of lifestyle to reduce stress.
Mild exercise on a regular basis as approved by the physician.
Not discontinuing medicine, even if the patient feels well.
Taking proper dosage of medication on time, as prescribed, without skipping any dose.
If medication is forgotten, not doubling the dose.
Taking medication with a full glass of water, on an empty stomach, 1 h before or 2 h after meals, so that it will be absorbed more efficiently (unless stomach upset occurs or the physician prescribes otherwise).
Avoiding taking any other medication, including OTC medicines, unless approved by the physician.
Discarding expired medicines and renewing the prescription.
Avoiding comparisons with other patients on similar drugs.
Contacting the physician immediately with any concerns regarding medicines.

See Table 25.1 for a summary of the cardiac glycoside and antiarrhythmics.

Antihypertensives

Antihypertensives (hypotensives) are numerous in the treatment and management of all degrees of hypertension. In cases of mild hypertension, the initial treatment regimen usually includes diet modification (low salt or low sodium), weight reduction when indicated, mild exercise program (e.g., walking or swimming), cessation of smoking, and stress reduction planning. In addition, the thiazide diuretics (see Chapter 15) are frequently prescribed to prevent sodium retention and edema, and for their hypotensive (blood pressure-lowering) effects. Antihypertensive drugs do *not* cure hypertension; they only control it. After withdrawal of the drug, the blood pressure will return to levels similar to those before treatment with medication, if all other factors remain the same. If antihypertensive therapy is to be terminated for some reason, the dosage should be gradually reduced, as abrupt withdrawal can cause rebound hypertension.

Drugs given to lower blood pressure act in various ways. The drug of choice varies according to the degree of hypertension (mild, moderate, or severe), other physical factors (especially other cardiac or renal complications), and effectiveness in individual cases. Frequently, antihypertensives are prescribed on a trial basis and then the dosage or medication is changed; and sometimes antihypertensives are combined for greater effectiveness and to reduce side effects. The health care worker must be observant of vital signs and side effects in order to assist the physician in the most effective treatment of hypertension on an individual basis.

Thiazide diuretics (see Chapter 15) are sometimes used alone to treat mild hypertension. Thiazides are also frequently combined with other antihypertensives to potentiate the hypotensive effects.

Side effects of antihypertensives are common, and the health care worker must be observant of changes in vital signs and adverse side effects. The most common side effect of the antihypertensives is *hypotension,* especially postural hypotension. Another side effect common to many of the antihypertensives is *bradycardia.* Exceptions include hydralazine (Apresoline), which can cause tachycardia.

BETA-ADRENERGIC AND CALCIUM BLOCKERS

There are numerous antihypertensives, and they vary in action. Included are beta-adrenergic blockers, such as propranolol (Inderal) and atenolol (Tenormin), and calcium blockers, such as diltiazem (Cardizem) and nifedipine (Procardia) (see Antiarrhythmic Agents for information on side effects, etc.).

METHYLDOPA

Another antihypertensive used for moderate to severe hypertension is methyldopa (Aldomet), an adrenergic inhibitor. It is usually administered with a diuretic. It is the drug of choice for hypertension in pregnant women because of safety to the fetus.

Side effects can include:

Hypotension and drowsiness

Anemia or leukopenia—rare

GI symptoms, including nausea, vomiting, diarrhea, constipation, and sore tongue

Sexual dysfunction

Liver disorders

Nasal congestion

Contraindications or extreme caution applies to:

Liver disorders

Dialysis patients

Blood dyscrasias

Interactions may occur with:

Levodopa (can cause CNS effects and psychosis)

Lithium

HYDRALAZINE

Hydralazine (Apresoline), a vasodilator, is frequently used in the treatment of moderate to severe hypertension, especially in patients with congestive heart failure, because it *increases* heart rate and cardiac output. The drug is generally used in conjunction with a diuretic and another hypotensive agent, for example, a beta-blocker.

Side effects can include:

Tachycardia and palpitations

Headache and flushing

Orthostatic hypotension

GI effects, including nausea, vomiting, diarrhea, and constipation

Blood abnormalities

Allergic reactions (e.g., asthma)

Contraindications include pregnancy.

ACE INHIBITORS

A newer type of hypotensive is the angiotensin-converting enzyme (ACE) inhibitor for example, captopril or enalapril. Inhibition of ACE lowers blood pressure by *decreasing vasoconstriction.* They are frequently effective with hypertension resistant to other drugs, and are used alone or in combination with a diuretic.

Side effects of ACE inhibitors can include:

Rash or photosensitivity

Loss of taste perception

Blood dyscrasias

Renal impairment

Severe hypotension
Cough or nasal congestion
Hyperkalemia

Contraindications or extreme caution applies to:

Renal impairment
Collagen disease, for example, lupus or scleroderma
Heart failure
Diabetes—increased risk of hypoglycemia

Interactions of ACE inhibitors apply to:

Diuretics—potentiate hypotension; watch blood pressure (BP) closely
Vasodilators; watch BP closely
Potassium-sparing diuretics—hyperkalemia risk
NSAIDs—antagonize effects of ACE inhibitors
Antacids—decrease absorption
Digoxin—possible digitalis toxicity
Lithium—risk of lithium toxicity

See Table 25.2 for a summary of the antihypertensives.

PATIENT EDUCATION

For all antihypertensives, patients should be instructed regarding:

Immediate reporting of any adverse side effects, especially slow or irregular heartbeat, dizziness, weakness, breathing difficulty, gastric distress, and numbness or swelling of extremities.

Taking medication on time as prescribed by the physician; *not* skipping a dose or doubling a dose; *not* discontinuing the medicine, even if the patient is feeling well, without consulting the physician first.

Rising slowly from reclining position to reduce lightheaded feeling.

Taking care in driving a car or operating machinery if medication causes drowsiness (ask the physician, nurse, or pharmacist about the specific medication, since medicines differ and individual reactions differ; older people are more susceptible to this effect).

Potentiation of adverse side effects by alcohol, especially dizziness, weakness, sleepiness, and confusion.

Reduction, or cessation, of smoking to help lower blood pressure.

Importance of diet in control of blood pressure; following the physician's instructions regarding appropriate diet for the individual, which may include a low-salt or low-sodium or weight-reduction diet if indicated.

Avoiding hot tubs and hot showers, which may cause weakness or fainting.

Mild exercise, on a regular basis, as approved by the physician.

TABLE 25.2. ANTIHYPERTENSIVES

Generic Name	Trade Name	Dosage
Beta-Adrenergic Blockers		
propranolol	Inderal	10–30 mg PO qid
metoprolol	Lopressor	50–100 mg PO tid
atenolol	Tenormin	50 mg PO qd
timolol	Blocadren	10 mg PO bid
Calcium Blockers		
diltiazem	Cardizem	60 mg tid
nifedipine	Procardia, Adalat, Procardia XL	30–60 mg qd short-acting PO puncture capsule ER swallow intact 30-90 mg qd
verapamil	Calan, Isoptin	40 mg bid or tid
amlodipine	Norvasc	2.5–5 mg qd
ACE Inhibitors		
captopril	Capoten	25–50 mg PO bid or tid
enalapril	Vasotec	5–10 mg bid
benazepril	Lotensin	Dose varies
Other Antihypertensives		
methyldopa	Aldomet	250–500 mg PO bid
clonidine	Catapres	0.1–0.8 mg PO
prazosin	Minipress	1.0–20 mg PO qd
hydralazine	Apresoline	10–50 mg qid

Note: This is only a representative list of the most commonly used drugs in this eategory. There are others.

Coronary Vasodilators

Coronary vasodilators are used in the treatment of angina. When there is insufficient blood supply (ischemia) to a part, the result is acute pain. The most common form of angina is angina pectoris, chest pain resulting from decreased blood supply to the heart muscle. Obstruction or constriction of the coronary arteries results in angina pectoris. Vasodilators are administered to dilate these blood vessels and stop attacks of angina or reduce the frequency of angina when administered prophylactically.

Coronary vasodilators used in the treatment and prophylactic management of angina include nitrates, beta-blockers, and calcium blockers.

The nitrates used most commonly for relief of acute angina pectoris, as well as for long-term prophylactic management, are nitroglycerin and isosorbide (Isordil, Sorbitrate).

Nitroglycerin is available in several forms and can be administered in sublingual tablets allowed to dissolve under the tongue or intrabuccal tablets allowed to dissolve in the cheek pouch for relief of acute angina pectoris. If relief is not attained after a single dose during an acute attack, additional tablets may be administered at

5-min intervals, with *no more than 3 doses given in a 15-min period.* If chest pain is not relieved after 3 doses, a physician should be contacted at once because unrelieved chest pain can indicate acute myocardial infarction.

Nitroglycerin is also available in timed-release capsules and tablets, and in a solution that must be diluted carefully according to the manufacturer's instructions for IV administration. Nitroglycerin tablets and capsules must be stored *only in glass containers* with tightly fitting metal screw tops away from heat. Plastic containers can absorb the medication, and air, heat, or moisture can cause loss of potency. Impaired potency of the SL tablets can be detected by the patient if there is an absence of the tingling sensation under the tongue common to this form of administration.

For long-term prophylactic management of angina pectoris, nitroglycerin is frequently applied topically as a transdermal system. One type of nitroglycerin that is absorbed through the skin is Nitrol ointment, applied with an applicator-measuring (Appli-Ruler) paper. Usual dosage is 0.5-2 inches applied every 8 h. The ointment is spread lightly (not massaged or rubbed) over any nonhairy skin area, and the applicator paper is taped in place. Care must be taken to avoid touching the ointment when applying (accidental absorption through the skin of the fingers can cause headache). If nitroglycerin ointment is discontinued, the dose and frequency must be decreased gradually to prevent sudden withdrawal reactions. See Figure 9.1 for ointment application technique.

Another topical nitroglycerin product, which has longer action, is in transdermal form (e.g., Nitro-Dur or Transderm-Nitro). The skin patch is applied every 24 h to clean, dry, hairless areas of the upper arm or body. Do not apply below the elbow or knee. The sites should be rotated to avoid skin irritation and raw, scarred, or callused areas should be avoided. Dosage varies widely, from 2.5–15 mg patches. *Check prescribed dosage carefully. Remove old patch.*

Nitroglycerin is also available as a spray for relief of acute angina pectoris.

Another nitrate used for acute relief of angina pectoris and for prophylactic long-term management is isosorbide. It is available in sublingual, PO, or chewable tablets, and in timed-release capsules.

A newer nitrate, erythrityl tetranitrate (Cardilate), is sometimes used for long-term prophylactic management of angina pectoris. It is administered orally or sublingually. It is not used for acute relief of angina attacks.

Side effects of the nitrates can include:

Headache (usually diminishes over time)

Postural hypotension, including dizziness, weakness, and syncope *(patients should be sitting during administration of fast-acting nitrates)*

Transient flushing

Blurred vision and dry mouth (discontinue drug with these symptoms)

Hypersensitivity reactions, enhanced by alcohol, including nausea, vomiting, diarrhea, cold sweats, tachycardia, and syncope

Contraindications or extreme caution applies to:

Glaucoma

GI hypermotility or malabsorption (with timed-release forms)

Intracranial pressure

Severe anemia

Hypotension

Interactions of nitrates may occur with alcohol, which potentiates hypotensive effects.

For long-term prophylactic treatment of angina pectoris, beta-blockers, such as propranolol (Inderal), and calcium blockers, such as nifedipine (Procardia) and verapamil (Isoptin), are frequently used. (See Antiarrhythmic Agents for information on side effects, etc.)

PATIENT EDUCATION

Patients receiving coronary vasodilators (nitrates) should be instructed regarding:

Administering fast-acting tablets (sublingual or buccal) while sitting down because the patient may become lightheaded.

Rising slowly from a reclining position.

Not drinking alcohol while taking these medicines, which can cause serious drop in blood pressure.

Using timed-release capsules or tablets to prevent attacks (they work too slowly to help once an attack has started).

Taking timed-release capsules or tablets on an empty stomach with a full glass of water.

Allowing sublingual tablets to dissolve under the tongue or in the cheek pouch and not chewing or swallowing them.

Chewing chewable tablets thoroughly and holding them in the mouth for 2 min without any food or water in the mouth.

Repeating sublingual, buccal, or chewable tablets in 5–10 min for a maximum of 3 tablets (if no relief of chest pain within 15–30 min, call the physician at once).

Not discontinuing medication suddenly if administered for several weeks (dosage must be reduced gradually under physician's supervision).

Sensations to be expected, including facial flushing, headache for a short time, lightheadedness upon rising too suddenly (if these symptoms persist or become more severe, or other symptoms occur, such as irregular heartbeat or blurred vision, notify the physician at once).

Preventing attacks of angina by administering a sublingual or chewable tablet before physical exertion or emotional stress. (It is preferable to avoid physical or emotional stress when possible.)

See Chapter 9 for patient education regarding administration of nitroglycerin ointment or patch.

Antilipemic Agents

Those patients with elevated serum cholesterol and increased low-density lipoprotein (LDL) concentrations are at greater risk of atherosclerotic coronary disease and myocardial infarction. The initial treatments of choice include dietary management (e.g. restriction of total and saturated fat and cholesterol intake), weight control, and appropriate exercise. If these measures are inadequate, drug therapy may be added. All antilipemic agents have potentially serious adverse side effects. Sometimes two or three agents are combined. Three commonly used agents include niacin, lovastatin, and/or a bile acid sequestrant, for example, cholestyramine (Questran), and gemfibrozil (Lopid).

Side effects of all antilipemics include GI upset. Additionally, cholestyramine can cause:

Constipation

Acidosis and increased urinary calcium excretion

Rash and irritation of skin, tongue and anal region

GI bleeding or bleeding gums

Interactions with cholestyramine can reduce absorption of all drugs, including fat-soluble vitamins and folic acid.

Side effects of niacin, in addition to GI effects, include:

Flushing, especially of the face, and pruritus (aspirin can be given 30 minutes prior to niacin to combat this effect; extended-release preparations also help)

Jaundice or liver damage is possible.

Interaction of niacin with beta-blockers or calcium blockers potentiates hypotensive effects.

Side effects of lovastatin, in addition to GI upset, can include:

Liver damage

Muscle cramps, weakness, or *myopathy,* which can lead to acute renal failure

Eye problems, for example, cataracts, especially with long-term use

Headache, dizziness, insomnia, lethargy

Interaction of lovastatin with immunosuppressive drugs or other antilipemic drugs increases risk of myopathy and renal failure.

Contraindications or extreme caution for all antilipemics applies to:

Gallbladder, liver, or kidney disease

Diabetes or gout

Peptic ulcer or allergy

Hypotension

Pregnant, lactating, or women of childbearing age

> **PATIENT EDUCATION**
>
> Patients on antilipemic therapy should be instructed regarding:
>
> Continuing diet (low fat, low cholesterol) and aerobic exercise.
>
> Taking medicine with meals to reduce GI upset.
>
> Reporting side effects to the physician immediately, especially muscle pain, weakness, or bleeding.
>
> With cholestyramine, high-fiber diet and/or a stool softnener, fat-soluble vitamin/folic acid supplements, and not taking other meds within 4 hours.
>
> Expecting facial flushing with niacin.

Vasoconstrictors

Vasoconstrictors are adrenergic in action (see Chapter 13). Drugs such as norepinephrine (Levophed) or metaraminol bitartrate (Aramine) constrict blood vessels, resulting in increased systolic and diastolic blood pressure. These drugs, administered IV, are used mainly in the treatment of shock, short term only.

Side effects can include:

Headache (may be a symptom of hypertension)
Weakness, dizziness, tremor, and pallor
Respiratory difficulty or apnea
Pain in the cardiac area
Palpitation, bradycardia, cardiac arrhythmias
Necrosis of tissues

Cautions with Levophed or Aramine include:

Close monitoring of IV site
Close monitoring of blood pressure and other vital signs

Anticoagulants

Anticoagulants are divided into two general groups: coumarin derivatives and heparin. The action of these two classes is quite different. However, their purpose is the same: to prevent formation of clots or decrease the extension of existing clots in such conditions as venous thrombosis, pulmonary embolism, and coronary occlusion. Also, many patients with artificial heart valves, mitral valve disease, and/or chronic atrial fibrillation receive anticoagulants to prevent embolism/thrombosis. Patients on anticoagulants, especially elderly patients, should be constantly observed for bleeding complications, such as cerebrovascular accidents (CVAs).

The coumarin derivatives and heparin do not dissolve clots; they only interfere with the coagulation process as a prophylaxis.

COUMARIN DERIVATIVES

Coumarin derivatives (e.g., Coumadin) are administered *orally*. The coumarin derivatives alter the synthesis of blood coagulation factors in the liver by interfering with the action of vitamin K. The *antidote* for serious bleeding complications during coumarin therapy is vitamin K. In some cases, fresh, frozen plasma is also given for bleeding complications. The action of the coumarin derivatives is slower than that of heparin, and therefore these drugs are generally used as follow-up for long-term anticoagulant therapy. Measurement of the prothrombin time (PT) is the most commonly used laboratory method of monitoring therapy with coumarin derivatives. The PT serves as a guide in determining dosage.

Interactions of coumarin derivatives with *many* drugs have been reported. Concurrent administration of any other drug should be investigated, and the following drugs should be *avoided* if possible. Some of the drugs that may *increase* response to coumarin derivatives include:

Anabolic steroids
Chloral hydrate and alcohol (acute intoxication)
Disulfiram
All NSAIDs, including aspirin
Tricyclic antidepressants
Thyroid drugs
Thiazides and quinidine

Some of the drugs that may *decrease* response to coumarin derivatives include:

Alcohol (chronic alcoholism)
Barbiturates
Estrogen (including oral contraceptives)
Corticosteroids

There are many other interactions. *Always check before administering any other medicine.*

HEPARIN

Heparin is not absorbed from the GI tract and must be administered *intravenously* or *subcutaneously*. Heparin acts on thrombin, inhibiting the action of fibrin in clot formation. The *antidote* for serious bleeding complications during heparin therapy is protamine sulfate. When administered IV, the action of heparin is immediate. A dilute flushing solution of heparin is also used to maintain patency of indwelling venipuncture devices used to obtain blood specimens and of catheters used for arterial access (arterial lines). Be sure to check that it is a *dilute flushing* solution before injection, and not full-strength heparin. However, 0.9% sodium chloride (normal saline) injection alone is used to flush *peripheral* venipuncture devices, for example, PRN adapters. Heparin is *not* used to flush these devices because of possible drug incompatibilities and laboratory test interferences.

When heparin is administered subcutaneously, especially if the patient is discharged and the medication will be administered at home, be sure to stress *patient education:*

1. Administer the heparin subcutaneously in the fat pad along the lower abdomen.
2. Rotate injection sites.
3. Do *not* rub the site with an alcohol sponge. Merely hold the sponge on the site *gently* for a few seconds.
4. Be sure there is no bleeding from the site.
5. Review additional cautions in Patient Education listed below.

Measurement of the activated partial thromboplastin time (APTT) is the most common laboratory test for monitoring heparin therapy. When long-term anticoagulant therapy is begun with coumarin derivatives, there is a short-term overlap period in which both heparin and coumarin derivatives are administered concurrently.

Interactions of heparin with aspirin and other NSAID, or with thrombolytic agents, for example, streptokinase or urokinase, may increase the risk of hemorrhage.

Side effects of all anticoagulants can include:

Major hemorrhage

Minor bleeding (e.g., petechiae, nosebleed, and bruising)

Blood in urine (hematuria) or stools (melena)

Contraindications of anticoagulants include:

GI disorders and ulceration of GI tract

Hepatic and renal dysfunction

Blood dyscrasias

Pregnancy

After stroke may increase risk of fatal cerebral hemorrhage

See Table 25.3 for a summary of the coronary and peripheral vasodilators and the anticoagulants.

TABLE 25.3. CORONARY VASODILATORS, ANTILIPEMIC AGENTS, AND ANTICOAGULANTS

Generic Name	Trade Name	Dosage
Coronary Vasodilators[a]		
Nitrates		
nitroglycerin	Nitrostat tabs S.L.	1–3 tabs q 5 min × 3 maximum in 15 min
	Nitrogard tabs buccal	1–3 tabs q 5 min × 3 maximum in 15 min
	Nitro-Bid caps E.R.	1.3–9 mg q8h
	Nitro-Bid, Nitrol oint 2%	1–2 inches q8h
	Transderm-Nitro, Nitro-Dur, others	1 transdermal patch 2.5–15 mg qd, rotate site
isosorbide, dinitrate	Isordil, Sorbitrate, S.L., chewable	2.5–10 mg × 3 maximum in 30 min Prophylactic 10–20 mg tid or qid ac Timed-release 20–40 mg q6–12h
isorbide monitrate	Monoket, Ismo	Prophylactic 10–20 mg tid, ISMO bid
erythrityl tetranitrate	Cardilate	Prophylactic PO or SL 10 mg tid or 6× qd
Antilipemic Agents		
cholestyramine	Questran	4 g tid ac. Mix powder with water, milk, or juice. Chew bars well. Force fluids
niacin	Nicobid, Slo-Niacin	Dose varies with response, take with meals
lovastatin	Mevacor	20–80 mg qd with meals
gemfibrozil	Lopid	Dose varies, bid ac
Anticoagulants		
coumarin derivatives	Coumadin, Dicumarol	PO dose varies, based on PT results
heparin	Heparin	IV, SC, dose varies
Platelet Inhibitors		
dipyridamole	Persantine	79–100 mg qid with coumarin
aspirin	Aspirin SR, Ecotrin, Ascriptin, many others	160–325 mg qd

Notes: Beta-blockers and calcium blockers are also administered prophylactically for angina pectoris, and can be given concurrently with the nitrates.

Other antilipemic agents are available. Some reduce triglycerides as well.

[a]For prevention and treatment of angina pectoris.

PATIENT EDUCATION

It is *very important* that patients on anticoagulant therapy be instructed regarding:

Careful daily observation of skin, gums, urine, and stools, and *immediate* reporting of any signs of bleeding.

Avoiding sports and activities that may cause bleeding.

Immediate reporting to the physician of any falls, blows, or injuries (internal bleeding is always a possibility).

Special care with shaving (electric razor only) and with teeth brushing or dental floss.

Wearing an identification tag or carrying a card indicating use of anticoagulant.

Immediate reporting of severe or continued headache or backache, dizziness, joint pain or swelling, tarry stools, abdominal distention, vomiting of material resembling coffee grounds, or nosebleed.

Avoiding other medications without the physician's approval, especially OTC aspirin, anti-inflammatory drugs, and antacids.

Avoiding alcohol.

Platelet Inhibitor Therapy

DIPYRIDAMOLE (PERSANTINE)

Persantine is a nonnitrate coronary vasodilator that inhibits platelet aggregation (clumping). It is used with coumarin anticoagulants in the prevention of postoperative thromboembolic complications of cardiac valve replacement.

Side effects of dipyridamole (Persantine), usually transient, can include:

Headache, dizziness, weakness

Nausea, vomiting, diarrhea

Flushing, rash

Caution with the elderly.

ASPIRIN

Because of its ability to inhibit platelet aggregation (clumping), aspirin has been investigated extensively for use in the prevention of thrombosis. Patients with prosthetic heart valves usually receive aspirin, or dipyridamole, with an oral anticoagulant to reduce the incidences of thrombosis.

Aspirin therapy, usually 160–325 mg daily, has also been used after myocardial infarction or recurrent transient ischemic attacks (TIAs) to reduce the risk of recurrence of attacks. Aspirin has also been used to reduce the risk of myocardial infarction in patients with unstable angina. However, aspirin therapy is not recommended for those without clinical signs of coronary heart disease because of an increased risk of hemorrhagic stroke associated with long-term aspirin therapy. Patients should be instructed not to start aspirin therapy without consulting a physician first. Patient education should include instruction regarding measures to reduce risk factors for coronary heart disease and stroke, that is, abstinence from all forms of tobacco, weight control, low-fat and low-cholesterol diet, and aerobic exercise on a regular basis.

Because of gastric irritation, aspirin should be administered with food or milk. Film-coated tablets, enteric-coated tablets and buffered aspirin preparations are available to reduce gastric irritation.

Aspirin is contraindicated for anyone with bleeding disorders. See Chapter 19 for a description of other side effects, contraindications, and interactions.

Worksheet For Chapter 25

CARDIOVASCULAR DRUGS

Note the drugs listed according to category and complete all columns. Learn generic trade names as specified by instructor.

Classifications and Drugs	Purpose	Side Effects	Contraindications or Cautions	Patient Education
Cardiac Glycosides 1. digoxin				
Antiarrhythmics 1. propranolol (a beta-adrenergic blocker with other uses) 2. verapamil (a calcium adrenergic blocker with other uses) 3. lidocaine 4. procainamide 5. quinidine				
Antilipemic Agents 1. cholestyramine 2. niacin 3. lovastatin 4. gemfibrozil				

Classifications and Drugs	Purpose	Side Effects	Contraindications or Cautions	Patient Education
Antihypertensives (Hypotensives) (see previous page for beta-blockers and calcium blockers) 1. methyldopa 2. prazosin 3. hydralazine				
ACE Inhibitors 4. captopril 5. enalapril				
Vasodilators (Coronary) 1. nitroglycerin Tabs SL Ointment Patch 2. isosorbide (Isordil)				
Anticoagulants 1. coumarin derivatives 2. heparin				
Platelet Inhibitors 1. aspirin 2. dipyridamole				

A. Case Study for Cardiovascular Drugs

Wilbur Worthington, a 65–year–old patient, has been treated in the hospital for cardic arrhythmias with tachycardia. He will be discharged on Lanoxin and Calan and will need the following patient information.

1. Side effects of Lanoxin can include all of the following EXCEPT
   a. Double vision
   b. Appetite loss
   c. Diarrhea
   d. Palpitations
2. Older adults on Lanoxin are also more prone to the following EXCEPT
   a. Sedation
   b. Confusion
   c. Mental disorder
   d. Insomnia
3. The following drugs can increase risk of digitalis toxicity and arrhythmias EXCEPT
   a. Diuretics
   b. Antacids
   c. Quinidine
   d. Decongestants
4. Calan does all of the following EXCEPT
   a. Dilates coronary arteries
   b. Increases heart contractions
   c. Blocks calcium
   d. Lowers blood pressure
5. Calan can have all of the following side effects EXCEPT
   a. Diarrhea
   b. Postural hypotension
   c. Bradycardia
   d. Vertigo

B. Case Study for Cardiovascular Drugs

Homer Grange is diagnosed with hypertension and elevated cholesterol with increased LDL. The following information will be helpful.

1. The following antihypertensives can cause bradycardia EXCEPT
   a. Tenormin
   b. Procardia
   c. Apresoline
   d. Aldomet
2. The following advice would be appropriate EXCEPT
   a. Stop smoking
   b. Rise slowly
   c. Reduce salt intake
   d. Stop medicine when better
3. What medicine is often prescribed with anithypertensives?
   a. Antacids
   b. NSAIDs
   c. Diurectis
   d. Hypnotics
4. Lovastatin, an antilipemic, can cause all of the following EXCEPT
   a. Muscle cramps
   b. Edema
   c. Liver damage
   d. GI upset

5. Advice for patients on antilipemic therapy should include all of the following EXCEPT
   a. Weight control
   b. Take medicine ac
   c. Low fat diet
   d. Appropriate exercise

CHAPTER **26**

Respiratory System Drugs and Antihistamines

OBJECTIVES

Upon completion of this chapter, the student should be able to:

1. Describe uses of and precautions necessary with oxygen therapy.
2. Explain the purpose of carbon dioxide inhalations.
3. Define bronchodilator, mucolytic, expectorant, antitussive, antihistamine, and decongestant.
4. Classify a list of respiratory system drugs according to action.
5. List uses, side effects, and contraindications for bronchodilators and antitussives.
6. Explain appropriate patient education for those receiving respiratory system drugs.
7. Describe the action and uses of the antihistamines and decongestants.
8. List the side effects, contraindications, and interactions of the antihistamines and decongestants.

Therapeutic measures for respiratory distress include oxygen, respiratory stimulants, bronchodilators, corticosteroids, mucolytics, expectorants, and antitussives.

Oxygen

Oxygen is used therapeutically for hypoxia (insufficient oxygen). Some of the conditions for which oxygen is indicated are heart and lung diseases, carbon monoxide poisoning, and some central nervous conditions with respiratory difficulty or failure. Oxygen may be administered by endotracheal intubation, nasal cannula, masks, tents, and hoods.

Side effects of oxygen delivered at too high a concentration or for prolonged periods of time can include:

Hypoventilation, particularly with COPD (chronic obstructive pulmonary disease), may cause CO_2 retention and acidosis

Confusion

Changes in the alveoli of the lungs

Blindness (in premature infants)

Cautions apply to:

Patients with COPD (high O_2 concentrations may cause hypoventilation or apnea).

Danger of fire when oxygen is used. Oxygen is not flammable but does support combustion. Smoking, matches, and electrical equipment that may spark (e.g., electric razors, hair dryers) are not allowed in rooms where oxygen is in use.

Respiratory Stimulants

Respiratory stimulants include:

- Caffeine citrate in the treatment of neonatal apnea
- Theophylline administered IV and orally to stimulate respiration in infants and patients with Cheyne-Stokes respiration
- Carbon dioxide inhalations to increase both depth and rate of respiration (e.g., in treatment of hyperventilation or hiccups)

Bronchodilators

Bronchodilators act by relaxing the smooth muscles of the bronchial tree, thereby relieving bronchospasm and increasing the vital capacity of the lungs. Bronchodilators are used in the symptomatic treatment of acute respiratory conditions such as asthma, as well as many forms of COPD. Classifications of bronchdilators include the sympathomimetics (adrenergics), the parasympatholytics (anticholinergics), and the xanthine derivatives.

SYMPATHOMIMETICS

Sympathomimetics (adrenergics) are potent bronchodilators that increase vital capacity and decrease airway resistance. The adrenergics work on the smooth muscle in the lungs to cause relaxation. However, they also can affect the entire sympathetic nervous system. The adrenergics may produce serious side effects and manufacturer's directions should be followed carefully regarding dosage and administration. Examples include albuterol, epinephrine, terbutaline, and others listed in Table 26.1.

TABLE 26.1. BRONCHODILATORS, CORTICOSTEROIDS, AND ASTHMA PROPHYLACTICS

Generic Name	Trade Name	Dosage
Sympathomimetics		
albuterol sulfate	Ventolin, Proventil	MDI 2 puffs q4–6h Aerosol O.5 cc 0.5% sol/3 cc NS Tabs ER 2–4mg
terbutaline sulfate	Brethaire, Brethine, Bricanyl	SC 1 mg/ml Tabs 2.5–5 mg
epinephrine	Primatene, Bronkaid Mist, Adrenalin	MDI 2 puffs q3h IM or SC 1:1000 sol 0.1–0.5 ml **Watch dose carefully!**
isoproterenol	Isuprel	MDI 2 puffs q4–6h SL tabs 10–20 mg IV 1:50,000 sol 0.5–1 ml Aerosol 0.5 ml 5% sol/3 cc NS
metaproterenol sulfate	Alupent	Tabs 10–20 mg Aerosol 0.3 cc 5% sol/3 cc NS MDI 2 puffs q4h
bitolterol mesylate	Tornalate	MDI 2 puffs q4–6h
pirbuterol acetate	Maxair	MDI 1–2 puffs/q4–6h
ephedrine	Ephedrine	Caps 25–50 mg ER Tabs 12.5–25 mg q4 IV 10–25 mg
isoetharine HCl	Bronkosol, Bronkometer, Arm-A-Med	Aerosol O.5 ml 1% sol/3 cc NS MDI 2 puffs q4h
salmeterol	Serevent	2 puffs q12h
Parasympatholytics		
atropine sulfate	Atropine	Aerosol 0.3–0.5 mg/3cc NS qid
ipatropium bromide	Atrovent	MDI 1–2 puffs qid Aerosol 1 unit dose (500 µg/2.5 NS) qid
Xanthines[a]		
aminophylline	Aminophylline DF, Truphylline, Phyllocontin	IV 20 mg/ml slowly Tabs 100–200 mg Caps ER 225 mg
theophylline	Theodur, Bronkodyl, Elixophyllin, Slo-bid Gyrocaps	Caps ER 100–300 mg
dyphylline	Dilor, Luffyllin	Tabs 200–400 mg Oral liq 33–53 mg/5 ml
oxtriphylline	Choledyl	Oral liq 50–100 mg/5 ml Tabs ER 100–600 mg
Corticosteroids		
beclomethasone	Beclovent, Vanceril	MDI 2 puffs q3–4h
dexamethasone	Decadron	MDI 2–3 puffs q3–4h
flunisolide	Aerobid	MDI 2 puffs bid
triamcinolone	Azmacort	MDI 2 puffs q3–4h
Asthma Prophylaxis		
cromolyn sodium	Intal	20 mg per treatment qid
nedrocromil sodium	Tilade	MDI 2 puffs qid

[a]Dosage based on response and drug levels.

Side effects of the adrenergics include potentiation of theophylline effects with increased risk of toxicity, especially:

GI—nausea, vomiting, decreased appetite
CNS stimulation—nervousness, tremor, dizziness
Cardiac irregularities—tachycardia, palpitations, arrhythmias, angina
Hypertension
Hyperglycemia

Cautions:

First administration should be observed by medical personnel for hypersensitivity reactions.
Patients should contact physician if decreased effectiveness occurs
Patient should be monitored closely, if administering oral inhaled adrenergics with other oral inhaled bronchodilators, for cardiovascular effects
Patients on beta-blocking drugs (Inderal) will have a significant decrease in the effectiveness of adrenergic drugs
Patients with cardiovascular or kidney disorders, diabetes, or seizure disorders

PARASYMPATHOLYTICS

Parasympatholytics (anticholinergics) achieve bronchodilation by decreasing the chemical that promotes bronchospasm. Parasympatholytics block the parasympathetic nervous system and can cause drying of pulmonary secretions. Adequate hydration should be encouraged to avoid mucus plugging. Examples are atropine and atrovent. See Table 26.1 for dosage.

Side effects:

Cardiac effects: changes in heart rate, palpitations
CNS stimulation: headache, drowsiness, dizziness, confusion, agitation
Thickened secretions and mucus plugging

Cautions: Not indicated for patients with unstable cardiac status, history of heart attacks, glaucoma, or drug sensitivity

XANTHINES

Xanthine derivatives, such as theophylline and aminophylline, and others listed in Table 26.1, cause bronchodilation by indirectly increasing the chemical that causes bronchodilation. Because different individuals metabolize xanthines at different rates, appropriate dosage must be determined by carefully monitoring the patient's response, tolerance, and blood concentrations. For faster absorption, oral forms may be taken with a full glass of water on an empty stomach. To reduce gastric irritation, take with meals. IM injection is contraindicated. Xanthines are commonly administered with other respiratory system drugs such as adrenergics and parasympatholytics.

Side effects of theophyllines can be mild, or severe with acute toxicity including:

GI distress: nausea, vomiting, epigastric pain, abdominal cramps, anorexia, or diarrhea

CNS stimulation: nervousness, insomnia, irritability, headache, tremors, seizures (can be fatal)

Cardiac effects: palpitation, tachycardia, arrhythmias, *especially with rapid IV administration*

Urinary frequency (mild diuresis)

Hyperglycemia

Caution: when administering theophylline applies to:

Cardiovascular, kidney, pulmonary, or liver dysfunction

Diabetes, peptic ulcer, or glaucoma

Children and elderly—more prone to toxicity

IV injection—*must be done slowly*—see cardiac side effects

Patients undergoing influenza immunization or who have influenza

Pregnancy and lactation

Interactions occur with:

Digitalis or other cardiac drugs, which may increase potential for toxicity

Oral anticoagulant action increased

Cimetidine, allopurinol, propranolol, erythromycin, oral contraceptives, and beta-blockers, which increase theophylline levels

Smoking, barbiturates, phenytoin, and rifampin, which decrease theophylline effectiveness

Corticosteroids

Synthetic corticosteroids are used to relieve inflammation, reduce swelling, and suppress symptoms in acute and chronic reactive airway disease (asthma and some COPD). Corticosteroids should be administered systemically (IV) in the acute or emergency setting. In the nonacute setting, corticosteroids may be administered by metered-dose inhaler (MDI) or aerosol. Inhaled corticosteroids have less systemic side effects than oral or IV administration.

Side effects of inhaled corticosteroids

Throat irritation and dry mouth

Hoarseness

Coughing

Oral fungal infections—patient should be encouraged to rinse mouth with water after administration

Contraindications and extreme caution with corticosteroids include:

Viral, bacterial, or fungal infections
Hypertension or congestive heart failure
Diabetes
Hypothyroidism or cirrhosis
Renal failure

See Chapter 23 for further information about corticosteroids and see Table 26.1 for summary of corticosteroids.

Asthma Prophylaxis

A prophylactic for asthma, cromolyn (Intal), is not classified with the other medications mentioned previously. It is described as a mast-cell stabilizer. Cromolyn has no value in the treatment of acute attacks of asthma. Patients with severe, perennial bronchial asthma are required to have a prior pulmonary function test to determine the probability of a satisfactory response to this therapy. Some patients are able to discontinue corticosteroids and have better response to bronchodilator drugs given concomitantly. Cromolyn has also been used in the prevention of exercise-induced bronchospasm. Some patients do not respond to this therapy. Cromolyn is available as a powder or solution for inhalation or a nasal solution. To be effective, the manufacturer's directions must be followed carefully.

Side effects of cromolyn can include:

Throat irritation, cough, bronchospasm with the powder
Nose burning, stinging, sneezing with nasal solution
Nausea or headache

Caution applies to:

Those with cardiovascular disorders
Proper use on a regular schedule

Mucolytics and Expectorants

Mucolytics, such as acetylcysteine (Mucomyst), liquefy pulmonary secretions. Expectorants, such as guaifenesin and others listed in Table 26.2, increase secretions, reduce viscosity, and help to expel sputum. Adequate fluid intake also helps loosen and liquefy secretions. A combination mucolytic-expectorant is iodinated glycerol (Organidin). Various expectorants are commonly combined in cough syrups for symptomatic management of coughs associated with upper respiratory infections, bronchitis, pharyngitis, influenza, measles, or coughs provoked by sinusitis. Expectorants should not be used for self-medication or persistent or

TABLE 26.2. MUCOLYTICS AND EXPECTORANTS

Generic Name	Trade Name	Dosage
Mucolytic		
acetylcysteine	Mucomyst	Aerosol 3–5 ml 10% sol adrenergic may be added for bronchospasm
Expectorants		
guaifenesin	Robitussin	Sol 1–2 tsp q3–4h
iodinated glycerol	Organidin	Elix 1–2 tsp qid Tabs 30 mg 2 qid Sol 20 gtt qid
potassium iodide	SSKI, Pima Syrup	1–2 tsp q4–6h

Note: Expectorants are frequently combined with other drugs, for example, antihistamines, decongestants, and antitussives in over-the-counter cough syrups.

chronic coughs such as that associated with smoking or COPD. A persistent cough may be indicative of a serious condition. If cough persists for more than a week or is recurrent, or accompanied by a fever, a physician should be consulted.

Side effects of the expectorants can include:

Nausea and vomiting

Stomatitis

Runny nose

Drowsiness

Contraindications or caution applies to:

Patients with ineffective or inadequate cough

Some asthmatics (prone to bronchospasm)

Cardiovascular disease and hypertension

Diabetes

Thyroid abnormalities—potassium iodide contraindicated

Pregnancy or lactation

See Table 26.2 for a summary of the mucolytics and expectorants.

Antitussives

Antitissives are medications to prevent coughing in patients not requiring a productive cough. Coughing, a reflex mechanism, helps eliminate secretions from the respiratory tract. A dry, nonproductive cough can cause fatigue, insomnia, and, in some cases, pain to the patient (e.g., pleurisy and fractured ribs). Narcotic antitussives may be used to relieve these patients but have limited use because of respiratory depressant action and bronchial constriction (e.g., morphine). Codeine, a narcotic with fewer side effects, is frequently used, but is addictive with long-term use. Codeine is added to some cough syrups, as is hydrocodone, another narcotic (e.g., Triaminic-DH).

Many over-the-counter cough syrups are available that combine several drugs, for example, antitussives with expectorants, antihistamines and decongestants. Patients should be cautioned to seek advice from a professional person familiar with each ingredient, such as a physician, pharmacist, nurse, or medical assistant. Some ingredients would be contraindicated in certain conditions. For example, antitussives and antihistamines would make it more difficult to expel secretions and thereby worsen conditions such as COPD. Products containing decongestants can cause serious adverse side effects in those with cardiovascular or thyroid conditions.

Side effects of narcotic antitussives can include:

Respiratory depression
Constipation
Urinary retention
Sedation and dizziness
Nausea and vomiting

Contraindications for narcotic antitussives apply to:

Addiction-prone patients
Asthma
COPD

Nonnarcotic antitussives (e.g., dextromethorphan) are more frequently used because they do not depress respirations, do not cause addiction, and have few side effects. Dextromethorphan is frequently combined with other drugs, such as sedatives and decongestants, in cough syrups.

Contraindications include:

Asthma
COPD
Caution with children, some CNS side effects reported, especially large doses

Interactions—dextromethorphan is incompatible with:

Penicillin
Tetracycline
Salicylates
Phenobarbital
Monoamine oxidase inhibitors (MAOIs)

See Table 26.3 for a summary of the antitussives.

TABLE 26.3. ANTITUSSIVES

Generic Name	Trade Name	Dosage	Comments
Narcotic			
codeine	Codeine, Tussar, Dihistine	Sol or tabs 10–20 mg q4–6h	Any cough medicine containing a controlled substance is not for extended use; can develop physical dependence and tolerance; watch for side effects
hydrocodone bitartrate	Triaminic-DH, Lorcet, Dolacet, Bancap	Caps 5–10 mg q4–6h	
Nonnarcotic			
benzonatate	Tessalon	Caps 100–200 mg tid	
dextromethorphan	Benylin, Robitussin	Sol 10–20 mg q4h Sol 30 mg q6–8h	Note incompatabilities
diphenhydramine	Benadryl	Caps 25–50 mg q4–6h	

PATIENT EDUCATION

Patients taking antitussives should be instructed regarding:

Starting with a low dose of antitussive and increasing the dose only if cough supression does not occur.

Caution with those operating machinery because of sedative effect.

Antihistamines

Antihistamines, such as diphenhydramine (Benadryl), competitively antagonize the histamine$_1$ receptor sites. Through this action, the antihistamines combat the increased capillary permeability and edema, inflammation, and itch caused by sudden histamine release.

Antihistamines are not curative, but provide *symptomatic relief of allergic symptoms caused* by histamine release. They are also used as adjunctive treatment of anaphylactic reactions *after* the acute symptoms (e.g., laryngeal edema and shock) have been controlled with epinephrine and corticosteroids.

Antihistamines are used to treat the symptoms of allergies (e.g., rhinitis, conjunctivitis, and rash). However, when antihistamines are used to reduce nasal secretions in the common cold, the consequent thickening of bronchial secretions may result in further airway obstruction, especially in those with COPD and asthma.

Some antihistamines are used in the symptomatic treatment of vertigo associated with pathology of the middle ear or in the prevention and treatment of motion sickness (see Chapter 16).

Side effects of the antihistamines are anticholinergic in action and include:

Drying of secretions, especially of the eyes, ears, nose, and throat

Sedation, dizziness, and hypotension, especially in the elderly

Muscular weakness and decreased coordination

Urinary retention and constipation

Visual disorders

Paradoxical excitement, insomnia, and tremors, especially in children

GI—nausea, vomiting, anorexia

Contraindications or extreme caution applies to:

COPD and asthma

Persons operating machinery or driving a car

Elderly patients

Cardiovascular disorders

Benign prostatic hypertrophy (BPH)

Infants, pregnancy, and lactation

Seizure disorders

Interactions of antihistamines may occur with:

Potentiation of CNS depression with tranquilizers, analgesics, hypnotics, alcohol, and muscle relaxants

Potentiation of anticholinergic effect with MAOIs

Phenothiazine antihistamines, which antagonize the vasopressor effect of epinephrine

---

PATIENT EDUCATION

Patients taking antihistamines should be instructed regarding:

Avoiding frequent or prolonged use of antihistamines, which may cause increased bronchial or nasal congestion and dry cough.

No self-medication (check with the physician first) in those with COPD or cardiovascular disorders, BPH, the elderly, and children.

Caution with those operating machinery because of sedative effect.

No mixing with alcohol or any other CNS depressant drugs.

Other structurally unrelated antihistamines include astemizole (Hismanal) and terfenadine (Seldane). These drugs are *selective* histamine receptor antagonists and have fewer CNS effects, for example, less sedation, than other antihistamines. They are used to provide symptomatic relief of seasonal allergic rhinitis, for example, hay fever.

Serious adverse *cardiac effects* of Hismanal and Seldane can include:

Life-threatening arrhythmias associated with higher than recommended dosage or higher serum levels

Contraindicated with:

Renal and hepatic impairment—metabolism affected with impaired elimination leading to dangerous levels

Erythromycin and certain antifungal agents, for example, ketoconazole which affect metabolism

Children under 12

PATIENT EDUCATION

Patients taking Hismanal and Seldane should be instructed regarding:

Avoiding any other drug, including OTC, without consulting physician first.

The danger of serious cardiac arrhythmias with more than recommended dosage or with cummlative effects.

Reporting symptoms such as fainting, dizziness, or palpitations to physician immediately.

Decongestants

Several adrenergic drugs, for example, phenylephrine (Neosynephrine) or pseudoephedrine (Sudafed), act as decongestants. These drugs constrict blood vessels in the respiratory tract, resulting in shrinkage of swollen mucous membranes and helping to open nasal airway passages. However, these drugs, both oral and nasal, should be used only on a short-term basis because rebound congestion may occur within a few days. Decongestants are frequently combined with antihistamines, analgesics, caffeine, and/or antitussives. Many of these products are available over the counter and, by combining several drugs, the possibility of adverse side effects is increased, especially without adequate medical supervision.

Side effects of decongestants can include:

Anxiety, nervousness, tremor, seizures

Palpitations, hypertension, headache, cerebral hemorrhage

Reduced cardiac output and reduced urine output

Electrolyte imbalance

Contraindications or extreme caution with decongestants applies to:

Cardiovascular disorders

Hyperthyroid or diabetes

Elderly,—especially those with glaucoma or BPH

Pregnancy or lactation

Interactions may occur with:

Potentiation of adverse side effects with other adrenergics, ergot, digitalis, tricyclics, some antihistamines, MAOIs, alcohol

Diuretics, for example, furosemide, may decrease effectiveness of decongestants

---

PATIENT EDUCATION

Patients taking decongestants should be instructed regarding:

Using decongestants for only a few days to avoid rebound congestion.

Avoiding when cardiac or thyroid conditions or diabetes are present.

Discontinuing with side effects such as nervousness, tremor, palpitations, or headache.

Avoiding combining with any other medications without consulting physician.

PATIENT EDUCATION

Patients taking respiratory system drugs should be instructed regarding:

Care in taking medications only as prescribed and required.

Avoiding combining respiratory system drugs with other prescription or OTC drugs or alcohol, which could potentiate CNS stimulation or depression, resulting in serious adverse side effects.

Avoiding self-medication when cardiac, thyroid, or CNS conditions are present

Liberal intake of fluids, which is encouraged to help liquefy secretions.

Benefit from desensitization therapy and air-conditioned environmental control for patients with allergic conditions.

Avoiding air pollution (e.g., smoke-filled rooms).

Exercises (e.g., swimming) that increase lung capacity and help reduce the necessity for medication.

Proper use of inhalers when prescribed. (See administration with inhalers in Chapter 9.)

See Table 26.4 for a summary of the antihistamines and decongestants.

Smoking Cessation Aids

Smoking cessation aids (see Table 26.5), Nicorrette gum, Nicoderm patch are used to slowly lower the level of nicotine while the patient participates in a behavior modification program for smoking cessation.

TABLE 26.4. ANTIHISTAMINES AND DECONGESTANTS

Generic Name	Trade Name	Dosage
Antihistamines		
astemizole	Hismanal	Tabs 10 mg qd
azatadine	Optimine	Tabs 1 mg bid
brompheniramine	Dimetane	Elix 2 mg/5 ml q4–6h Tabs 4 mg q4–6h ER tabs 8–12 mg q8–12h
chlopheniramine	Chlor-Trimeton, Teldrin, Aller-Chlor	Elix 2 mg/5 ml q4–6h Tabs 4 mg 4–6h Tabs 8–12 mg bid
clemastine	Tavist	Tabs 1.34 mg bid
diphenhydramine	Benadryl	Elix 25–50 mg q4–6h Tabs 25–50 mg q4–6h IM or IV 10–50 mg q4–6h
doxylamine	Unisom, (Nitetime Sleep-Aid)	Tabs 7.5–12.5 mg q4–6h
loratadine	Claritin	Tabs 10 mg qd
promethazine	Phenergan	Elix 6.25–50 mg/5 ml q4–6h Tabs 12.5–50 mg in PM IM or IV 25–50 mg/ml Supp 12.5–50 mg
terfenadine	Seldane	Tabs 60 mg bid
Decongestants		
oxymetazoline HCL	Afrin, Allerest	Sol 0.05% 2–3 sprays
phenylephrine	Neosynephrine, Nostril	Sol 0.125–0.25% 1–3 drops/sprays
phenylpropanolamine HCl	Rhinocaps, Genex	Caps 20 mg q4h
pseudoephedrine HCl	Sudafed, Novafed, Efidac	Caps 120 mg q12h Sol or tabs 30–60mg q4–6h Tabs extended release 120 mg q12h

Note: This is a representative list. Many prescription and over-the-counter drugs have combinations of antihistamines and decongestants. These combinations sometimes also include antitussives.

TABLE 26.5. SMOKING CESSATION AIDS

Generic Name	Trade Name	Dosage
nicotine	Nicorette	10–12 pieces of gum/day of 2 mg/piece not to exceed 30 pieces/day
	Nicoderm, Habitrol	1st dose 21 mg patch/day, 4–8 wk 2nd dose 14 mg patch/day, 2–4wk 3rd dose 7 mg patch/day, 2–4wk

Side effects:

Mechanical problems with chewing gum, especially if patient has dentures

Cardiac irritability

Chewing too fast—may cause lightheadedness, nausea, vomiting, throat and mouth irritation

Cautions:

Patients with dental problems that might be exacerbated by chewing gum

Drug abuse and/or overdependence

Overdosage

Pregnancy and lactation

Patients should be warned not to smoke

Worksheet for Chapter 26

RESPIRATORY DRUGS

Note the drugs listed according to category and complete all columns. Learn generic or trade names as specified by instructor.

Classifications and Drugs	Purpose	Side Effects	Contraindications or Cautions	Patient Education
Bronchodilators Theophyllines				
1. Aminophyllin				
2. Theo-Dur				
3. Bronkodyl				
Adrenergics				
1. epinephrine (Primatene, Bronkaid)				
2. ephedrine				
3. Alupent				
4. Isuprel				
5. Tornalate				
6. Serevent				
7. Ventolin				

Classifications and Drugs	Purpose	Side Effects	Contraindications or Cautions	Patient Education
Corticosteroids 1. beclomethasone (Vanceril) 2. dexamethasone (Decadron) 3. triamcinolone (Azmacort)				
Asthma Prophylaxis cromolyn (Intal)				
Mucolytics and Expectorants 1. Mucomyst 2. Robitussin				
Antitussives 1. codeine 2. dextromethorphan (Romilar, Benylin) 3. Tessalon 4. Benadryl				
Antihistamines 1. Seldane, Hismanal 2. Benadryl				
Decongestants 1. Neosynephrine 2. Sudafed 3. Afrin				

A. Case Study for Respiratory Medications

Fred Farmer, a 68-year-old man with a history of COPD, complains of increased shortness of breath and nasal congestion. His Theo-Dur prescription ran out last week and was not refilled. He has been using Alupent inhaler more frequently without relief, and also taking an OTC decongestant.

1. The following descriptions apply to Theo-Dur EXCEPT:
   - a. Xanthine
   - b. Corticosteroid
   - c. Bronchodilator
   - d. Diuretic effect

2. Side effects of Theo-Dur can include the following EXCEPT
   - a. GI distress
   - b. Nervousness
   - c. Sedation
   - d. Tachycardia

3. The following statements are true of Alupent EXCEPT
   - a. Adrenergic action
   - b. Potentiates theophylline
   - c. Dilates bronchioles
   - c. Can be used PRN q2h

4. Side effects of Alupent can include the following EXCEPT
   - a. Palpitations
   - b. Hyperglycemia
   - c. Hypotension
   - d. Tremor

5. Side effects of decongestants can include the following EXCEPT
   - a. Anxiety
   - b. Insomnia
   - c. Headache
   - d. Hypotension

B. Case Study for Respiratory Medications

Mae Wright, a 44-year-old asthmatic, began using a Beclovent inhaler a week ago. Today, she complains of a thick white coating on her tongue. She has also been taking OTC Benadryl for a runny nose.

1. What class of drug is Beclovent?
   - a. Adrenergic
   - b. Xanthine
   - c. Corticosteroid
   - d. Antihistamine

2. Side effects of Beclovent can include the following EXCEPT
   - a. Increased heart rate
   - b. Oral fungal infections
   - c. Dry mouth
   - d. Hoarseness

3. What should Ms. Wright be reminded to do after using her Beclovent inhaler?
   - a. Hold her breath for 1 minute
   - b. Gargle with mouthwash
   - c. Rest for several minutes
   - d. Rinse mouth with water

4. Antihistamines are used to treat all of the following EXCEPT
   - a. Rhinitis
   - b. Conjunctivitis
   - c. Rash
   - d. Asthma

5. Side effects of antihistamines can include all of the following EXCEPT
   a. Dizziness
   b. Mucus plugs
   c. Urinary frequency
   d. Sedation

CHAPTER 27

Preoperative Medications and Local Anesthetics

OBJECTIVES

Upon completion of this chapter, the student should be able to:

1. List the most common components of preoperative injections and give examples of each.
2. Describe side effects and cautions with preoperative medications.
3. Identify two medications that are incompatible with others in the same syringe.
4. Differentiate the five methods of administration of local anesthetics.
5. Describe side effects and cautions with local anesthetics.
6. Explain the interactions of epinephrine with local anesthetic.
7. List the important aspects of patient education with preoperatives and local anesthetics.

Preoperative Medications

Midazolam (Versed) is a benzodiazepine. It is used preoperatively to relieve anxiety, provide sedation, light anesthesia and amnesia of operative events. Because of its more rapid onset of sedative effects and more pronounced anxiolytic effects during the first hour following administration, it is considered the drug of choice with short surgical procedures. Midazolam is usually administered IM and the duration of amnesia is about 1 hour. It has also been used IV or orally for preoperative sedation and to relieve anxiety with good results.

Midazolam is also used IV for *conscious sedation* and relief of anxiety, either alone or in combination with an opioid, for example, meperidine, for short-term procedures such as, endoscopy cardiac catheterization or coronary angiography. Midazolam is also used IV for induction of general anesthesia, along with an opioid. This potent sedative requires individualized dosage with adjustment for age, weight, clinical condition, and procedure.

Side effects of midazolam (Versed) can include:

Depressed respiration with large doses, especially geriatric patients and those with COPD (chronic obstructive pulmonary disease)

Paradoxical reactions (agitation or involuntary movements) occur occasionally

Nausea and vomiting occasionally

Cautions with Versed:

Watch for apnea, hypoxia, and/or cardiac arrest

Respiratory status should be monitored continuously during parenteral use

Facilities and equipment for respiratory and cardiovascular support should be readily available

Vital signs should be monitored carefully for changes in blood pressure or decrease in heart rate

Patients with electrolyte imbalance, renal impairment, congestive heart failure, and children are at increased risk of complications

Contraindicated in pregnancy and comatose patients.

Interactions of Versed apply to:

CNS depressants, including alcohol, potentiate possibility of respiratory depression

Cimetidine (Tagamet) and ranitidine (Zantac) can potentiate respiratory depression

Other preoperative medications, given before general anesthetics, commonly include a combination of an *anticholinergic* or antiemetic, with one or more of the following: sedative hypnotic or an opioid, for example, meperidine.

Anticholinergics (see Chapter 13) most commonly used as preoperative medications include atropine and glycopyrrolate (Robinul). They reduce the secretions of the mouth, pharynx, bronchi, and GI tract and reduce gastric activity. Anticholinergics, as preoperative medication, also are used to prevent cholinergic effects during surgery, such as hypotension or bradycardia, and some cardiac arrhythmias associated with general anesthetics or vagal stimulation. However, only *atropine* acts as a bronchodilator and reduces the incidence of laryngospasm that can occur during general anesthesia.

Side effects of the anticholinergic preoperative medications can include:

Drying of all secretions

Decreased GI and genitourinary motility, constipation, and urinary retention

Flushing

Cardiac arrhythmias and tachycardia

Confusion and/or excitement, especially with the elderly and infants

Blurred vision

Contraindications or caution applies to:

COPD

Gastric ulcer and hiatal hernia

GI infections and ulcerative colitis

Angle-closure glaucoma

BPH (benign prostatic hypertrophy and renal disorders

Myasthenia gravis

Cardiovascular disease

Elderly patients and infants

Interactions with potentiation of sedation occurs with CNS depressants

---

PATIENT EDUCATION

Patients receiving preoperative medications should be instructed regarding:

Side effects to expect (e.g., dry mouth, blurred vision, sleepiness, weakness, and dizziness).

Remaining in bed after preoperative medication is given to prevent falls or injury.

Antiemetics given preoperatively to prevent postoperative nausea and vomiting, and sometimes given postoperatively as well, include promethazine (Phenergan) and ondansetron (Zofran).

Phenergan is a phenothiazine derivative with potent antihistamine properties. It produces sedation, and also has antiemetic and anticholinergic effects, as well as tranquilizing properties. It is usually given with an opioid analgesic preoperatively.

Side effects of promethazine are anticholinergic and include:

Drowsiness, dizziness, dry mouth, blurred vison

Potentiation of CNS depression

Paradoxial agitation, nervousness, confusion possible

Contraindications or caution with promethazine apply to:

Cardiovascular disease

Impaired liver or peptic ulcer

COPD and asthma (cough reflex suppressed)

Children—may precipitate extrapyramidal effects (dystonia) and CNS stimulation (confusion)

Elderly—require reduced dose

Seizure disorders

Administration: Promethazine may be given deep IM or *well dilated* in a freely flowing IV infusion. *Never* give subcutaneously because of irritation and possible tissue necrosis. Watch IV closely for possible infiltration with tissue damage. Check for compatibility before mixing in a syringe or IV.

Interactions of promethazine with:

CNS depressants—potentiate sedation, watch for overdose, especially with the elderly

Epinephrine—may antagonize vasopresser effect

Some drugs may be incompatible chemically. Check compatibility list before mixing in syringe.

Zofran is a selective blocking agent of serotonin receptors with strong antiemetic properties. It is administered by IV injection only, 4 mg given slowly over 2 to 5 minutes. It is given immediately before induction of general anesthesia. It is usually given along with a barbiturate hypnotic (e.g., pentobarbital sodium) and opioid (e.g., fentanyl).

Side effects of ondansetron (Zofran), reported in less than 2%, of cases, can include: Headache and dizziness

See Table 27.1 for summary of preoperative medications, anticholinergics, antimetics, sedative, sedative-hypnotic, and opioids.

Other medications administered concurrently with the anticholinergics and/or antiemetics preoperatively include sedative-hypnotic barbiturates such as pentobarbital (never combine in a syringe with any other drug). Opioids, such as meperidine (Demerol) 50–100 mg, are usually combined in a syringe with the anticholinergics to reduce the number of injections given concurrently. Check compatibilities. Preoperative medications are usually adminstered intramuscularly 30–60 minutes before the start of anesthesia, according to directions of the anesthesiologist.

TABLE 27.1. PREOPERATIVE MEDICATIONS

Generic Name	Trade Name	Dosage
Anticholinergics		
atropine	Atropine	0.4–0.6 mg SC, IM, IV
glycopyrrolate	Robinul	0.2 mg SC, IM, IV
Antiemetics		
ondansetron	Zofran	4 mg IV over 2–5 min
promethazine	Phenergan	25–50 mg deep IM or IV
Sedative and Sedative Hypnotic		
midazolam	Versed	5 mg IM, IV dose varies
pentobarbital sodium	Pentobarbital Sodium	Deep IM or slow IV, dose varies
Opioids		
meperidine	Demerol	50–100 mg IM
fentanyl	Fentanyl Citrate	50–500 μg IM or IV
combinations	Fentanyl and Droperidol, Innovar	50–100 mg IM, **monitor respirations**

Another opioid with strong analgesic, sedative, and anxiolytic properties is fentanyl citrate. It can be used IM preoperatively, or by slow IV injection as a supplement to general anesthesia. It is sometimes combined with Droperidol for certain procedures.

Caution: Because of potential respiratory depression, fentanyl should only be used in a monitored setting with assisted ventilations available.

Reduced dosage and *extra precaution* required for fentanyl:

Cardiovascular or pulmonary disease
Liver dysfunction
Geriatrics (older than 65)

Contraindicated in pregnancy or young children

Light anesthesia for short-term surgical and endoscopy procedures is sometimes achieved by intravenous administration of diazepam (Valium) 10–20 mg (never combined in a syringe with any other drug). (See Chapter 20.)

Caution: Too rapid IV administration may cause hypotension and/or respiratory depression. However, Versed is usually the drug of choice for these procedures, instead of Valium.

Local Anesthetics

Local anesthetics are administered to produce temporary loss of sensation or feeling in that specific area only. Local anesthetics may be administered by the following five methods:

1. *Infiltration anesthesia.* Achieved by injecting the local anesthetic solution into the skin, subcutaneous tissue, or mucous membranes of the area to be anesthetized. It is used in minor surgical and dental procedures (e.g., procaine or lidocaine).
2. *Direct topical anesthesia.* Achieved by application of the local anesthetic directly to the surface of the area to be anesthetized. It is used for temporary relief of painful eye, ear, nose, and throat or dental conditions or to reduce the discomfort of minor procedures (e.g., cocaine solution, *never* injected, is applied to nasal mucosa before nasal surgery; benzocaine lozenges or gels are for throat or mouth pain; benzocaine otic drops are for ear pain; Nupercaine ointment is for hemorrhoids, episiotomy, or minor skin lesions; ethyl chloride spray is for very short surgical procedures such as incision and drainage of carbuncles).
3. *Peripheral nerve block (regional anesthesia).* Achieved by injecting a local anesthetic solution into or around nerves or ganglia supplying the area to be anesthetized (e.g., face or extremities).

4. *Spinal anesthesia.* Achieved by injecting local anesthetic solutions intrathecally (into the subarachnoid space of the spinal canal) either in the lumbar region or lower (saddle block), depending on the area to be anesthetized. Spinal anesthesia is used for abdominal surgery or obstetrics.

5. *Epidural anesthesia.* Produced by injecting local anesthetic solution into the epidural space just outside the spinal cord, for example, caudal (sacral) anesthesia, frequently used in obstetrics.

Although local anesthetics do not produce loss of consciousness, there is some degree of systemic absorption. CNS and cardiovascular effects are possible, depending on the sensitivity of the individual and the amount and type of local anesthesia used. Epinephrine may be added to the local anesthetic solution, constricting peripheral blood vessels to prolong the duration of action, and therefore adrenergic effects are possible (e.g., palpitations, tachycardia, and anxiety). Hypersensitivity reactions with anaphylaxis are possible, and therefore resuscitative procedures, drugs, and equipment should always be available when local anesthetics are administered. Obtaining a history of allergy before administration is essential.

Side effects of local anesthetics can include:

Hypersensitivity reaction, edema, and anaphylaxis
Hypotension and cardiac arrest (not as likely when epinephrine is added)
Respiratory difficulties (especially with high spinals)
CNS depression or excitation and seizures

Contraindications or extreme caution applies to:

Cardiovascular disease
Hyperthyroidism
Hepatic disorders
Pregnancy
History of allergy, asthma
Elderly patients

Interaction of local anesthetics with *epinephrine* not only prolongs the duration of the anesthesia but also helps localize the anesthesia, thus decreasing systemic effects.

PATIENT EDUCATION

Patients receiving topical anethetics should be instructed regarding:

Accurate reporting of allergies or other physical conditions prior to local anesthetic.
Prompt reporting of any side effects during local anesthesia (e.g., palpitations, nervousness, vertigo, and weakness).
Reassurance about the safety of the procedure both before and during the administration of local anesthetics.

See Table 27.2 for a summary of the local anesthetics.

TABLE 27.2. LOCAL ANESTHETICS

Generic Name	Trade Name	Dosage
benzocaine	Chloraseptic, Americaine, Anbesol	Lozenges, sol, aerosols, gels, pastes
cocaine	Cocaine	Topical sol (never inject) for ENT
dibucaine	Nupercainal	Ointment, cream
diclonine HCl	Dyclone, Sucrets	Topical sol (never inject), lozenges
ethyl chloride	Ethyl Chloride	Spray
lidocaine[a]	Xylocaine	0.5%, 1%, 1.5%, 2%, higher with spinals
procaine[a]	Novocaine	1%, 2%, higher with spinals
tetracaine HCL	Pontocaine	1%, 10–15 mg, spinal Ophthalmic sol 0.5%, topical sol 0.2%

Note: Other local anesthetics are available. This is a representative list.

[a]Available plain or in combination with epinephrine (very important to note difference).

Worksheet for Chapter 27

PREOPERATIVE MEDICATIONS AND LOCAL ANESTHETICS

Note the drugs listed according to category and complete all columns. Learn generic or trade names as specified by instructor.

Classifications and Drugs	Purpose	Side Effects	Contraindications or Cautions	Patient Education
Preoperative Medications: Drying Agents Anticholinergics 1. atropine				
2. Robinul				
Antiemetics 1. ondansetron (Zofran)				
2. promethazine (Phenergan)				

Classifications and Drugs	Purpose	Side Effects	Contraindications or Cautions	Patient Education
Sedatives and Opioids				
1. midazolam (Versed)				
2. pentobarbital				
3. meperidine				
4. fentanyl				
Local Anesthetics				
1. benzocaine				
2. cocaine				
3. ethyl chloride				
4. Xylocaine, Novocain				

A. Case Study for Preoperative Medications

Jan Howard has been scheduled for bronchosopy in the outpatient department. The physician has said that she will receive Versed. She needs to know what to expect.

1. Versed will produce all of the following EXCEPT
    a. Memory loss
    b. Sedation
    c. Reduced anxiety
    d. Loss of consciousness

2. Versed can be administered in the following ways EXCEPT
    a. IM
    b. By mouth
    c. Spinal
    d. IV

3. The following will be monitored continuously EXCEPT
    a. Respiratory status
    b. Electrolyte level
    c. Blood pressure
    d. Cardiac rate

4. Versed is most frequently combined with which one?
    a. Hydroxyzine
    b. Diphenhydramine
    c. Meperidine
    d. Cemetidine

5. The amnesia effects will last approximately how long?
    a. 2 hours
    b. 1 hour
    c. 4 hours
    d. 24 hours

B. Case Study for Local Anesthetics

Gwen Eastwood has been scheduled for removal of a ganglionic cyst on her hand. She will receive a local anesthetic in the outpatient department. The following information is important.

1. Which drug will probably be injected locally?
    a. Cocaine
    b. Pontocaine
    c. Xylocaine
    d. Ethyl Chloride

2. Which drug may be added to prolong duration of anesthesia?
    a. Norepinephrine
    b. Epinephrine
    c. Neostigmine
    d. Pilocarpine

3. This adjuvant drug, mentioned above, might cause the following effects EXCEPT
    a. Palpitations
    b. Tachycardia
    c. Sedation
    d. Anxiety

4. Before local anesthetics, it is most important to check for a history of all of the following EXCEPT
    a. Asthma
    b. Diabetes
    c. Allergies
    d. Cardiac arrhythmias

5. She should be told that she will be monitored closely for all of the following EXCEPT
   a. Level of analgesia
   b. Level of consciousness
   c. Blood pressure
   d. Cardiac rate

CHAPTER **28**

Drugs and Geriatrics

OBJECTIVES

Upon completion of this chapter, the student should be able to:

1. Define polypharmacy.
2. List at least 15 drugs that are inappropriate for older people.
3. Describe four factors that may lead to cumulative effects in the elderly.
4. Name at least five categories of drugs that frequently cause adverse side effects in older adults.
5. List at least 10 drugs which can cause mental problems in the elderly.
6. Describe the dangers and side effects associated with NSAID therapy.
7. List side effects and cautions for gastrointestinal drugs.
8. Explain patient education for NSAID and GI drugs.
9. Describe patient education for all patients on long-term drug therapy.
10. List the responsibilities of health care personnel in preventing complications of drug therapy.

Today people are living longer and are taking more medications. Consequently, there has also been an increase in serious complications resulting from drug reactions. It has been estimated that more than 200,000 adults over the age of 60 are hospitalized yearly as the result of adverse drug effects. Therefore, it is imperative that the health care community works together to reverse this dangerous trend.

The aging process is an individualized matter. Because of genetic or environmental factors, or good health practices, for example, exercise, healthy diet, and mental stimulation, some older individuals may not feel or appear particularly different. However, we need to realize that there are gradual changes in body composition and organ function as we grow older. These changes can affect the reaction to drugs and make the individual more sensitive to a wide variety of medications.

A recent study by Harvard Medical School researchers looked at medicines prescribed for individuals over 65 years of age. The panel of experts in geriatrics and pharmacology found, "a disturbingly high level of potentially inappropriate prescribing for older people. Over the course of one year, almost one quarter of older Americans were unnecessarily exposed to potentially hazardous prescribing."

The panel found the following medicines less effective or not as safe as other readily available alternatives.

Drugs That May Be Inappropriate for Older People

Butazolidin	Norflex
Dalmane	Persantine
Darvon/Darvocet	Robaxin
Diabinese	Seconal
Elavil	Soma
Flexeril	Talwin
Indocin	Valium
Librium	Vasodilan
Meprobamate	

Complex changes of aging involve both anatomic and physiologic factors that affect how drugs are processed in the body (see Chapter 3). The four processes that drugs undergo in the body—that is, absorption, distribution, metabolism (biotransformation), and excretion—are all altered as the body ages. The end result of this slowed process can be a buildup of drugs in the system, leading to dangerous or toxic levels.

Cumulative effects of drugs in the elderly can be due to:

Inadequate absorption—slowed GI motility or reduced fluid intake

Impaired distribution—circulatory dysfunction

Slower metabolism—hepatic dysfunction

Impaired excretion—renal dysfunction, constipation or poor exchange of gases in the lungs

Because the increase in the amount of drug circulating in the system is often gradual, the consequences of an "overdose" may not be recognized. Family, friends, and even patients themselves may conclude that their symptoms are just due to "old age."

Some medicines that are perfectly safe for a 30-year-old may produce unexpected results in a person over 50 or 60. An example is digoxin (Lanoxin). An elderly person still on the same dose that was appropriate 10 or 20 years earlier may experience side effects such as loss of appetite, weakness, personality changes, nightmares, confusion, or even hallucinations. In addition, digoxin can interact with many other drugs, sometimes slowing clearance of the drug from the system, which could result in cumulative effects, including possible dangerous arrhythmias.

Some drugs in the following categories frequently cause adverse side effects, especially among older adults:

Tranquilizers, antipsychotics, sedatives, and hypnotics

Antidepressants, especially tricyclics

High blood pressure and cardiac drugs

Glaucoma eyedrops (beta blocker)

Antimotility and antispasmodic drugs

Antiulcer drugs (e.g., Tagamet)

Many medications can cause mental problems in older people. One government study found that more than 150,000 elders had experienced *serious mental impairment either caused or worsened by drugs.* Many medications can cause anxiety, depression, confusion, disorientation, forgetfulness, hallucinations, nightmares, or impaired mental clarity, *especially in the elderly.* Drugs that can cause mental impairment in older adults include:

Aldomet	Mellaril
Artane	Pamelor
Benadryl	Phenergan
Bentyl	Prednisone
Cogentin	Pro-Banthine
Compazine	Quinidine
Corgard	Reglan
Dalmane	Sinemet
Desyrel	Sinequan
Dilantin	Tagamet
Ditropan	Tegretol
Donnatol	Tenormin
Elavil	Thorazine
Haldol	Timoptic
Inderal	Tofranil
Lopressor	Xanax

Other CNS drugs also impair mental function. This is a representative list of the most frequently used drugs. In addition, all antipsychotics can cause tardive dyskinesia and/or parkinsonism. Alcohol can also potentiate adverse effects of many drugs.

Many CNS drugs and antihypertensives can also cause dizziness or impair motor function, which increases the risk of falls. These drugs can also impair sexual functioning, reducing the quality of life.

Many older people suffer from arthritis and take over-the-counter nonsteroidal anti-inflammatory drugs (NSAIDs), frequently without adequate supervision. Anyone taking NSAIDs should be cautioned about the real danger of serious complications. Every year there are over 70,000 hospitalizations and more than 7,000 deaths from drug-induced bleeding ulcers or perforations. Particularly in the elderly, there may be no warning signs of pain and the first symptoms of trouble may be a "silent" bleed that could lead to fatal GI hemorrhage.

Side effects of all NSAIDs and corticosteroids (e.g., prednisone) can include:

Indigestion, heartburn, abdominal pain

Nausea, vomiting, and anorexia

Flatulence, diarrhea or constipation

Silent ulceration (no symptoms of gastrointestinal problems)

Other possible side effects of NSAIDs (including aspirin):

Prolonged bleeding time

Liver toxicity and kidney dysfunction

Bronchospasm (especially with asthma)

Visual or hearing problems (e.g. tinnitus)

See Chapter 21 for a list of NSAIDs and interactions.

Misoprostol (Cytotec) is sometimes given for the prevention of NSAID-induced gastric ulcers, but may cause severe diarrhea.

PATIENT EDUCATION FOR NSAID THERAPY

Patients should be instructed regarding:

Administration with food.

Not exceeding dosage prescribed by physician.

Not taking aspirin, alcohol, or any other drugs at the same time because they may potentiate GI or bleeding problems.

The possibility of "silent" bleeding.

Reducing dosage of NSAIDs and substituting acetaminophen for pain, if possible at least part of the time.

Trying exercise and heat for pain control, as approved by physician.

Gastrointestinal problems, for example, indigestion, heartburn, and constipation, are frequent complaints of older adults. Consequently, a common practice is the taking of over-the-counter remedies without adequate awareness of potential side effects or implications.

PATIENT EDUCATION FOR GASTROINTESTINAL MEDICINES

Side effects of antacids can include constipation (with aluminum or calcium carbonate products), diarrhea (with magnesium antacids), acid rebound, belching or flatulence (with calcium carbonate).

Avoid prolonged use (no longer than 2 weeks) of OTC antacids without medical supervision because of the danger of masking symptoms of GI bleeding or GI malignancy.

Avoid taking antacids within 2 hours of any other drug because of numerous interactions (see Chapter 16).

Antiulcer drugs, for example, Tagamet, can cause mental confusion, especially in the elderly.

Avoid frequent use of strong cathartics, which can lead to laxative dependence and loss of normal bowel function. Instead, increase fluids and high-fiber diet and regular bowel habits. If laxatives are necessary, use bulk laxatives (e.g., psyllium) or stool softeners.

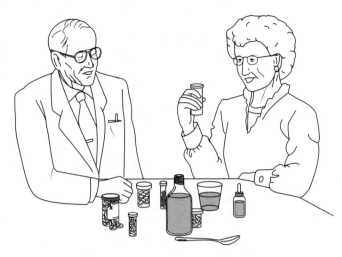

Figure 28.1 Polypharmacy. *"My internist prescribed the red pill, my cardiologist the white one, my allergist the blue one, and the ophthalmologist the eyedrops."*

Individuals at any age, but especially the elderly, may be the victims of *polypharmacy,* that is, excessive use of drugs or prescriptions for many drugs given at one time (see Fig. 28.1). Polypharmacy increases the risk of dangerous interactions with potentially serious adverse side effects. Health care workers should take every opportunity to educate their patients regarding their medicines, the purpose for them, possible side effects, potential dangers, and interactions between medicines. Anyone receiving medicines should be monitored on an ongoing basis to determine continuing effectiveness and possible cumulative or adverse effects. Medicines should be reviewed regularly to determine feasibility of reducing dosage or possibly substituting a more effective or safer medicine.

PATIENT EDUCATION

Geriatric patients should be instructed regarding:

Making a list of *all* medicines (with dosage). Include pain medicine, eyedrops, and topical medications. This list should be carried in wallet and/or be readily available at all times.

The purpose for their medicines, side effects, and interactions.

Reporting side effects to physician immediately.

The importance of seeing their physician on a regular basis, every 6 months to a year or more often, to reevaluate the need for and effectiveness of the drug.

Not stopping the medicine or changing the dose without consulting the physician. Abrupt withdrawal can be dangerous with some medicines.

Asking the physician to prescribe a generic or less expensive alternate if the cost of the medicine is prohibitive. Sometimes social service departments can assist the patient in securing expensive medicines that are imperative to the patient's health.

If there is a problem with remembering to take medicines, ask the pharmacist to recommend a pillbox organizer or chart with dosage times.

All health care workers must be aware of their responsibilities in preventing complications of drug therapy in patients of any age, but especially the old and the very young, who are more vulnerable. The following guidelines should be helpful:

- Educate yourself, your patients and their families regarding adverse side effects, cumulative effects, and interactions.
- With each newly prescribed drug, note diagnoses, allergies, and other medications.
- Monitor long-term drug use for effectiveness and physiological or mental changes. Do periodic lab tests as appropriate (e.g., digitalis levels).
- *Question* any inappropriate medicine or dosage. You have a moral, ethical, and legal responsibility to do what is best for the patient.
- Document all adverse side effects, calls to the physician, and action taken.

A. Case Study for Drugs and Geriatrics

Harry Elder, a 75-year-old man, has a diagnosis of hypertension, angina, arteriosclerosis, GERD (gastroesophageal reflux disease), and BPH. He is receiving Lanoxin, Inderal, Xanax, Lopressor, Pepcid, and Dalmane.

1. He is at risk for cumulative effects with his diagnoses and the following conditions EXCEPT
   a. Impaired excretion
   b. Hepatic dysfunction
   c. Circulatory dysfunction
   d. Slowed GI motility

2. Side effects of Lanoxin can include the following EXCEPT
   a. Confusion
   b. Weakness
   c. Palpitations
   d. Anorexia

3. All of the drugs he is taking have the potential for causing mental impairment, depression, or confusion EXCEPT
   a. Inderal
   b. Xanax
   c. Lopressor
   d. Pepcid

4. All of the drugs he is taking have the potential for causing weakness or dizziness EXCEPT
   a. Lanoxin
   b. Dalmane
   c. Pepcid
   d. Xanax

5. Serious interactions with toxicity are possible with his drugs and the following EXCEPT
   a. Antihistamines
   b. Antacids
   c. Alcohol
   d. Analgesics

B. Case Study for Drugs and Geriatrics

Grace Grey, an 83-year-old resident of a nursing home, has a diagnosis of arthritis, diabetes, organic brain syndrome, and gastritis. Her medicines include Prednisone, Naprosyn, Diabinese, Haldol, Tagamet, Ditropan, Metamucil, and Compazine PRN.

1. Side effects of corticosteriod and/or NSAIDs can include all of the following conditions EXCEPT
   a. GI distress
   b. Incontinence
   c. Bleeding
   d. Ulcers

2. Her medicines that could cause confusion include the following EXCEPT
   a. Diabinese
   b. Tagamet
   c. Ditropan
   d. Compazine

3. Haldol can cause all of the following EXCEPT
   a. Confusion   c. Weakness
   b. Depression   d. Diarrhea

4. Which oral antidiabetic agent is contraindicated in the elderly?
   a. Micronase   c. Diabinese
   b. Tolinase   d. Glucotrol

5. Which is the only laxative which should be taken daily?
   a. Dulcolax   c. Milk of Magnesia
   b. Agoral   d. Metamucil

Note: A **Comprehensive Review Exam** for Part II can be found at the end of the
        text on page 499.

        Answers to this comprehensive exam are available in the Instructor's
        Guide.

Summary

The health care worker has a great responsibility in the administration of medications and when advising others regarding drug therapy. As the elderly population increases and many more new drugs are developed and prescribed, more knowledge is required regarding cumulative effects and interactions. Moral, ethical, and legal issues of drug therapy are raised with increasing frequency. Therefore, it is imperative that the health care worker keep abreast of changes in drug therapy practices. Complete knowledge and judgment are necessary for effective administration and adequate patient education. The following guidelines should prove useful for safe drug therapy:

- Always research new drugs before administration to determine side effects, interactions, and cautions.
- Assess the patient before administration for allergies, general condition, and possible contraindications, and after administration for results and adverse effects.
- Question any inappropriate drugs, dosages, or possible interactions.
- Responsibilities of Drug Administration are discussed further in Chapter 7.

Comprehensive Review Exam for Part I

1. Drug standards regulate all of the following factors in drug preparation EXCEPT
   - a. Strength
   - b. Purity
   - c. Color
   - d. Quality

2. All of the following facts are true of the Pure Food and Drug Act EXCEPT
   - a. For consumer protection
   - b. Listed approved drugs
   - c. Set minimal standards
   - d. Passed in 1776

3. The Food and Drug Administration regulates all of the following drug factors EXCEPT
   - a. Prescription labeling
   - b. Shape of tablet
   - c. Effectiveness
   - d. Safety

4. Which of the following drugs is *not* a controlled substance?
   - a. Marijuana
   - b. Valium
   - c. Codeine
   - d. Thyroid

5. Which statement is *not* true of controlled drugs?
   - a. Listed by schedule
   - b. Refilled PRN
   - c. May cause dependence
   - d. Sometimes illegal

6. Which is *not* a good source of drug information?
   - a. PDR
   - b. USP/NF
   - c. Drug insert
   - d. News magazine

7. Which statement is true of the generic name of a drug?
   - a. Assigned by drug company
   - b. Written in capital letters
   - c. Common name
   - d. Same as trade name

8. The term OTC refers to drugs:
   - a. Often times controlled
   - b. Requiring prescription
   - c. For sale to anyone
   - d. Officially certified

9. Which of the following conditions is *not* commonly listed as a *contraindication* for drug administration?
   a. Obesity
   c. Pregnancy
   b. Allergy
   d. Lactation

10. Before giving a new drug, you must know all of the following EXCEPT
    a. Interactions
    c. Side effects
    b. Contraindications
    d. Usual price

11. An antibiotic with *photosensitivity* listed as a side effect could cause:
    a. Deafness
    c. Blindness
    b. Sunburn
    d. Kidney damage

12. Which is *not* a source of drugs?
    a. Minerals
    c. Animals
    b. Gases
    d. Laboratory

13. Which is *not* a process that drugs go through in the body?
    a. Tolerance
    c. Metabolism
    b. Distribution
    d. Excretion

14. Which of the following patient characteristics is *not* a factor affecting the processing of drugs in the body?
    a. Weight
    c. Mental state
    b. Age
    d. Skin color

15. Drug toxicity from cumulative effects may result from all of the following EXCEPT
    a. Low metabolism
    c. High blood pressure
    b. Poor circulation
    d. Kidney malfunction

16. Which term does *not* describe an adverse or unexpected result from a drug?
    a. Idiosyncrasy
    c. Placebo effect
    b. Anaphylaxis
    d. Teratogenic effect

17. Which route of administration is used most often?
    a. Topical
    c. Injection
    b. Sublingual
    d. Oral

18. Which is *not* a form of parenteral administration?
    a. Inhalation
    c. Dermal patch
    b. Rectal
    d. Injection

19. Which type of medication can be crushed and mixed with food to facilitate administration?
    a. Timed-release capsule
    c. Scored tablet
    b. Lozenge
    d. Enteric-coated tablet

20. Which is *not* a topical form of administration?
    a. Ointment
    c. Eyedrops
    b. Intradermal
    d. Vaginal cream

21. Which is the most rapid form of administration?
    a. PO
    c. IM
    b. IV
    d. SC

22. Which is the least accurate system for measuring medication?
    a. Metric   c. Household
    b. Apothecary

23. Which is the most frequently used system for measuring medicine?
    a. Apothecary   c. Household
    b. Metric

24. Medication orders must contain all of the following EXCEPT
    a. Dosage   c. Medication name
    b. Route   d. Patient's address

25. The prescription blank for a controlled substance must contain all of the following EXCEPT
    a. Physician's DEA number   c. Frequency
    b. Name of drug company   d. Number of refills

26. Which type of equipment is least accurate in measuring medicine?
    a. Medicine cup   c. Teaspoon
    b. Minim glass   d. Syringe

27. Responsibilities of the health care worker include all of the following EXCEPT
    a. Patient education   c. Judgment
    b. Current information   d. Prescribing

28. Which is *not* appropriate action after administration of medication?
    a. Assessment   c. Evaluation
    b. Research concerning meals d. Documentation

29. Which is the *least* helpful information in dispensing medication?
    a. Allergies   c. Health history
    b. Handicaps   d. Patient's occupation

30. If a medication error is made, all of the following actions are required EXCEPT
    a. Report to physician   c. Note on patient record
    b. File incident report   d. Apologize to patient

31. Before giving any medicine, it is essential to review the five Rights of Medication Administration, including all of the following EXCEPT
    a. Right amount   c. Right drug company
    b. Right drug   d. Right time schedule

32. Documentation of a controlled drug given PRN for pain requires all of the following EXCEPT
    a. Note on narcotic record   c. Note of effectiveness
    b. Note of trade name   d. Note on patient record

33. Which one is *not* used for administration by the gastrointestinal route?
    a. Nasogastric tube   c. Rectal suppository
    b. Oral inhaler   d. Timed-release capsule

34. Which one is *not* an advantage of the oral route over other routes?
    a. Speed
    b. Safety
    c. Economy
    d. Convenience
35. If a medication is ordered PO and the patient is NPO, which action is *most* appropriate?
    a. Give medication by injection
    b. Give medication rectally
    c. Omit medication and note on chart
    d. Consult the person in charge
36. Oral medications are usually best administered with which fluid?
    a. Fruit juice
    b. Milk
    c. Water
    d. Hot tea
37. When preparing cough syrup, which is the most appropriate action?
    a. Shake the bottle
    b. Dilute with liquid
    c. Hold label side down
    d. Hold medicine cup at eye level
38. Which of the following is *not* required for administration of rectal suppository?
    a. Lubricant
    b. privacy
    c. Bed elevated
    d. Disposable glove
39. Which parenteral route is *least* likely to be used for systemic effects?
    a. Transdermal
    b. Topical
    c. Sublingual
    d. Inhalation
40. Which route has the slowest action?
    a. Transcutaneous
    b. Inhalation
    c. Sublingual
    d. Injection
41. After instilling eyedrops, which is the most appropriate action?
    a. Rub eyelid vigorously
    b. Press inner canthus
    c. Close eyelid quickly
    d. Discard eyedropper
42. Which is *not* appropriate for intradermal injection?
    a. Tuberculin syringe
    b. 21-gauge, 1-inch needle
    c. Wheal formation on skin
    d. 0.1–0.2 ml solution
43. Which is *not* true of intramuscular injections?
    a. Skin held taut
    b. 1½-inch needle usual
    c. 45-degree angle of needle
    d. Can be Z-track
44. Which one of these intramuscular injection sites is used for infants?
    a. Dorsogluteal
    b. Ventrogluteal
    c. Deltoid
    d. Vastus lateralis
45. Ipecac to induce vomiting would be indicated in poisoning with which substance?
    a. Ammonia
    b. Strychnine
    c. Lighter fluid
    d. Aspirin
46. Ipecac would be contraindicated in patients with all of the following conditions EXCEPT
    a. Semiconscious
    b. Hypertension
    c. Diabetes
    d. Cardiac

47. If there is doubt about the type of poison, toxicology tests will be done on all of the following EXCEPT
    a. Urine   c. Blood
    b. Stool   d. Emesis

48. Which group is *least* at risk of accidental poisoning?
    a. Infants   c. Healthy adults
    b. Elderly

49. Patient education to prevent poisoning includes all of the following advice EXCEPT
    a. Label all medications and   c. Always read medicine labels
       poisons
    b. Discard medications in toilet   d. Keep medications at bedside

Calculate the correct dosage for administration in the following problems. Label your answers. Remember that syringes are not marked in fractions; therefore, when computing dosages for administration, you must convert all fractions to decimals and round off to one decimal place.

50. You are to give 7,500 U of heparin SC. The vial is labeled 10,000 U/ml. How many milliliters should you give?

51. You are to give 10 ml of Phenergan cough syrup with codeine. The bottle is labeled 10 mg of codeine in 5 ml of cough syrup. How much codeine would the patient receive in each prescribed dose?

52. The medicine bottle label states that the strength of each tablet in the bottle is 0.25 mg. The physician has ordered that the patient is to receive 0.5 mg. How many tablets should you give?

53. The physician has ordered 20 mg of meperidine to be given. On hand is medication containing 50 mg/ml. How many milliliters should you give?

54. To convert pounds to kilograms (Kg), you would divide the number of pounds by what number?

Comprehensive Review Exam for Part II

1. Deficiency of potassium may result in:
   a. Diarrhea
   b. Petechiae
   c. Cardiac arrhythmias
   d. GI bleeding

2. Which would be least likely to require vitamin or mineral supplements?
   a. Executive secretary
   b. Nursing mother
   c. Adolescent
   d. Alcoholic

3. The following statements are true of vitamin C EXCEPT
   a. Destroyed by heat
   b. Unstable with antacids
   c. Found in citrus fruits
   d. Large supplements helpful

4. Which condition will slow absorption of topical medication?
   a. Heat
   b. Moisture
   c. Macerated skin
   d. Callused skin

5. The following statements are true of resistance to antibiotics EXCEPT
   a. Caused by too frequent use
   b. Caused by incomplete treatment
   c. Decreased with use of combination drugs
   d. Decreased with use of antacids concurrently

6. All of the following drugs are used in the initial treatment program for tuberculosis EXCEPT
   a. Isoniazid
   b. Rifampin
   c. Fluconazole
   d. Pyrazinamide

7. Most antibiotics are best administered:
   a. With fruit juice
   b. With antacids
   c. 1 h ac
   d. 1/2 h pc

8. Allergic hypersensitivity can be manifested in all of the following ways EXCEPT
   a. Diarrhea
   b. Rash
   c. Hives
   d. Anaphylaxis

9. Which of the following would be most likely to develop a penicillin reaction?
   a. Premature infant
   b. Cancer patient
   c. Diabetic
   d. Allergic asthmatic

10. The following statements are true of atropine EXCEPT
    a. Used as a mydriatic
    b. Used as a cycloplegic
    c. Treatment for glaucoma
    d. Can cause blurred vision

11. The following statements are true of corticosteroid ophthalmic ointment EXCEPT
    a. Can delay healing
    b. Used short term
    c. Anti-inflammatory
    d. Used for infections

12. The following instructions are appropriate for those taking loop diuretics, for example, Lasix or Bumex, EXCEPT
    a. Avoid alcohol
    b. Report rash
    c. Take at bedtime
    d. Limit exposure to sun

13. The following side effects are possible with thiazide diuretics EXCEPT
    a. Hypokalemia
    b. Hypoglycemia
    c. Increased uric acid
    d. Muscle weakness

14. The thiazides are used to treat all of the following conditions except:
    a. Hypertension
    b. Congestive heart failure
    c. Gout
    d. Edema

15. Which term does *not* describe a purpose for antineoplastic drugs?
    a. Cytotoxic
    b. Analeptic
    c. Palliative
    d. Remission

16. Which is *not* a frequent side effect of antineoplastic drugs?
    a. Jaundice
    b. Diarrhea
    c. Ulcers of mucosa
    d. Nausea and vomiting

17. Which side effect is *not* associated with atropine?
    a. Diaphoresis
    b. Confusion
    c. Blurred vision
    d. Urinary retention

18. Which side effect is *not* associated with epinephrine?
    a. Palpitations
    b. Lethargy
    c. Tachycardia
    d. Tremor

19. Which is *not* an action of cholinergic drugs?
    a. Increased peristalsis
    b. Lowered intraocular pressure
    c. Reduced salivation
    d. Bladder contraction

20. Drugs that can cause mental impairment in the elderly include all of the following EXCEPT
    a. Tagamet
    b. Naprosyn
    c. Benadryl
    d. Ditropan

Jim J. is admitted to the emergency room with a history of insecticide poisoning (cholinergic action). Questions 21 and 22 are related to Jim's situation:

21. Jim's symptoms might include all of the following EXCEPT
    a. Facial flushing
    c. Diarrhea
    b. Diaphoresis
    d. Nausea

22. His treatment would most likely include which drug?
    a. Prostigmin
    c. Atropine
    b. Adrenalin
    d. Isuprel

23. Which statement is *not* true of Lomotil?
    a. Slows peristalsis
    c. Has drying effect
    b. Contains atropine
    d. Used for food poisoning

24. Which laxative would be used for chronic constipation?
    a. Milk of Magnesia
    c. Ex-Lax
    b. Dulcolax
    d. Metamucil

25. Which medication is *not* an antiemetic?
    a. Phenergan
    c. Dramamine
    b. Imodium
    d. Compazine

26. The most likely prescription for frequent gas pains is:
    a. Milk of Magnesia
    c. Mylicon
    b. Colace
    d. Metamucil

27. Which statement is *not* true of the nonsteroidal anti-inflammatory drugs?
    a. Alleviate pain of arthritis
    c. Used long term sometimes
    b. Raise prostaglandin levels
    d. Reduce joint swelling

28. Which drug is *not* a muscle relaxant?
    a. Robaxin
    c. Delalutin
    b. Valium
    d. Flexeril

29. Which is *not* a likely side effect with narcotic use?
    a. Constipation
    c. Urinary retention
    b. Tachycardia
    d. Blurred vision

30. Which drug does *not* potentiate the CNS depression effect of analgesics and hypnotics?
    a. Alcohol
    c. Corticosteroids
    b. Antihistamines
    d. Muscle relaxants

31. Which is the most common side effect of prolonged use of haldoperidol (Haldol)?
    a. Hypertension
    c. Diaphoresis
    b. Diarrhea
    d. Parkinsonism

32. Which statement is *not* true of the tricyclic antidepressants?
    a. Rapidly effective
    c. Tranquilizing effect
    b. Cause dry mouth
    d. Anticholinergic action

33. Which statement is *not* true of the minor tranquilizers?
    a. For psychosomatic disorders
    c. May cause photosensitivity
    b. Relieve nausea and vomiting
    d. Useful long term

34. Adjuvant drugs that can enhance analgesic effect when combined with opioids include all of the following EXCEPT
    a. Elavil
    b. Effexor
    c. Dilantin
    d. Tofranil
35. All of the following have GI bleeding as a possible side effect EXCEPT
    a. Ibuprofen
    b. Prolisec
    c. Prednisone
    d. Naprosyn
36. Which medication is used to treat febrile convulsions in children?
    a. Dilantin
    b. Mysoline
    c. Zarontin
    d. Phenobarbital
37. Which is a purpose of the anticonvulsants?
    a. Reduce seizures
    b. Sedate the patient
    c. Cure epilepsy
    d. Treat parkinsonism
38. Which is *not* an antiparkinsonian drug?
    a. Cimetidine
    b. Cogentin
    c. Sinemet
    d. Symmetrel
39. Which condition is *not* treated with estrogen?
    a. Breast engorgement
    b. Prostatic cancer
    c. Threatened abortion
    d. Severe menopausal symptoms
40. Which condition is *not* treated with testosterone?
    a. Enuchoidism
    b. Androgen deficiency
    c. Cryptorchidism
    d. Metastatic breast cancer
    e. Prostate cancer
41. Which is *not* a possible side effect of corticosteroids?
    a. Delayed healing
    b. Peptic ulcer formation
    c. Reduced resistance to infection
    d. Hypoglycemia
42. Midazolam (Versed), a preoperative medication, can cause all of the following EXCEPT
    a. Slow respiration
    b. Tachycardia
    c. Amnesia
    d. Sedation
43. The following statements are true of isoproterenol (Isuprel) EXCEPT
    a. May cause hypoglycemia
    b. May cause palpitations
    c. May be given sublingually
    d. Used with inhaler
44. The following statements are true of codeine used as an antitussive EXCEPT
    a. May depress respirations
    b. Useful with COPD
    c. May be addictive
    d. Classified as narcotic
45. Which of the following stimulates respirations?
    a. Valium
    b. Robaxin
    c. Butazolidin
    d. Carbon dioxide
46. Which is *not* a symptom of hypoglycemia?
    a. Tremor
    b. Dry skin
    c. Irritability
    d. Weakness
    e. Drowsiness

COMPREHENSIVE REVIEW EXAM FOR PART II   **503**

47. Which is *not* a symptom of hyperglycemia and diabetic acidosis?
    a. Nausea and vomiting   d. Sweating
    b. Fruity breath   e. Excessive thirst
    c. Lethargy

48. The antihistamines, Seldane and Hismanal, can cause cardiac arrhythmias under the following conditions EXCEPT
    a. With erythromycin   c. With liver disease
    b. With ketoconazole   d. With penicillin

49. All of the following might be a symptom of digitalis toxicity EXCEPT
    a. Cardiac arrhythmia   c. Urinary retention
    b. Blurred vision   d. GI disturbance

50. Which of the following antihypertensives is *least* likely to cause bradycardia?
    a. Reserpine   c. Apresoline
    b. Inderal   d. Catapres

Glossary

Absorption.   Passage of a substance through a body surface into body fluids or tissues.

Acetylcholine.   Mediator of nerve impulses in the parasympathetic system.

Addiction.   Physical and/or psychological dependence on a substance, especially alcohol or drugs, with use of increasing amounts (tolerance) and withdrawal reactions.

Adjunct.   Addition to the course of treatment.

Adjuvant.   A drug added to a prescription to hasten or increase the action of a principal ingredient.

Adsorbent.   Substance that leads readily to absorption.

Allergic reaction.   Response of the body resulting from hypersensitivity to a substance (e.g., rash, hives, and anaphylaxis).

Alopecia.   Loss or absence of hair.

Ampule.   Glass container with drug for injection, must be broken at the neck to withdraw drug in solution.

Analeptic.   A drug used to stimulate the central nervous system, especially with poisoning by CNS depressants.

Anaphylaxis.   Allergic hypersensitivity reaction of the body to a foreign substance or drug. Mild symptoms include rash, itching, and hives. Severe symptoms include dyspnea, chest constriction, cardiopulmonary collapse, and death.

Angina pectoris.   Severe chest pain resulting from decreased blood supply to the heart muscle.

Anorexia.   Loss of appetite.

Antagonism.   Opposing action of two drugs in which one decreases or cancels out the effect of the other.

Antidote.   Substance that neutralizes poisons or toxic substances.

Antimuscarinics.   Drugs that block cholinergic stimuli at muscarinic receptors. A type of anticholinergic. Also called parasympatholytics.

Antineoplastic.   Agent that prevents the development, growth, or spreading of malignant cells.

Antioxidant.   Agent that prevents or inhibits oxidation or cell destruction in damaged or aging tissues. A compound that fights against the destructive effects of free radical formation.

Antipyretic.   Medication to reduce fever.

Asymptomatic.   No evidence of clinical disease.

Ataxia.   Defective muscular coordination, especially with voluntary muscular movements (e.g., walking).

Bactericidal.   Destroying bacteria.

Bacteriostatic.   Inhibiting or retarding bacterial growth.

Biotransformation.   Chemical changes that a substance undergoes in the body.

Bipolar disorder.   Manic-depressive mental disorder in which the mood fluctuates from mania to depression.

Blood dyscrasia.   A condition in which any of the blood constituents are abnormal or are present in abnormal quantity.

BPH.   Benign prostatic hypertrophy.

Bradycardia.   Abnormally slow heartbeat.

Bradykinesia.   Abnormally slow movement.

Broad spectrum.   Antibiotic effective against a large variety of organisms.

Buccal.   In the cheek pouch.

Calculus.   Stone.

Cardiotonic.   Increasing the force and efficiency of contractions of the heart muscle.

Cardioversion.   Correcting an irregular heartbeat (arrhythmia). Usually accomplished by electrical shock (e.g., defibrillation).

Catecholamines.   Mediators released at the sympathetic nerve endings (e.g., epinephrine and norepinephrine).

Chemotherapy.   Chemicals (drugs) with specific and toxic effects upon disease-producing organisms.

Clonic.   Spasm marked by alternate contraction (rigidity) and then relaxation of muscles.

Coanalgesic.   Nonopioid analgesic drugs that are combined with opioids for more effective analgesic action in relief of acute or chronic pain (e.g., NSAID or acetaminophen).

Coenzyme.   Enzyme activator.

Concomitant.   Taking place at the same time.

Contraindication.   Condition or circumstance that indicates that a drug should not be given.

COPD.   Chronic obstructive pulmonary disease.

Cryptorchidism.   Undescended testicles.

Cumulative effect.   Increased effect of a drug that accumulates in the body.

Cycloplegic.   Drug that paralyzes the muscles of accommodation for eye examinations.

Cytotoxic.   Destroys cells.

Dependence.   Acquired need for a drug after repeated use; may be psychological with craving and emotional changes or physical with body changes and withdrawal symptoms.

Diplopia. Double vision.

Drug. Chemical substance taken into the body that affects body function.

Dystonic reaction. Spasm and contortion, especially of the head, neck, and tongue, as an adverse effect of antipsychotic medication.

Emetic. Agent that induces vomiting.

Endogenous. Produced or originating within a cell or organism.

Endorphin. Endogenous analgesics produced within the body.

Enteric coated. Tablet with a special coating that resists disintegration by the gastric juices and dissolves in the intestines.

Enuresis. Urinary incontinence; bed-wetting.

Eunuchism. Lack of male hormone resulting in high-pitched voice and absence of beard and body hair.

Euphoria. Exaggerated feeling of well-being and elation.

Euthyroid. Normal thyroid function.

Excretion. Eliminating waste products of drug metabolism.

Extrapyramidal. Disorder of the brain characterized by tremors, parkinsonlike symptoms, or dystonic twisting of body parts, sometimes associated with prolonged use of antipsychotic drugs.

Flatulence. Excessive gas in the digestive tract.

Free radicals. Unbound compounds that attack and damage the cells or initiate growth of abnormal cells, resulting in conditions such as cancer or atherosclerosis.

Gastroesophageal reflux disease (GERD). A backward flow of gastric secretions into the esophagus causing inflammation and discomfort. GERD is treated with drugs to accelerate gastric emptying.

Generic name. General, common, or nonproprietary name of a drug.

Gingivitis. Inflammation of the gums characterized by redness, swelling, and tendency to bleed.

Glossitis. Inflammation of the tongue.

Glycosuria. Sugar in the urine.

Gout. Form of arthritis in which uric acid crystals are deposited in and around joints.

Hepatotoxicity. Damage to the liver as an adverse reaction to certain drugs.

Homeostasis. Body balance, state of internal equilibrium.

Hypercalcemia. Abnormally high blood calcium.

Hyperglycemia. Abnormally high blood sugar.

Hyperpyrexia. Extreme elevation of body temperature.

Hypersensitivity. Allergic or excessive response of the immune system to a drug or chemical.

Hypoglycemia. Abnormally low blood sugar.

Hypokalemia. Abnormally low blood potassium.

Hypoxia. Deficiency of oxygen.

Idiopathic. Condition without a known cause.

Idiosyncracy. Unusual reaction to a drug, other than expected.

Immunosuppressive. Decreasing the production of antibodies and phagocytes and depressing the inflammatory reaction.

Indications. List of conditions for which a drug is meant to be used.

Interactions. Actions that occur when two or more drugs are combined, or when drugs are combined with certain foods.

Intra-articular (intracapsular). Injected into the joint.

Intradermal (ID). Injected into the layers of the skin.

Intramuscular (IM). Injected into the muscle.

Intravenous (IV). Injected into the vein.

Ischemia. Holding back of the blood; local deficiency of blood supply due to obstruction of circulation to a part (e.g., heart or extremities).

Keratolytic. An agent that promotes loosening or scaling of the outer layer of the skin.

Korsakoff's psychosis. Disorder characterized by polyneuritis, disorientation, mental deterioration, and ataxia with painful foot drop, usually associated with chronic alcoholism.

Lability. State of being unstable or changeable.

Legend drug. Available only by prescription.

Leukopenia. Abnormal decrease in white blood cells, usually below 5,000.

Local. Affecting one specific area or part.

Lozenge (troche). Tablet that dissolves slowly in the mouth for local effect.

Megadose. Abnormally large dose.

Metabolism. Physical and chemical alterations that a substance undergoes in the body.

Miotic. Drugs that cause the pupil to contract.

Mortar and pestle. Glass cup with glass rod used to crush tablets.

Myalgia. Tenderness or pain in the muscles.

Mydriatic. Drug that dilates the pupil.

Myelosuppression. Inhibiting bone marrow function.

Myopathy. Abnormal condition of skeletal muscle.

Nebulizer (vaporizer). Apparatus for producing a fine spray or mist for inhalation.

Nephrotoxicity. Damage to the kidneys as an adverse reaction to certain drugs.

Neurotransmitters. Substances that travel across the synapse to transmit messages between nerve cells.

Nystagmus. Involuntary rhythmic movements of the eyeball.

Objective. Referring to symptoms observed or perceived by others.

Oligospermia. Deficient sperm production.

Orphan drug. A drug or biological product for the diagnosis, treatment, or prevention of a rare disease or condition, that is, one affecting less than 200,000 persons in the United States, or greater than 200,000 persons where the cost of developing the drug is probably not recoverable in the United States.

Osteomalacia. Softening of the bones due to inadequate calcium and/or vitamin D.

Ototoxicity. Damage to the eighth cranial nerve resulting in impaired hearing or ringing in the ears (tinnitus); adverse reaction to certain drugs.

Over-the-counter drug (OTC). Medication available without a prescription.

Palliative. Referring to alleviation of symptoms.

Paradoxical. Opposite effect from that expected.

Paraphilia. A psychosexual disorder in which unusual or bizarre imagery or acts are necessary for realizations of sexual excitement.

Parenteral. Any route of administration not involving the gastrointestinal tract (e.g., injection, topical, and inhalation).

Pedophilia. Sexual attraction to children.

Pellagra. A disease caused by deficiency of niacin (nicotinic acid), characterized by skin, gastrointestinal, mucosal, neurologic, and mental symptoms.

Photosensitivity. Increased reaction to sunlight with danger of sunburn; adverse reaction to certain drugs.

Placebo. Inactive substance given to simulate the effect of another drug; physical or emotional changes that occur reflect the expectations of the patient.

Placebo effect. Relief from pain as the result of suggestion without active medication.

Polypharmacy. Excessive use of drugs or prescription of many drugs given at one time.

Potentiation. Increased effect; action of two drugs given simultaneously is greater than the effect of the drugs given separately.

Priapism. Prolonged penile erection.

Proliferation. Rapid reproduction.

Prototype. Model or type from which subsequent types arise (e.g., an example of a drug that typifies the characteristics of that classification).

Psychomotor epilepsy. Also known as temporal lobe epilepsy because of the area in the brain that is involved; characterized by temporary impairment of consciousness, confusion, loss of judgment, and abnormal acts, even crimes and hallucinations, but no convulsions.

REM. Rapid eye movement, or dream, phase of sleep.

Selective distribution. Affinity or attraction of a drug to a specific organ or cells.

Somogyi effect. Hyperglycemic rebound, usually a result of frequent overdoses of insulin, which causes an accelerated release of glucagon.

Status epilepticus. Continual attacks of convulsive seizures without intervals of consciousness.

Stomatitis. Inflammation of the mucous membranes of the mouth.

Subcutaneous (SC). Beneath the skin.

Subjective. Perceived by the individual, not observable by others.

Sublingual (SL). Under the tongue.

Superinfection. A new infection with different resistant bacteria or fungi. Usually associated with certain types of antibiotic therapy.

Synergism. Action of two drugs working together for increased effect.

Synthetic.   Prepared in the laboratory by artificial means.

Systemic.   Affecting the whole body or system.

Tachycardia.   Abnormally fast heartbeat.

Tachypnea.   Abnormal rapidity of respiration.

Tardive dyskinesia.   Slow, rhythmical, stereotyped, involuntary movements such as tics.

Temporal lobe epilepsy.   See **Psychomotor epilepsy.**

Teratogenic effect.   Effect of a drug administered to the mother that results in abnormalities in the fetus.

Thrombocytopenia.   Abnormal decrease in number of blood platelets.

Timed-release capsules (sustained-release or extended-release).   Capsules containing many small pellets that are dissolved over a prolonged period of time.

Tinnitus.   Ringing in the ears.

Tolerance.   Decreased response to a drug after repeated dosage; greater amounts of the drug are required for the same effect.

Tonic.   A persistent, involuntary muscular contraction.

Topical.   Applied to a specific area for a local effect to that area only (e.g., applied to skin or mucous membranes).

Toxicity.   Condition resulting from exposure to a poison or a dangerous amount of a drug.

Toxicology.   Study and detection of toxic substances, establishing treatment and methods of prevention of poisoning.

Trade name.   Name by which a pharmaceutical company identifies its product; brand name.

Transdermal (transcutaneous) delivery system.   Patch containing the medicine is applied to the skin; the drug is absorbed through the skin over a prolonged period of time.

Uricosuric.   Promoting urinary excretion of uric acid.

Vial.   Glass container with rubber stopper that must be punctured with a needle to withdraw a drug solution or to reconstitute a drug in powdered form.

Wernicke's syndrome.   Mental disorder characterized by loss of memory, disorientation, and confusion, usually associated with old age or chronic alcoholism.

Withdrawal.   Cessation of administration of a drug, especially a narcotic or alcohol, to which a person has become physiologically and/or psychologically addicted; withdrawal symptoms vary with the chemical used.

Xerophthalmia.   Dryness of the eyes.

Xerostomia.   Dryness of the mouth.

Index

Stelazine, 345
See also Trifluoperazine
Stimulant laxatives, 260
Stool softeners, 258
Streptomycin, 283, 284, 285
Subcutaneous injection, 50, 52, 135–136
Sublingual administration, 37, 55, 120
Sucralfate, 252–253, 257
Sucrets, 477
See also Diclonine
Sudafed, 463, 465
See also Pseudoephedrine
Sufenta, 318
Sulfadoxine, 291
Sulfasalazine, 295
Sulfasoxazole, 295
Sulfinpyrazone, 243
Sulfonamides, 292–293
Sulfonylureas, 394–395
Sulfur, 194
Sulindac, 366
Supplies for administration, 55–59
Surfak, 264
See also Docusate
Symadine, 295
See also Amantadine
Symmetrel, 295, 378, 380
See also Amantadine
Sympathomimetics, 206, 307–308, 454–456
Synarel, 419
Synergism, 35
Synthetic sources of drugs, 28–29
Synthroid, 389, 391
See also Levothyroxine
Syntocinon, 418
See also Oxytocin
Syringes
Carpuject prefilled, 129, 130
insulin, 59, 129
parts of, 127
standard, 57, 59, 128, 129
tuberculin, 59, 128, 129
Systemic effect, 29, 119–120

TACE, 409
See also Chlorotrianisene
Tacrine, 29
Tagamet, 35, 251, 257, 485
See also Cimetidine
Talbutal, 326
Talwin, 318, 484
See also Pentazocine

Tambocor, 432, 434
See also Flecainide
Tamoxifen, 220, 224
Tapazole, 390, 391
See also Methimazole
Tavist, 465
See also Clemastine
Tegretol, 322, 323, 375, 485
See also Carbamazepine
Tegrin, 194
See also Coal tar
Teldrin, 465
See also Chlorpheniramine
Temazepam, 325, 326
Tempra, 319
See also Acetaminophen
Tenormin, 434, 436, 439, 485
See also Atenolol
Tensilon, 210
See also Edrophonium
Teratogenic effect, 38
Terbutaline, 416–417, 418
Terbutaline sulfate, 454, 455
Terfenadine, 462–463, 465
Terramycin, 285
See also Oxytetracycline
Tessalon, 461
See also Benzonatate
Testosterone, 404, 405
Testred, 405
See also Methlytestosterone
Tetracaine, 309, 477
Tetracyclines, 31, 35, 279, 285
THC, 351–352
See also Marijuana
Theodur, 455
See also Theophyllines
Theophyllines, 454, 455, 456
Therapeutic dose, 36
Thiamine (Vitamin B_1), 168
Thiazides, 231–233, 436
Thioridazine, 345
Thiotepa, 219, 224
Thiothixene, 345
Thorazine, 342, 345, 485
See also Chlorpromazine
Thyroid, 389, 391
Ticar, 278
See also Ticarcillin
Ticarcillin, 275, 278
Tigan, 261, 264
See also Trimethobenzamide